Health
and
Behavior

**The Interplay of Biological,
Behavioral,
and
Societal
Influences**

Committee on Health and Behavior:
Research, Practice, and Policy
Board on Neuroscience and Behavioral Health

INSTITUTE OF MEDICINE

NATIONAL ACADEMY PRESS
Washington, D.C.

NATIONAL ACADEMY PRESS • 2101 Constitution Avenue, N.W. • Washington, DC 20418

NOTICE: The project that is the subject of this report was approved by the Governing Board of the National Research Council, whose members are drawn from the councils of the National Academy of Sciences, the National Academy of Engineering, and the Institute of Medicine. The members of the committee responsible for the report were chosen for their special competences and with regard for appropriate balance.

Support for this project was provided by Robert Wood Johnson Foundation, Contract No. 030324 and National Institutes of Health and Center for Disease Control, Contract No. N01-OD-4-2139, TO #38. The views presented in this report are those of the Institute of Medicine Committee on Health and Behavior: Research, Practice and Policy and are not necessarily those of the funding agencies.

Library of Congress Cataloging-in-Publication Data

Health and behavior : the interplay of biological, behavioral, and
societal influences / Committee on Health and Behavior, Research,
Practice, and Policy, Board on Neuroscience and Behavioral Health,
Institute of Medicine.
    p. ; cm.
Includes bibliographical references and index.
  ISBN 0-309-07030-9 (hardcover)
  1. Medicine and psychology. 2. Social medicine.
  [DNLM: 1. Health Behavior. 2. Attitude to Health. 3. Preventive
Health Services. 4. Socioeconomic Factors. W 85 H4338 2001] I.
Institute of Medicine (U.S.). Committee on Health and Behavior:
Research, Practice, and Policy.
  R726.5 .H43225 2001
  613'.01'9—dc21

                2001003541

Additional copies of this report are available for sale from the National Academy Press, 2101 Constitution Avenue, N.W., Box 285, Washington, D.C. 20055. Call (800) 624-6242 or (202) 334-3313 (in the Washington metropolitan area), or visit the NAP's home page at **www.nap.edu.**

For more information about the Institute of Medicine, visit the IOM home page at: **www.iom.edu.**

The serpent has been a symbol of long life, healing, and knowledge among almost all cultures and religions since the beginning of recorded history. The serpent adopted as a logotype by the Institute of Medicine is a relief carving from ancient Greece, now held by the Staatliche Museen in Berlin.

"Knowing is not enough; we must apply.
Willing is not enough; we must do."
—Goethe

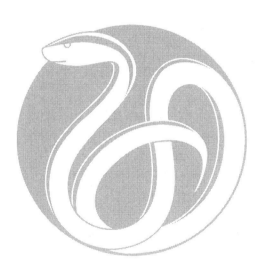

INSTITUTE OF MEDICINE

Shaping the Future for Health

THE NATIONAL ACADEMIES

National Academy of Sciences
National Academy of Engineering
Institute of Medicine
National Research Council

The **National Academy of Sciences** is a private, nonprofit, self-perpetuating society of distinguished scholars engaged in scientific and engineering research, dedicated to the furtherance of science and technology and to their use for the general welfare. Upon the authority of the charter granted to it by the Congress in 1863, the Academy has a mandate that requires it to advise the federal government on scientific and technical matters. Dr. Bruce M. Alberts is president of the National Academy of Sciences.

The **National Academy of Engineering** was established in 1964, under the charter of the National Academy of Sciences, as a parallel organization of outstanding engineers. It is autonomous in its administration and in the selection of its members, sharing with the National Academy of Sciences the responsibility for advising the federal government. The National Academy of Engineering also sponsors engineering programs aimed at meeting national needs, encourages education and research, and recognizes the superior achievements of engineers. Dr. William A. Wulf is president of the National Academy of Engineering.

The **Institute of Medicine** was established in 1970 by the National Academy of Sciences to secure the services of eminent members of appropriate professions in the examination of policy matters pertaining to the health of the public. The Institute acts under the responsibility given to the National Academy of Sciences by its congressional charter to be an adviser to the federal government and, upon its own initiative, to identify issues of medical care, research, and education. Dr. Kenneth I. Shine is president of the Institute of Medicine.

The **National Research Council** was organized by the National Academy of Sciences in 1916 to associate the broad community of science and technology with the Academy's purposes of furthering knowledge and advising the federal government. Functioning in accordance with general policies determined by the Academy, the Council has become the principal operating agency of both the National Academy of Sciences and the National Academy of Engineering in providing services to the government, the public, and the scientific and engineering communities. The Council is administered jointly by both Academies and the Institute of Medicine. Dr. Bruce M. Alberts and Dr. William A. Wulf are chairman and vice chairman, respectively, of the National Research Council.

DAVID SPIEGEL, Professor of Psychiatry and Behavioral Sciences, Department of Psychiatry, Stanford University School of Medicine, Stanford, California

Liaison to the IOM Board on Neuroscience and Behavioral Health

BEATRIX A. HAMBURG, Visiting Scholar, Department of Psychiatry, Cornell University Medical College, New York, New York

Liaison to the IOM Board on Health Promotion and Disease Prevention

ELENA O. NIGHTINGALE, Scholar-in-Residence, National Academy of Sciences, Washington, District of Columbia

Study Staff

TERRY C. PELLMAR, Director, Board on Neuroscience and Behavioral Health (since May 1999)

WENDY S. PACHTER, Study Director (until April 2000)

ALLISON L. FRIEDMAN, Senior Project Assistant (until December 1999)

AMELIA B. MATHIS, Project Assistant

LINDA V. LEONARD, Administrative Assistant (until September 2000)

LORA K. TAYLOR, Administrative Assistant (since October 2000)

CARLOS GABRIEL, Financial Associate (until December 2000)

JENNIFER CANGCO, Financial Associate (since January 2001)

ROBERT COPPOCK, Consultant

KATHLEEN R. STRATTON, Director, Board on Health Promotion Disease Prevention (until September 1999)

ROBERT M. COOK-DEGAN, Director, National Cancer Policy Board (until June 2000)

Preface

In 1982, the Institute of Medicine published a landmark study titled *Health and Behavior: Frontiers of Biobehavioral Research*. That study drew on the findings of six invitational conferences to provide a perspective on the frontiers of the biobehavioral sciences, their relevance to public health—particularly to decreasing the burden of illness—and their implications for science policy. The report stimulated research and training in the biobehavioral sciences, and although the report is now 18 years old, much of it is still current.

The Board on Neuroscience and Behavioral Health and the Board on Health Promotion and Disease Prevention of the Institute of Medicine were interested in updating the 1982 report because of the broad range of research and intervention activity it stimulated, and the growing recognition of the importance of behavior to health during the years since the original report. The Robert Wood Johnson Foundation, the Office of Behavioral and Social Science Research of the National Institutes of Health, and other Department of Health and Human Services sponsors, including the National Institute of Mental Health and the Centers for Disease Control, provided funding for a new study that would differ in several ways from the original report. First, the new study was not to be merely an update of the areas covered in the original report or diseases in which the contribution of behavior is recognized (such as HIV and AIDS), but instead was to identify factors involved in health and disease for which research is incomplete. Second, this study was to go beyond biobehavioral research to consider applications and cost-effectiveness.

The Institute of Medicine convened the Committee on Health and Behavior: Research, Practice and Policy in September 1998. The Committee comprised 12 members with experience in basic, clinical, and public health research; practice in settings ranging from public health to private practice and managed care; and experience with federal, local, and private policy. Committee members had specific expertise in internal, family, adolescent, and pediatric medicine; health policy; epidemiology and social epidemiology; family therapy; clinical and social psychology; law and ethics; health education; neuroendocrinology; and immunology and psychiatry.

The Committee refined its statement of task at the first meeting. The Committee decided that the health and behavior field had become much too large to study comprehensively in the time allotted. The Committee therefore agreed to focus primarily on new and promising developments in the field since 1982, based on the best available research, or, occasionally, on the Committee's assessment of where the field is heading. Committee members agreed that health and behavior should be broadly defined to include both behavioral and psychosocial factors as in the 1982 report, rather than limiting consideration to "health behaviors" such as eating, smoking and other substance use and abuse, and physical activity. This decision also reflected the sense of the Committee that since 1982 the social sciences have made new and exciting contributions to understanding health and behavior and that these have implications for interventions and policy. Psychosocial factors are the individual interpretations or understandings of social relationships, events, or status that reflect a combination of psychological and social variables and are internalized and affect biological factors.

The Committee also decided at the first meeting to consider "applications" of behavioral and psychosocial interventions rather than "practice." The significance of this change was to enable the Committee to think beyond traditional medical or other clinical practice to include programmatic and public health interventions.

The resulting charge to the Committee was to (1) update scientific findings about the links between biological, psychosocial and behavioral factors, and health; (2) identify factors involved in health and disease but for which research on these factors and effective behavioral and psychosocial interventions is incomplete; (3) identify and review effective applications of behavioral and psychosocial interventions in a variety of settings; (4) examine implementation of behavioral and psychosocial interventions, including guidelines and changes in provider behaviors; (5) review evidence of cost-effectiveness; and (6) make recommendations concerning further research, applications, and financing.

The Committee prepared papers on a variety of topics and deliberated in a series of five meetings, several of which were open to the public. Several experts in health and behavior were invited to address the Committee at meetings, and several more were invited to a workshop on health, communications, and behavior (see agenda in Appendix A). Additional information was obtained through six commissioned papers; a contribution by the Working Group on Family-Based Interventions in Chronic Disease; active participation in meetings by consultants in public health, health psychology and law; and comments on draft papers by a number of additional expert consultants prior to formal review (see Appendix B). The Committee noted great enthusiasm in the health and behavior field, and many busy experts were willing to give generously of their time and effort for little or no compensation. The Committee is grateful to all who provided assistance; those who served as consultants are acknowledged by name in Appendix B.

Reviewers

The report was reviewed by individuals chosen for their diverse perspectives and technical expertise in accordance with procedures approved by the National Research Council's Report Review Committee. The purpose of this independent review is to provide candid and critical comments to assist the authors and the Institute of Medicine in making the published report as sound as possible and to ensure that the report meets institutional standards for objectivity, evidence, and responsiveness to the study charge. The content of the review comments and the draft manuscript remain confidential to protect the integrity of the deliberative process. The committee wishes to thank the following individuals for their participation in the report review process:

Bobbie Berkowitz, University of Washington
Joel Dimsdale, University of California, San Diego
Lewis Kuller, University of Pittsburgh
Michael Marmot, University College, London Medical School
James Prochaska, University of Rhode Island
Sally Shumaker, Wake Forest University Medical School

Although the reviewers listed above have provided many constructive comments and suggestions, they were not asked to endorse the conclusions or recommendations nor did they see the final draft of the report before its release. The review of this report was overseen by Paul Cleary, Harvard Medical School and Maureen Henderson, University of Washington. Appointed by the National Research Council and Institute of Medicine, they were responsible for making certain that an independent examination of this report was carried out in accordance with institutional procedures and that all review comments were carefully considered. Responsibility for the final content of this report rests entirely with the authoring committee and the institution.

Contents

Health
and
Behavior

Executive Summary

Health-care professionals, patients, families, community leaders, and policy makers all struggle to understand interactions between health and behavior and to use that knowledge to improve the health status of individuals and populations. Health and behavior are related in myriad ways, yet those interactions are neither simple nor straightforward. Given the wide acknowledgment that cigarette smoking is linked to a variety of deadly diseases, for example, why do people start smoking? And given equally convincing evidence connecting excess weight with cardiovascular disease and other health problems, why are so many people far above their optimal weight? Does such unhealthy behavior indicate a simple lack of willpower? How does the social environment influence these behaviors? Does stress make people sick, or does illness produce stress? This report presents current knowledge about links between health and behavior, about the influence of the social environment on these behaviors, and about interventions to improve health through modifying behavior or personal relationships. It also addresses what must still be learned to answer questions like those above.

The committee entered into its endeavor expecting to discover and share what works and what does not regarding health and behavior. After diligently exploring the literature, the complexity of the issue became evident. The committee noted the vast array of interventions at various levels, with varying endpoints on different populations, with different methodologies. Each committee member brought to the table their own perspective about what would be most effective, but the data were inadequate to convince any of the experts of a best approach to shaping and maintaining behavior change. While conventional wisdom tells us that we need to do more exercise, eat less, avoid tobacco, wear seatbelts, and be careful with firearms, deciding what specific interventions to produce and sustain these changes presents a dilemma.

A critical obstacle to answering definitively the question of what works best is the difficulty of generalizing the findings of current studies. Many factors contribute to the problem: outcome measures among the studies differ, populations studied differ, and methodologies differ. For example, an intervention may be exceptionally effective on a highly motivated population but fail for the general public. Measurement of a behavioral outcome such as self-reported tobacco use is difficult to compare with an outcome measure such as change in sales of tobacco. Another obstacle is that there are no rigorous evaluations of interventions. Evaluations may assess short-term changes, but long-term effectiveness should also be assessed because maintaining behavior change has been shown to be difficult. Only with additional research and evaluation of interventions will the best approaches be found. This report presents the current level of understanding and demonstrates the limits of the currently available research.

In preparing this report, the Committee on Health and Behavior: Research, Practice and Policy examined recent scientific advances about the biological, psychological, and social determinants of health and about the nature of the interactions between health and behavior. It also looked at research addressing interventions intended to change health-related behavior, cognition, and emotions, or interactions with the social environment (i.e., psychosocial factors) with the aim of improving health. Finally, it considered how to translate this knowledge from research to application.

The committee approached its charge with a broad vision of a variety of basic and applied sciences. This broad approach facilitated the recognition of relationships among different determinants of health and from various scientific disciplines. The tradeoff is that some subjects were not treated in depth or at all in the report, although wherever possible references are provided for readers who would like more information. The overall findings and recommendations appear at the end of this summary.

DEFINITION OF BEHAVIOR

As in the 1982 Institute of Medicine report on Health and Behavior, this report uses the term "biobehavioral sciences" to encompass the many disciplines that contribute to behavior and health because it reflects the rich, dynamic, and interactive nature of the fields contributing to knowledge of health and behavior. The term biobehavioral sciences includes not only the behavioral sciences that conduct experimental analyses of animal and human behavior but is broadly inclusive of relevant sciences such as neuroanatomy, neurology, neurochemistry, endocrinology, immunology, psychology, psychiatry, epidemiology, ethnology, sociology, and anthropology, as well as the new interdisciplinary fields such as behavioral genetics, psychoneuroimmunology, and behavioral medicine.

DEFINITION OF HEALTH

Health is sometimes negatively defined as the absence of disease and injury, sometimes as a normative judgment referring to the average state of most people, and sometimes as a positive concept of well-being. This report uses "health" with the meaning of "positive health." Although disease is commonly regarded as either present or absent, most health problems fall on a continuum. Changing diagnostic thresholds—such as reducing the body mass index guide for overweight from 28 to 25—can abruptly change the health status for large numbers of people. Furthermore, current wellness or illness must be considered together with prospects for the future. The concept of "positive health," while controversial, derives from evidence that attitudes and behaviors enhance the body's resistance to and recovery from disease, illness, and surgical intervention.

RISK FACTORS

Individuals (and the physiological and psychological processes within them) develop and live in social systems. People influence and are influenced by their families, social networks, the organizations in which they participate, their communities, and their society. Interventions to improve health or to influence health-related behavior can occur at any one or several of those levels. A full understanding of the interactions between health and behavior requires consideration of the separate levels and the interplay among them.

Biobehavioral Factors

A growing body of evidence shows that the physiological systems associated with the response to stress are potent contributors to illness. The response to stressful challenges helps to maintain constant and appropriate internal conditions, called homeostasis. The stress response involves reactions to emergencies and a rapid and pervasive adjustment of internal states to prepare the organism for fight or flight, but long-term behavioral, physiological, and psychological factors contribute. The cumulative, converging effects of these various factors culminate in patterns shown in the physiological mediators of the stress response including the failure to shut them off when they are not needed. The cost to the body produced by overactive mediators is called allostatic load. Allostasis is the process of adaptation and connotes the maintenance of stability (or homeostasis) through change. Allostasis thus describes a process of adaptation to challenge; allostatic load is the wear and tear on the body as a result of repeated allostatic responses.

Allostatic load is more than chronic stress. It can also reflect a genetically or developmentally induced failure to cope efficiently with the normal challenges of daily life. Developmental influences are implicated in influencing individual susceptibility to stress-related disorders. Changes in balance among neurotransmitters in the brain from the time of early development through adulthood to old age can influence behavioral responses to potentially stressful situations, can alter the interpretation of stimuli, and might be associated with anxiety and depression. Research with laboratory animals indicates that early-life experiences strongly influence lifetime allostatic load. For example, in laboratory animals poor maternal care is associated with increased behavioral and stress hormone reactivity in adult life.

The immune system is highly integrated with other physiological systems. It is sensitive to virtually every hormone, and sympathetic, parasympathetic, and sensory nerves innervate the organs of the immune system. The nervous, endocrine, and immune systems communicate bidirectionally through common hormones, neuropeptides, and cytokines. Stress-induced activation of neuroendocrine pathways has been shown to modulate various physiological systems, including the immune system. Stress-induced modulation of the immune system has been linked to the expression of inflammatory, infectious, and autoimmune diseases.

Several psychological factors—including hostility, anger, depression, and vital exhaustion—have been associated with susceptibility to diseases such as coronary heart disease. Strong links have been identified between the trait of hostility and the incidence of and mortality from heart disease. Some hypothesize that people who are hostile have exaggerated cardio-vascular reactivity to stress and that this either contributes to the development of atherosclerosis or triggers acute events. However, hostility also is correlated with increased likelihood of smoking, with decreased likelihood of quitting smoking, and with lower socioeconomic status. Each of these will increase allostatic load. Depression affects about half of patients who experience myocardial infarction, predicts significantly poorer outcome with heart disease, and roughly doubles the risk of recurrent cardio-vascular events. Hope and optimism, in contrast, have been suggested as important components of psychological well-being and as factors that can contribute to good physical health. There is increasing evidence that these and other psychosocial factors are important determinants of physical health and disease.

People show large differences in resilience to and recovery from illness, injury, or surgery and in how they overcome adversity. Resilience, the ability to recover from adversity, is thought to result from cellular processes that protect and build cells and tissues—processes that involve some reserve capacity and resistance to the damaging effects of stressors—but relatively little is known about its physiological basis and psychosocial influences. Another important construct is *coping*, the volitional management of stressful events or conditions and regulation of cognitive, behavioral, emotional, and physiological responses to stress. Successful coping is facilitated by a cognitive style characterized by realistic optimism—the tendency to anticipate positive outcomes. Conversely, pessimistic thinking is associated with coping that involves avoidance and social withdrawal, which are related to higher symptoms of anxiety and depression.

Behavioral Factors

Several behaviors that exert a strong influence on health are reviewed in this report: tobacco use, alcohol abuse, physical activity and diet, sexual practices, and disease screening. Although epidemiologic data on the relationships between these behaviors and various health outcomes were available in the early 1980s, many refinements in knowledge have occurred since then. Causal conclusions have been strengthened by more sophisticated research designs, dose/response relationships have been clarified, the influence of many of these behaviors on overall public health has been quantified, and scientific guidelines have been formulated.

One example of behavioral influences on health is the impact of diet and physical activity on obesity, a serious risk factor in many diseases such as heart disease and diabetes. Although overweight and obesity are increasing among all sociodemographic groups in the United States, the prevalence is influenced by specific sociocultural variables, including gender, ethnicity, socioeconomic status, and education. Obesity in children and adolescents also is increasing and, because it often persists into adulthood, enhances the risk of chronic disease later in life. Contributing to this epidemic is the fact that relatively few Americans participate in regular physical activity. Furthermore, an increasing proportion of the population is eating outside the home, consuming larger portions of higher calorie and higher fat foods.

Preventing weight gain in the first place reduces the likelihood that conditions such as hypertension and diabetes will develop. Because treatment of obesity has poor long-term success, and lost weight often is regained, avoiding weight gain is preferable. Since many dietary habits are established during childhood, educating school-aged children about nutrition has been demonstrated to help establish healthy eating habits early in life. Weight loss in adults is beneficial but difficult to maintain and requires permanent lifestyle changes that combine good dietary habits, decreased sedentary behavior, and increased physical activity. Changes in the physical and social environment can help people maintain the necessary long-term lifestyle changes both for diet and for physical activity. Physical activity does not need to be vigorous to be beneficial to health. For people who are inactive, even small increases have been associated with measurable health benefits. Weight loss accompanied by proper diet can promote health: for example, diets low in saturated fatty acids and cholesterol and higher in polyunsaturated fat are associated with low risks of coronary heart disease.

Social Factors

Most behaviors are not randomly distributed in the population, but are socially patterned and often occur together. Many people who drink also use tobacco. Those who follow health-promoting dietary practices also tend to be physically active. People who are poor, have low levels of education, or are socially isolated are more likely to engage in a wide array of risk-related behaviors and less likely to engage in health-promoting ones. Understanding why unhealthy behaviors are more prevalent among those with lower social standing requires recognizing that behaviors once thought of as falling exclusively within the realm of individual choice occur in a social context. The social environment influences behavior by shaping norms; enforcing patterns of social control (which can be health promoting or health damaging); providing or not providing environmental opportunities to engage in particular behaviors; and reducing or producing stress, for which engaging in specific behaviors might be an effective short-term coping strategy. Furthermore, environments place constraints on individual choice.

Lower mortality, morbidity, and disability among socioeconomically advantaged people have been observed for hundreds of years, using various indicators of socioeconomic status and multiple disease outcomes. A solid body of evidence at the individual level shows that social integration, the quality of social ties, and extent of social support are critical in influencing disease processes and mortality. At the population level, research shows that patterns of social cohesion and social capital are related to health outcomes.

Researchers examining social relationships in early and later life describe the importance of deep, meaningful, loving human connections and of affect in intimate relationships. Individuals on positive relationship pathways (positive ties with parents during childhood, intimate ties with spouse during adulthood) are less likely to exhibit high allostatic load than are those on negative relationship pathways. Relational strengths also appear to offer protection against cumulative economic adversity. Strong social relations, however, do not always improve a person's health status. Evidence documents the adverse consequences of divorce and bereavement, deficits in belongingness, and loneliness. Caregivers of relatives with progressive dementia exhibit impaired wound-healing compared with controls matched for age and family income. Social conflicts have been shown to increase susceptibility to infection. Social isolation and loneliness are associated with physiological changes involving blood pressure, catecholamines, and aspects of cellular and humoral immune function.

A social network is the web of social relationships and and the structural characteristics of that web. Prospective cohort studies in the United States, Scandinavia, and Japan consistently show that people who are isolated or disconnected from others are at increased risk of dying prematurely. Epidemiological evidence consistently supports the notion that social ties, especially intimate ties and emotional support provided by them, promote increased survival and better prognosis among people after myocardial infarction or with serious cardiovascular disease. Generally, social networks are related more strongly to mortality than to the incidence or onset of disease.

Perhaps the most striking finding that emerges from the analyses of social environmental influences is the graded and continuous nature of the association between income and mortality, with differences persisting well into the middle-class range of incomes. The fact that socioeconomic differences in health are not confined to segments of the population that are materially deprived in the conventional sense suggests strongly that socioeconomic differences are not simply a function of absolute poverty. Moreover, because causes of death that are purportedly not amenable to medical care show socioeconomic gradients similar to those of potentially treatable causes, differential access to health care programs and services cannot be solely responsible for these differentials in health. Finally, because the gradient in morbidity and mortality persists even between middle class and well-to-do men and women, and even in societies in which material conditions are very good, it seems unlikely that gradients are due solely to material circumstances per se. It has become evident that community socioeconomic status independently influences mortality. Understanding the dynamics of why some populations have particular risk distributions leads to different etiologic questions than does focusing on the reasons some individuals are in the extremes of the risk distribution. Pursuing a population-based strategy, rather than a high-risk strategy, leads to different research questions and policy approaches.

HEALTH-RELATED INTERVENTIONS

Interventions must recognize that people live in social, political, and economic systems that shape behaviors and access to the resources they need to maintain good health. This report approaches interventions with an ecologic or social-systems perspective that places the person in his or her primary social context and observes how he or she interacts with other important factors to affect and be affected by disease outcomes. The ecologic perspective emphasizes the importance of family, organizations, communities, and society as a whole.

Individual Behavior

Growing evidence suggests that effective programs oriented toward individual health behaviors require a multifaceted approach to helping people adopt, change, and maintain healthful behavior. Maintaining a particular behavior over time might require different strategies than will establishing that behavior in the first place. Models of behavior change have been developed to guide strategies to promote healthy behaviors and facilitate effective adaptation to and coping with illness. The models are useful constructs for thinking about behavioral change and designing interventions. Each model has its own focus on specific behavioral attributes and its own set of limitations. Given the particular difficulty in maintaining behavior changes, the relapse of behaviors that have been eliminated (or "extinguished") by an intervention is of particular interest. Research into the classical conditioning model shows that extinction of behaviors does not involve unlearning, but rather new learning that does not overwrite the original behavior. While original learning of a behavior readily extends to new contexts of physical, social, and emotional environments, extinction does not. Those findings suggest that the effectiveness of an intervention to reduce or eliminate a health risk, such as cigarette-smoking, will be limited to the extent that it is bound to the context in which it is delivered.

Education and counseling can promote primary prevention measures (e.g., preventing tobacco use, choosing a healthy diet). Interventions aimed at secondary prevention behaviors can influence early detection of illness. For instance, willingness to self-examine and participate in screening procedures is important for detection and treatment of cancer. Counseling by a primary care physician can be effective in changing the behaviors of patients. Effectiveness is improved by the recognition that different patients have different needs. Some patients respond favorably to printed materials and some to coaching via telephone-based counseling, but some cannot change health-related behavior without one-on-one structured education and counseling supplemented by frequent reinforcement from their physicians. Multiple modalities of support are used in the practices that are most heavily committed to encouraging beneficial behavior change and that target individual patients. However, engaging busy practices to reach into new health promotion endeavors rather than to focus on delivery of acute care is challenging. Health-care systems and practices in the United States are moving toward a continuous improvement model of identifying problems and testing interventions, instead of the traditional methods of identifying faulty practices by investigating clinical cases that have unsatisfactory outcomes. Little research funding in the past has been applied to systematic evaluation of fundamental (systemic) changes in clinical practices that might support health-enhancing behavior change in defined populations.

Psychosocial interventions can improve people's coping skills and provide emotional support, thereby improving quality of life and medical outcomes among the chronically ill. Poor adjustment to illness can substantially increase the cost of medical care. Thus, providing appropriate psychotherapeutic and psychopharmacologic treatment for the the chronically ill not only can improve coping and reduce patient discomfort but also can make the delivery of medical care more efficient. For example, there is evidence that psychosocial interventions can improve quality of life, psychological adjustment, health status, and survival of cancer patients. The mechanisms through which psychosocial interventions exert their effect are unknown, but it has been suggested that depression exacerbates symptoms and that psychotherapy augments the immune response.

In response to mounting evidence that behaviors, such as tobacco use and consumption of high-fat diets, are risk factors for chronic diseases, several studies target interventions for medically at-risk individuals. Other interventions arise from the concept of population-attributable risk, which measures the amount of disease in the population that can be attributed to a given exposure. A large number of people exposed to a small risk might generate more cases than will a small number exposed to a high risk, so that when risk is widely distributed in the population, small changes in behavior across an entire population can yield larger improvements in population-attributable risk than would larger changes among a smaller number of high-risk individuals.

Population-based intervention trials in a community, worksite, or school often focus on changing individual behavior for primary prevention of disease. Several early population-based community intervention studies tracked changes in morbidity and mortality and showed some success. Subsequent intervention studies, however, had insufficient funding to follow participants for long enough or in sufficient numbers to determine long-term costs and consequences of the interventions for survival. Instead of quality of life, or disease incidence, these programs used behavior change as the primary outcome because evidence strongly linked behavior to morbidity and mortality. In addition, the smaller community-wide studies were less likely to achieve the necessary intensity and breadth to show significant intervention effects. Workplace interventions for individual behavior change have been increasing in the past 15 years. The interventions range from intensive group behavioral counseling sessions and supervised exercise prescriptions to simple, broad approaches such as mailed self-help materials and newsletters. Although several of the programs achieved statistically significant effects, the quality of the studies was generally inadequate to make judgments about the effectiveness of the interventions. Schools also provide a setting for behavior-change interventions. Interventions at this level have met with varied success. Recognition of multilevel influences on smoking in youths, for example, has led to multifaceted interventions, including schoolwide media campaigns in combination with individual approaches. Reviews of youth smoking-control interventions generally conclude that social influence interventions can curb smoking onset, although with a somewhat guarded picture of their efficacy. School-based interventions for physical activity in the 1980s and 1990s were found to improve student knowledge and psychosocial factors but were less likely to change behavior significantly. The more extensive multicomponent interventions typically had better results. Some programs were able to show a sustained difference in physical activity between experimental and control schools for several years.

Families

Another level of intervention for health-related behavior change focuses on the family. Family relationships have greater emotional intensity than do most other social relationships, and evidence suggests a substantive, positive association between the specific bonds within families and chronic-disease management and outcomes.

Chronic disease is a long-term stressor for patients and their families. Significant changes are required of the patient and family members in day-to-day activities and in the way they relate to one another. Parents, spouses, and other family members are frequently the patient's primary source of support, and their ability to meet the patient's needs is often compounded by the distress that illness generates among other family members. In addition, family members frequently provide important channels of community resources to patients.

Family relationships also determine the capacity for regulation of emotional and psychological processes. Stable, secure, and mutual family relationships enhance disease management behavior by permitting a sharing of the burdens associated with disease. Family members often determine important contextual factors that affect health-related behavior, such as diet and exercise.

Most family-based, clinical-intervention research has concerned chronic diseases of childhood and adolescence (e.g., insulin-dependent diabetes, asthma). Interventions have focused more on adherence to treatment and metabolic control than on family-behavior variables or family processes themselves. However, a few studies demonstrate improved family relationships associated with better health outcomes. Family-focused intervention studies of dementia in the elderly (especially Alzheimer's disease) are increasing, but relatively less attention has been directed to family-focused interventions for diseases of adulthood. The available data suggest that recognizing and attending to the family relationship context adds considerably to improving the health and well-being of patients and family members struggling with the management of a chronic disease.

Organizations

Formal and informal organizations constitute another framework for describing interactions between behavior and health. Organizations are important components of social and physical environments, and they exert considerable influence over the choices people make, the resources they have to aid them in those choices, and the factors in the workplace that could influence health status (e.g., work overload, exposure to toxic chemicals). As employees, consumers, customers, clients, and patients, people are influenced by the organizations to which they belong.

Well-evaluated interventions at the organizational level are scarce. Some worksite health promotion programs include employee participation in planning the efforts ranging from soliciting employee input through surveys or focus groups to having employee groups take full responsibility for implementation. Evaluation of these interventions is limited, and results have been mixed. Another strategy relies on training key figures in the organizations in methods for creating a supportive organizational culture and developing a comprehensive health promotion program. Again, the interventions and assessments are limited. One important aspect of organizational interventions is the occupational safety and health (OSH) programs that address the influence of physical (e.g., noise, extreme temperatures), chemical, ergonomic, and psychosocial work hazards on employee health. Strategies to enhance compliance with universal precautions among health-care workers provide a case in point: although descriptive research clearly indicates the influence of organizational safety climate and work task design on compliance rates, most interventions have targeted only individual employee knowledge, attitudes, and behaviors for change. Organizations have also intervened to reduce on-the-job psychosocial stressors. Programs that focused solely on individual-level coping enhancement—even when they involved substantial resources—were less effective than programs that attempt to change work organization, task structure, or communication patterns in worksites.

Communities

Communities also provide an important level of intervention for improvement of health. A community need not be a geographic area, but instead might be a unit of identity. A community of identity can exist within a defined geographic neighborhood or, for example, as a graphically dispersed ethnic or professional group in which there is a shared sense of identity. Communities are also "units of solution" that include members with the knowledge, skills, and expertise necessary to solve problems. Community-level interventions can reduce the social, structural, and environmental stressors that degrade health status and that are beyond the ability of any single person to control or change. Community-level interventions also can strengthen the situational factors, such as social support, community empowerment, community capacity, and social cohesion, that have been shown to protect against deleterious effects of stress.

Community interventions present a complex set of challenges. In general, they emphasize the social, cultural, economic, and political context of communities of identity and involve the community in the control and development of the process for which full specification of goals and objectives is not possible at the beginning. The very nature of these interventions and the necessary commitment to the long time-frame required to bring about major community-level changes preclude application of traditional evaluation designs and methods to assess effectiveness. Lessons from experiences with community interventions include

- the importance of the community, rather than an outside organizer, in defining needs and priorities;

- the need for an initial and continuing community diagnosis and assessment to identify and build on community strengths and resources;
- the flexible implementation of theories and methodologies, tailoring them to a particular community context;
- the importance of using participatory and empowering approaches to evaluate community- level change interventions;
- the necessity of long-range planning and developing diversified bases of funding.

Emphasis is needed on public health interventions that involve communities of identity with the goal of collectively identifying resources, needs, and solutions that can influence community-level variables.

Society

There is an inverse relationship between social class and a variety of diseases. Even beyond the stressors associated with low income, social structure clearly shapes people's daily lives. There are many ways in which the effects of income extend beyond purchasing power. People in middle-class neighborhoods have proportionally more pharmacies, restaurants, banks, and specialty stores; low-income areas have more fast-food restaurants, check-cashing stores, liquor stores, and laundromats.

Many social, economic, political, and cultural factors are associated with health and disease for which changes in individual health behaviors alone are not likely to result in improved health and quality of life. Public health laws provide a number of approaches to prevent injury and disease and to promote the population's health. First, government interventions can be aimed at individual behavior—through education, deterrence, or incentives. Health communications campaigns are designed to educate and persuade people to make healthier choices. The government can deter risk behaviors by imposing civil and criminal penalties (e.g., seatbelt and motorcycle helmet laws) or by creating incentives for individual behavior change (e.g., imposing taxes on tobacco or alcohol). Second, the government can require safer product design (e.g., passive restraints in cars, trigger locks on handguns, or childproof caps on medicines). Finally, the law can change the informational, physical, social, or economic environment to facilitate safer behavior. Such approaches can include accurate labeling and instructions (e.g., on foods, pharmaceutical products, or nutritional supplements); restrictions on commercial advertising of hazardous products and activities (e.g., tobacco, alcoholic beverages, gambling); and creation of housing and building codes to prevent injury and disease (e.g., sanitation, lead paint) and to make environments safer (e.g., guards on upper-level apartment windows, median barriers on highways, regulations for safe disposal of toxic substances).

AN INTERVENTION CASE STUDY: TOBACCO

Tobacco control provides a good illustration of the translation of research to application. This example was selected because there is substantial evidence that tobacco use causes ill health, public health interventions and clinical effectiveness have been evaluated, and cost-effectiveness studies are available. Many approaches have been used to decrease the prevalence of tobacco use. Despite the multitude of interventions, it is still not possible to conclude what works and what does not. Some general conclusions can be drawn.

At the individual level, there have been reviews of thousands of studies on clinical interventions to reduce tobacco use. The findings suggest that counseling and pharmacotherapies are effective. Community-based interventions have shown variable success. Many of them have been directed toward youth in the belief that they would have the greatest impact for the future. Some very well designed intervention trials, however, conclude that the approaches used were ineffective. A review of government-level approaches to tobacco use prevention and cessation revealed that single approaches via clean air laws, price increases, counter-advertising, enforcement of existing laws restricting youth access, and others may be effective with some people. However, a combination of these approaches has the greatest possibility of success.

In summary, there is limited evidence that any single step is effective in reducing tobacco use. Although a number of studies have been published, many if not most suffer from design flaws that fail adequately to consider co-factors existing in the community. The conclusion of the committee is that a multi-pronged approach including (but not limited to) education, clinical intervention, price increases, restricted access to tobacco, clean air laws, and counter-advertising must be used. In current tobacco users, counseling and pharmacotherapies have the greatest potential.

FINDINGS AND RECOMMENDATIONS

Finding 1: Health and disease are determined by dynamic interactions among biological, psychological, behavioral, and social factors. These interactions occur over time and throughout development. Cooperation and interaction of multiple disciplines are necessary for understanding and influencing health and behavior.

Recommendation 1: Funding agencies should direct resources toward interdisciplinary efforts for research and intervention studies that integrate biological, psychological, behavioral, and social variables. The investigations that will be most productive will reflect an understanding of the complexity and interconnections of disciplines. Collaborations across disciplines need to be encouraged and expanded.

Finding 2: A fundamental finding of the report is the importance of the interaction of psychosocial and biological processes in health and disease. Psychosocial factors influence health directly through biological mechanisms and indirectly through an array of behaviors. Social and psychological factors include socioeconomic status, social inequalities, social networks and support, work conditions, depression, anger, and hostility.

Recommendation 2: Research efforts to elucidate the mechanisms by which social and psychological factors influence health should be encouraged. Intervention studies are needed to evaluate the effectiveness of modifying these factors to improve health and prevent disease. Such intervention studies should span the breadth of all phases of clinical trials, from feasibility studies to randomized double-blind studies. Community-based participatory research should also be conducted. Research should include all levels of intervention, from individual to family, community, and society.

Finding 3: Behavior can be changed: behavioral interventions can successfully teach new behaviors and attenuate risky behaviors. Maintaining behavior change over time, however, is a greater challenge. Short-term changes in behavior are encouraging, but improved health outcomes will often require prolonged interventions and lengthy follow-up protocols.

Recommendation 3: Funding for health-related behavioral and psychosocial interventions should support realistically long-duration efforts.

Finding 4: Individual behavior, family interactions, community and workplace relationships and resources, and public policy all contribute to health and influence behavior change. Existing research suggests that interventions at multiple levels (individual, family, community, society) are most likely to sustain behavioral change.

Recommendation 4: Concurrent interventions at multiple levels (individual, family, community, and society) should be encouraged to promote healthy behaviors. Assessments of coordinated efforts across levels are needed. Such efforts should address the psychosocial factors associated with health status (e.g., access to healthy foods or safe places to exercise) as well as individual behavior.

Finding 5: Initiating and maintaining a behavior change is difficult. Evidence indicates that it is easier to generalize a newly learned behavior than to change existing behavior. The old adage "an ounce of prevention is worth a pound of cure" is valid in the context of behavior and health as well.

Recommendation 5: Resources should be allocated to the promotion of health-enhancing behavior and primary prevention of disease. This should be a priority for public health and health care systems.

Finding 6: The goals of public health and health care are to increase life expectancy and improve health-related quality of life. Many behavioral intervention trials document the capacity of interventions to modify risk factors, but relatively few measured mortality and morbidity. However, ramifications of interventions are not always apparent until they are fully evaluated, and unexpected consequences can result.

Recommendation 6: Intervention research must include appropriate measures (including biological measures) to determine whether the strategy has the desired health effects.

Finding 7: Changing unhealthy behavior is not simply a matter of "willpower." Individual behavior has biological underpinnings and consequences and is influenced by the social and psychological contexts in which it occurs. While biological interventions and exhortations to individuals to change their behaviors are easier to administer, changes in social factors, policies, and norms are necessary for improvement and maintenance of population health. Much can be learned as states change cigarette taxes, create controls on public advertising for various products, and increase or decrease opportunities for exercise during the school day or as communities implement or eliminate walking and bicycle paths. Such social and policy decisions are rich opportunities for learning about behavior change and health.

Recommendation 7: Program planners and policy makers need to consider modifying social and societal conditions to enable healthy behavior and social relationships. Interventions must be evaluated to enable continuous improvement of programs and policies. Research in these domains should be rigorous and scientific, but method should not dominate substance. Longitudinal research designs, natural experiments, quasi-experimental methods, community-based participatory research, and development of new research methods are necessary to advance knowledge in these areas.

1

Introduction

Recent decades have seen increasing attention to the contribution of psychosocial factors, particularly behavior, to enhancing or compromising health. *Healthy People* (U.S. Department of Health, Education, and Welfare, 1979) and *Health and Behavior: Frontiers of Research in the Biobehavioral Sciences* (IOM, 1982; hereafter referred to as the 1982 report) identified and integrated a range of research and identified promising areas, or "scientific opportunities," for future development. Cigarette smoking, excessive alcohol consumption, other substance abuse, unhealthy dietary habits, sedentary lifestyles, and nonadherence to effective medication regimens were among the health-compromising behaviors identified and targeted for modification or prevention with consequent benefit to the public health. The 1982 report recognized that "both access to health care and regard for its advice are behaviorally influenced" (IOM, 1982: 25) and that "the burden of illnesses and disabilities in the United States and the world is closely related to social, psychological, and behavioral aspects of the way of life of the population" (IOM, 1982: 49-50).

The 1982 report was influential in creating opportunities for research and was almost prescient in its statements about areas that have developed greatly since that time. For example, large-scale studies of social risk factors, such as social class or socioeconomic status, have contributed to our understanding of population health in many ways (Chapter 4). Further research has supported most of what was presented in the 1982 report, but exciting progress has been made in the new areas, such as psychoneuroimmunology (Chapter 2).

Times have changed since 1982, with consequent changes in perspective. It is now acknowledged, for example, that cardiovascular disease is an important killer of women as well as of men, necessitating research and improvements in practice. National concern about the public health consequences of tobacco use has led to a wide range of interventions and the evaluation of approaches. The emergence of new medical and public health problems, such as human immunodeficiency virus (HIV) and other infectious diseases, since the 1982 report has again demonstrated the importance of behavior to health and has led to the application of information about health and behavior to new problems as well as to the development of new knowledge itself.

Finally, advances in methods and conceptual models since 1982 have enriched and challenged the biobehavioral sciences—the fields that have contributed knowledge and application in the areas of health and behavior addressed in this report.

DEFINITION OF BEHAVIOR

The 1982 *Health and Behavior* report adopted the term *biobehavioral sciences* to encompass the many disciplines that contribute to behavior and health. After considerable discussion, the Committee on Health and Behavior: Research, Practice and Policy also chose to use this term, as defined in 1982, because it reflects the rich, dynamic, and interactive nature of the fields contributing to knowledge of health and behavior and because it is still current:

> The term *biobehavioral sciences* is used . . . to refer to the panoply of basic, applied, and clinical sciences that contribute to an understanding of behavior. It naturally includes the behavioral sciences that conduct experimental analyses of animal and human conduct. It also includes such basic sciences as neurology, neurochemistry, endocrinology, and neuroanatomoy, as well as the fields of psychology, ethology, sociology, and anthropology. One merit of a broadly inclusive terminology is that it encompasses the many changes in specialties and subspecialties that currently characterize the area. As overlapping areas of interest emerge, they often are labeled with compound names, such as behavioral genetics, psychoneuroimmunology, immunohistochemistry, or behavioral medicine. All are part of the biobehavioral sciences. (IOM, 1982)

Biopsychosocial is a related term used in this report to encompass consideration of variables from the biological, psychological, and social do-mains. An important characteristic of biopsychosocial or biobehavioral research is that it "involves the study of the interactions of biological factors with behavioral or social variables and how they affect each other (i.e., the study of bidirectional, multilevel relationships)" (Anderson, 1999).

DEFINITION AND MEASUREMENT OF HEALTH

Health is sometimes negatively defined as the absence of disease and injury, sometimes as a normative judgment referring to the average state of most people, and sometimes as a positive concept of well-being. Dis-ability and illness can be distinct from health or, together with health, represent different points on a continuum (Patrick and Erickson, 1993).

The various definitions of health, each emphasizing different con-cepts, have been debated for centuries. Precise biomedical or biological definitions (absence of abnormal biological markers or physiological ab-normalities) are useful because they offer opportunities for precise mea-surement, but they fail to capture all the attributes typically associated with health. On the other hand, the broad definition adopted by the World Health Organization in 1948 ("Health is a state of complete physi-cal, mental, and social well-being and not merely the absence of infir-mity") is comprehensive but difficult to apply.

Common epidemiologic measures, which emphasize morbidity and mortality, are incomplete. Morbidity data, for example, often omit infor-mation about mortality; mortality data typically do not include informa-tion about concurrent morbidity. Disease and disability affect multiple aspects of wellness. A comprehensive definition of health requires inte-gration of broader concepts of morbidity and mortality (IOM, 1998).

From a medical perspective, people are healthy if they are uninjured and free of disease, but a person with risk factors for disease might be considered unhealthy. As increasing numbers of people are screened or as technology improves, more disease is revealed (Black and Welch, 1997). New technologies might identify "diseases" that have little effect on life expectancy or quality of life. Pathology thus depends on the state of bio-medical knowledge and technology. Despite the appeal of the medical model, however, it can provide evidence that is in conflict with other indicators of health. The health care system defines the need for health care based on the technology available for assessment and treatment. But, when a patient feels distress, health care needs do not always correlate with health care system definitions (Evans and Stoddard, 1990).

Although disease usually is regarded as a binary variable—it is either present or absent—most health problems fall on a continuum. Changing the thresholds associated with a disease can thus change the number of people who would be considered sick. For example, in the past, "overweight" was defined as a body mass index greater than 28. When that threshold recently was reset at 25 (NHLBI, 1998), most of the adult U.S. population became classified as overweight. Similarly, new methods for assessing subthreshold depression greatly increased the number of people characterized as having that condition (Judd et al., 1996). Although slightly more than 5% of patients in general medical practice qualify for a diagnosis of depression, as defined by the American Psychiatric Association in its DSM-IV (APA, 1994), more than 25% meet the criteria for "subsyndromal" depression (Wells, 1996).

An alternative to the traditional biomedical model, the "outcomes model," emphasizes patient outcomes rather than disease pathologies. The biomedical model is predicated on finding specific biological problems; the outcomes model considers consequences from the perspective of the patient. Successful treatments improve quality of life or extend length of life. This might differ significantly from what would be considered successful treatment using strictly biomedical measures. One review (Fowler et al., 1994), for example, found that although many surgical procedures have no effect on life expectancy, they can help relieve symptoms and improve functional status. Outcomes assessment is useful to determine whether symptoms are, in fact, relieved. A growing body of work demonstrates that measures of wellness are significant predictors of longevity for patients with chronic illnesses (Coates et al., 1997; Idler and Benyamini, 1997; Kaplan et al., 1994). Typically, simple self-report measures of overall health status perform at least as well as physiological indicators do.

Contemporary definitions recognize that health is multidimensional. Spilker (1996) identified five major domains of life quality: physical status and functional ability, psychological status and well-being, social interactions, economic and vocational status and factors, and religious and spiritual status. Various health outcomes approaches assess different dimensions, and the dimensions themselves vary considerably in approach. An emerging consensus suggests that the concept of health must integrate mortality with multiple dimensions of life quality. Most attempts include physical and mental symptoms of behavioral and social functioning.

Symptoms could be as various as pain, cough, anxiety, or depressed mood. Physical functioning is typically measured by limited mobility or by confinement to bed or home. Social functioning is indicated by performance of usual social roles such as attendance at school, ability to work, or participation in recreational activities. The concept of health-related quality of life incorporates combinations of these attributes (Erickson et al., 1995; Patrick and Erickson, 1993).

Time

The concept of health implicitly includes a time dimension. Current wellness or illness must be considered together with prospects for the future. A person infected with HIV might seem healthy today, but might not be called healthy because he or she is at high risk for disease and premature death in the future. The failure to separate current health status from prognosis is a major conceptual obstacle to defining health. Both health and severity of illness should be assessed with respect to the two independent constructs of current function and prognosis (see NRC, 2000a).

Time also is essential in considering development throughout life. Prenatal and early postnatal development are particularly important for lifelong health and well-being. Not only do people of different ages have different health concerns, but the unique vulnerabilities and strengths of different periods of life have implications for health and behavior during each period as well as for those that follow. Research and practice in the field of health and behavior should be considered from the perspective of the entire lifespan (see NRC, 2000a; IOM, 2000).

Positive Health

The concept of positive health has evolved over the past 40 years, beginning with *Current Concepts of Positive Mental Health* (Jahoda, 1958). Recent definitions include at least four constructs: a healthy body; high-quality personal relationships; a sense of purpose in life; self-regarded mastery of life's tasks; and resilience to stress, trauma, and change (Ryff and Singer, 1998). Each component is associated with positive health outcomes. Those who are physically fit and have healthy habits are less likely to develop disability or die prematurely from chronic disease (Rowe and Kahn, 1998). People with high-quality personal relationships and supportive social networks tend to be more resistant to disease and to recover more quickly than those with poorer social relationships. Several epidemiologic studies show that supportive social relationships reduce the risk of death from cardiovascular disease (Berkman, 1995). The magnitude of the effect of social isolation on the risk of cardiovascular disease is comparable to that of elevated serum cholesterol or mild hypertension (Atkins et al., 1991). Positive psychological states are associated with better coping with severe stress attendant to acquired immune deficiency syndrome (AIDS), cancer, or arthritis (Folkman, 1997). Frankl (1992) demonstrated that a sense of purpose in life was associated with a greater likelihood of surviving Nazi concentration camps and of psychological recovery from that experience.

Although the concept of positive health is clearly important, it presents several challenges (NRC, 2000a). First, it is not clear whether positive health is incorporated into other definitions of health—particularly those that include both current function and prognosis. Most of the evidence supporting positive health per se is associated with better outcomes for those with healthy bodies, high-quality personal relationships, a sense of purpose, and high self-regard. Like people who refrain from smoking cigarettes or who have low serum cholesterol, those with positive psychological attributes could stay healthy longer than other people do or adapt better to health challenges.

Second, assessing positive health is difficult. Across cultures, socioeconomic status, and ethnic groups, people rate restrictions in activities associated with health conditions as less desirable than not having such restrictions (Patrick et al., 1985). The requirement to use a wheelchair is consistently rated as less desirable than is being able to walk freely (Kaplan, 1994). Such consensus is not evident, however, for attributes associated with good health. For example, there is much greater variability in ratings for the desirability of having a spouse, of participating in community activities, or of other aspects of social affiliation (Kaplan, 1985). There is considerable agreement regarding desirable aspects of physical functioning but there is little agreement regarding social components.

There is also a difficulty with the "algebra" of positive health. Current approaches regard optimal health as the condition of having no limitations on activity and being free of symptoms. This frames health in negative terms. Rather, the concept of positive health suggests that optimal health should be characterized by having a sense of purpose in life, of high-quality personal relationships, and high self-regard. The way in which "positive" and "negative" components interact to produce a given health status has not been described.

THE INTERSECTION OF HEALTH AND BEHAVIOR

In 1974, the Lalonde report presented a framework of the health field that went beyond providing medical care and identified human biology, environment, lifestyle, and health care organization as major elements. That report initially led to a focus on lifestyle, or individual behavior, as both the locus of responsibility and the target of clinical and community interventions. Later, Evans and Stoddart (1990), attempting to encompass the dimensions that individuals, care providers, and policymakers believe to be important, provided an even broader framework for determinants of health (Figure 1-1). One goal was to bridge the gap between the increasingly sophisticated knowledge of the relationships among multiple categories of conditions that influence health, and health policy that fo-

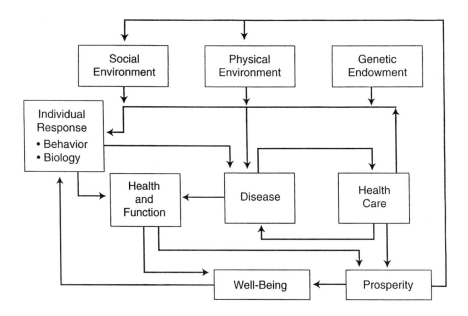

FIGURE 1-1 A model of the determinants of health. Source: Reprinted from R.G. Evans and G.L. Stoddart, 1990, Producing Health, Consuming Health Care, *Social Science and Medicine* 31:1347-1363, with permission from Elsevier Science Ltd, Kidlington, UK.

cused primarily on providing health care. The model shows that factors that include social and physical environment and genetic endowment also influence individual biological and behavioral determinants of health. This crucial point—that behavior is not simply individual choice but is shaped by multiple forces operating at different levels of organization—is developed further in this report.

Individuals influence and are influenced by their families, social networks, the organizations in which they participate (workplaces, schools, religious organizations), the communities of which they are part, and the society in which they live. Interventions to improve health or to influence behavior can occur at any one of those levels or at more than one. This ecologic framework suggests that, because all of the levels are in dynamic interaction (continually changing as a result of reciprocal influences), planned change is likely to be most effective if a comprehensive intervention targets all levels and if the likely consequences (for the other levels) of intervening at one level are recognized (Gottlieb and McLeroy, 1994; Stokols, 1992, 1996). Clearly, no one organization or intervention can address all components of this model. The framework therefore implies the need to bring together a range of individuals and organizations with a variety of skills and interests in efforts to promote or improve health.

Table 1-1 outlines multiple targets of change and strategies for intervention at each level (from individual to population). The targets and strategies are not comprehensive. The table provides an overview of how the ecologic approach can be used to examine change at various levels.

Interventions that target cigarette smoking provide some of the best examples, because interventions have occurred at most of these levels and rates of cigarette smoking have declined among adults in the United States. Without carefully planned research, however, it is impossible to know which intervention, or what combination of interventions, was necessary and sufficient to achieve that result. It is important to give people information through clinical or public health messages, but disapproval of smoking by family and friends, constraints on smoking in workplaces and other locations, lawsuits, congressional hearings, taxes, and advertising policies all confound efforts to attribute the result to a single intervention or level of intervention.

This report is not the first to propose an ecologic (see McLeroy et al., 1988) or contextual approach (see Ewart, 1991) to health and behavior. However, the committee has amassed evidence from many disciplines that points to the same conclusion: health and behavior are influenced by factors at multiple levels, including biological, psychological, and social. Interventions that involve only the person—for example, using self-control or willpower—are unlikely to change long-term behavior unless other factors, such as family relationships, work situation, or social norms, happen to be aligned to support a change. The committee hopes that this report will stimulate researchers, practitioners, program developers, and public and private policymakers to consider the multiple levels for assessments and interventions in health and behavior.

UNDERLYING ASSUMPTIONS

The committee agreed on the following assumptions:

• Biological, behavioral, and social factors such as genetic endowment, cognitive and emotional interpretations of experience, physical environment, social relationships, and socioeconomic status interact through multiple feedback mechanisms to influence individual health over time. Those interactions are often bidirectional, so cause-and-effect models, used alone, are likely to misrepresent relationships among them.

• Because health is not defined solely in biological terms but also is a function of psychological and social variables, many events or interventions traditionally considered irrelevant actually are quite important for the health status of individuals and populations.

STATEMENT OF TASK

An Institute of Medicine Committee on Health and Behavior: Research, Practice, and Policy was convened in 1998 to update the 1982 *Health and Behavior* report. Funded by the Robert Wood Johnson Foundation, the National Institutes of Health, and the Centers for Disease Control, the committee was charged with the following tasks: (1) update scientific findings about the links between biological, psychosocial and behavioral factors, and health; (2) identify factors involved in health and disease but for which research on these factors and effective behavioral and psychosocial interventions is incomplete; (3) identify and review effective applications of behavioral and psychosocial interventions in a variety of settings; (4) examine implementation of behavioral and psychosocial interventions, including guidelines and changes in provider behaviors;

TABLE 1-1 Ecological Approach to Health and Behavior Research and Practice[a]

Ecological Level	Change Process	Target of Change at Each Level	Strategies and Skills at Each Level
Individual	Physiological	HPA (hypothalamic-pituitary-adrenal) axis CNS (limbic and other systems) Immune system Metabolism Cardiovascular system	Physical activity Pharmacologic therapies Meditation Biofeedback Hypnosis Cognitive therapies
	Psychological	Developmental processes Knowledge Attitudes Beliefs Values Skills Behavior Self-concept, self-efficacy, self-esteem	Tests and measurements Role modeling Education Mass media Social marketing Skills development Resistance to peer pressure Patient counseling and education
Family, social networks	Psychosocial	Social networks Social support Families Workgroups Peers Neighbors	Extending social networks Changing group norms Strengthening families Social support groups Increasing social support

Organization	Norms Incentives Organizational culture Management styles Organizational structure Communication networks	Organizational development Incentive programs Coalition development Participatory action research Team development
Community	Economic opportunities Community resources Neighborhood organizations Community competencies Social and health services Organizational relationships Governmental structures Formal leadership Informal leadership	Community development Community coalitions Empowerment Conflict strategies Media advocacy Public advocacy Consciousness raising Social action Community-based participatory research
Population (societal)	Legislation Regulations Tax policy	Media advocacy Policy analysis Political change Lobbying Political organizing

aAdapted from Health Promotion in the Workplace, 2nd ed., by M.P. O'Donnell and J.S. Harris. Copyright 1993. Reprinted with permission of Delmar, a division of Thomson Learning.

(5) review evidence of cost-effectiveness; and (6) make recommendations concerning further research, applications, and financing.

The committee interpreted their charge with a focus on research rather than policy issues. The report is an overview and summary of available research aimed at a diverse audience. Even with this focus, the committee encountered limitations as to what it was able to address. After examining the evidence, it became clear that there are inadequate data to evaluate fully the cost-effectiveness of behavioral and psychosocial interventions in comparison with other ways of promoting health. Cost-effectiveness analysis attempts to determine ways of promoting good health—procedures, tests, medications, educational programs, regulations, taxes or subsidies, and combinations and variations of these—provide the most effective use of resources. Currently, there are few studies assessing which behavioral and psychosocial interventions contribute the most to good health that are set in this larger context and based on information that demonstrates that they are in the public interest. Comparing behavioral and psychosocial interventions with other ways of promoting health on the basis of cost-effectiveness requires additional research. This topic is only briefly reviewed in Chapter 7.

The committee began this endeavor expecting to discover and share what works and what does not regarding health and behavior. After diligently exploring the literature, the complexity of the issue became evident. The committee noted the vast array of interventions at various levels, with varying endpoints on different populations, with different methodologies. Each committee member brought to the table their own perspective about what would be most effective, but the data were inadequate to convince any of the experts of a best approach to shaping and maintaining behavior change. While conventional wisdom tells us that we need to do more exercise, eat less, avoid tobacco, wear seatbelts, and be careful with firearms, deciding what specific interventions produce these sustained changes presents a dilemma.

A critical obstacle to answering definitively the question of what works best is the difficulty of generalizing the findings of current studies. Many factors contribute to this problem: outcome measures among the studies differ, populations studied differ, and methodologies differ. For example, an intervention may be exceptionally effective on a highly motivated population but fail for the general public. Measurement of a behavioral outcome such as self-reported tobacco use is difficult to compare with an outcome measure such as change in sales of tobacco. Another obstacle is that there are no rigorous evaluations of interventions. Evaluations may assess short-term changes, but long-term effectiveness must enter the equation because maintaining behavior change has been shown to be difficult. Only with additional research and evaluation of interventions will the best approaches be found. This report illustrates the current level of understanding and demonstrates the limits of the currently available research. The example of tobacco in Chapter 8 aims to illustrate the complications inherent in the field.

BOUNDARIES OF THE STUDY

The field of health and behavior is very large. It includes, at minimum, the intersection of biological, social, and behavioral sciences with public health and medicine. The Committee, therefore, had to make hard choices about what to include and exclude from this report. The areas represented in this report are those in which Committee members either had expertise or found to be important enough to seek expert input with the resources available. While behaviors associated with the greatest burden of illness, such as tobacco use, seemed important to consider, the Committee also found it important to focus on health, not just morbidity and mortality. Stress and adaptation, psychosocial aspects of coping with illness, and resilience were deemed important by the Committee. The Committee chose to examine developments in biological, social, and behavioral determinants of health as well as the implications of these factors for intervention and research at the levels of individuals, families, communities, and populations. Issues in translation from research to application, including cost-effectiveness, were also considered.

A number of areas were excluded for a variety of reasons. Injury and substance abuse have been the subjects of recent IOM reports (IOM 1996, 1997a, 1999), so the Committee chose not to devote resources to these. Genetics, health, and behavior were the subject of a concurrent IOM study, and developments in genetics are occurring very quickly. The Committee therefore decided not to go into depth in that area, in which recent, excellent material is available (see Collins, 1999, for an overview of medical and societal implications of the human genome project; Carson and Rothstein, 1999, for various perspectives on behavioral genetics). Child and spousal abuse are difficult and controversial topics, and the Committee was not sufficiently constituted to consider these areas from the range of perspectives necessary to be thorough. While the report does discuss various aspects of obesity, the Committee found that the biology of metabolism and weight regulation—along with clinical and public health perspectives and interventions in this area—are developing, complex, and controversial, and therefore deserve much more attention than the Committee was able to pay here. The Committee recommends that resources be devoted to a comprehensive study of biological, social and psychological factors in obesity and weight regulation and to the effects of medical, public health, and advertising messages about weight. The role of advertising and social marketing is an important consideration in health and behavior and is the topic of a forthcoming IOM report (2001). That report focuses on communication of health messages to diverse populations. The role of diversity in health and disease is a critical concern that is also very relevant to the behavioral and societal influences. Recently, an IOM study was initiated to assess racial and ethnic differences in health care and to provide recommendations regarding interventions to eliminate these disparities (Committee on Understanding and Eliminating Racial and Ethnic Disparities in Health Care, IOM).

The Committee believes that lifespan and lifecourse development (Elder, 1996) are very important to the understanding of health and behavior. The Committee drafted materials and discussed differences in health and behavior across the lifespan, as well as the implications of early experience for later health at many of its meetings. The Committee concluded that it did not have the full range of necessary expertise or the resources to comprehensively address the complex intersection of lifespan and lifecourse development and health and behavior, though it is mentioned in various places in the report. At the first Committee meeting, David Hamburg, the chair of the 1982 study, told the Committee that lifespan development was the one area he most wished could have been addressed in the 1982 report. This Committee feels similarly about this report. Recent reports from the National Academies (IOM, 2000; NRC, 2000a,b,c) provide some discussion of health-related behavioral and social research at various points throughout life. The Committee agreed that development across the lifespan is an important determinant of health that deserves further attention.

Because the field of health and behavior is so extensive, the committee was unable to provide an exhaustive review for all covered topics. This is true, for example, in the description of interventions for behavior change at the various levels. Instead, the report presents a sampling of the many approaches that have been used. These provide the reader with a feel for the state of the science rather than an all-inclusive account of what has been done. For other topics such as the health behaviors described in Chapter 3, the committee relied heavily on existing comprehensive reviews, especially publications from United States government agencies, to provide an overview of the area and supplemented this with data from recent peer-reviewed articles. Other sections of the report carefully reviewed the current literature from peer-reviewed journals to provide a summary of topics that are not available elsewhere. The resulting report should not be considered to be a comprehensive analysis of all efforts in health and behavior but rather an overview that tries to convey a sense of the excitement and growth in this multidisciplinary field.

ORGANIZATION OF THE REPORT

The charge to the committee preparing this report included updating scientific findings about the links between biological, psychosocial, and behavioral factors and health since the 1982 report (IOM, 1982) and addressing the links between determinants of health and interventions based on them in a variety of settings.

Part One describes the status of knowledge regarding biological, behavioral, and social factors that affect health. To emphasize the importance of reciprocal interactions among those factors in the determination of the health status of individuals and populations, without implying that "everything is related to everything else," the report groups biobehavioral linkages with physiological evidence in Chapter 2, behavioral risk factors in Chapter 3, and social risk factors in Chapter 4.

Part Two addresses research and practice regarding interventions in health-related behavior. Chapter 5 discusses the interventions at the level of individual behavior and families. Chapter 6 reviews interventions at the levels of organization, community, and society. Chapter 7 addresses the evaluation of interventions and the dissemination of research findings and practical experience.

Part Three (Chapter 8) presents the principal findings and the committee's recommendations. It includes a description of experience with interventions aimed at reducing cigarette smoking because these interventions have been pursued at all of the levels addressed in this report.

REFERENCES

Anderson, N.B. (1999). Office of Behavioral and Social Sciences research definition of research areas: A definition of behavioral and social sciences research for the National Institutes of Health [Online]. Available: http://www1.od.nih.gov/obssr/def.htm [2000, April 5].

APA (American Psychiatric Association) (1994). *Diagnostic and statistical manual of mental disorders: DSM-IV.* Washington, DC: American Psychiatric Association.

Atkins, C.J., Kaplan, R.M., and Toshima, M.T. (1991). Close relationships in the epidemiology of cardiovascular disease. In W.H. Jones and D. Perlman (Eds.) *Advances in Personal Relationships, 3* (pp. 207–231). London: Jessica Kingsley Publishers.

Berkman, L.F. (1995). The role of social relations in health promotion. *Psychosomatic Medicine, 57,* 245–254.

Black, W.C. and Welch, H.G. (1997). Screening for disease. *American Journal of Roentgenology, 168,* 3–11.

Carson, R.A. and Rothstein, M.A. (Eds.) (1999). *Behavioral Genetics: The Clash of Culture and Biology.* Baltimore: Johns Hopkins University Press.

Coates A., Porzsolt F., and Osoba, D. (1997). Quality of life in oncology practice: Prognostic value of EORTC QLQ-C30 scores in patients with advanced malignancy. *European Journal of Cancer, 33,* 1025–1030.

Collins, F.S. (1999). The human genome project and the future of medicine. *Annals of the New York Academy of Science, 882,* 42–55.

Elder, G.H., Jr. (1996). Human lives in changing societies: Life course and developmental insights. In R.B. Cairns, G.H. Elder, Jr., and E.J. Costello (Eds.) *Developmental Science* (pp. 31–62). New York: Cambridge University Press.

Erickson, P., Wilson, R., and Shannon, I. (1995). *Years of Healthy Life. Healthy People 2000, Statistical Notes Number 7.* Washington, DC: USDHHS, Centers for Disease Control and Prevention, NCHS.

Evans, R.G. and Stoddart, G.L. (1990). Producing health, consuming health care. *Social Science and Medicine 31,* 1347–1363.

Ewart, C.K. (1991). Social action theory for a public health psychology. *American Psychologist 46,* 931–946.

Folkman, S. (1997). Positive psychological states and coping with severe stress. *Social Science Medicine 45,* 1207–1221.

Fowler, F.J., Jr., Cleary, P.D., Magaziner, J., Patrick, D.L., and Benjamin, K.L. (1994). Methodological issues in measuring patient-reported outcomes: The agenda of the Work Group on Outcomes Assessment. *Medical Care 32,* JS65–JS76.

Frankl, V. E. (1992). *Man's Search for Meaning: An Introduction to Logotherapy 4th edition.* Boston: Beacon Press.

Gottlieb, N.H., and McLeroy, K.R. (1994). Social health. In M.P. O'Donnell and J.S. Harris (Eds.) *Health Promotion in the Workplace* (pp. 459–493). Albany, NY: Delmar.

Idler, E.L. and Benyamini, Y. (1997). Self-rated health and mortality: A review of twenty-seven community studies. *Journal of Health and Social Behavior, 38,* 21–37.

IOM (Institute of Medicine) (1982). *Health and Behavior: Frontiers of Research in the Biobehavioral Sciences.* Hamburg, D.A., Elliott, G.R., and Parron, D.L. (Eds.) Washington, DC: National Academy Press.

IOM (Institute of Medicine) (1996). *Pathways of Addiction: Opportunities in Drug Abuse Research.* Washington, DC: National Academy Press.

IOM (Institute of Medicine) (1997). *Dispelling the Myths About Addiction: Strategies to Increase Understanding and Strengthen Research.* Washington, DC: National Academy Press.

IOM (Institute of Medicine) (1998). *Summarizing Population Health: Directions for the Development and Application of Population Metrics.* M.J. Field, and M.R. Gold (Eds.) Washington, DC: National Academy Press.

IOM (Institute of Medicine) (1999). *Reducing the Burden of Injury: Advancing Prevention and Treatment.* R.J. Bonnie, C.E. Fulco, and C.T. Liverman (Eds.).Washington, DC: National Academy Press.

IOM (Institute of Medicine) (2000) *Promoting Health: Intervention Strategies from Social and Behavioral Research.* B.D. Smedley and S.L. Syme (Eds.) Washington, DC: National Academy Press.

IOM (Institute of Medicine) (2001). *Speaking of Health: Assessing Health Communication. Strategies for Diverse Populations.* C. Chrvala and S. Scrimshaw (Eds.), Washington, DC: National Academy Press.

Jahoda, M. (1958). *Current Concepts of Positive Mental Health.* New York: Basic Books.

Judd, L.L., Paulus, M.P, Wells, K.B., and Rapaport, M.H. (1996). Socioeconomic burden of subsyndromal depressive symptoms and major depression in a sample of the general population. *American Journal of Psychiatry, 153,* 1411–1417.

Kaplan, R.M. (1985). Social support and social health. In I.G. Sarason and B.R. Sarason (Eds.) *Social Support Theory, Research, and Application* (pp. 95–113). The Hague: Martinus Nijhoff International Publisher.

Kaplan, R.M. (1994). Value judgment in the Oregon Medicaid Experiment. *Medical Care, 32,* 975–988.

Kaplan, R.M., Ries, A.L., Prewitt, L.M., and Eakin, E. (1994). Self-efficacy expectations predict survival for patients with chronic obstructive pulmonary disease. *Health Psychology, 13,* 366–368.

Lalonde, M.A. (1974). *New Perspectives on the Health of Canadians. A Working Document.* Ottawa: Information Canada.

McLeroy, K.R., Bibeau, D., Steckler, A., and Glanz, K. (1988). An ecological perspective on health promotion programs. *Health Education Quarterly, 15,* 351–377.

NHLBI (National Heart, Lung and Blood Institute) (1998). *Clinical Guidelines on the Identification, Evaluation, And Treatment of Overweight and Obesity in Adults: The Evidence Report.* U.S. Department of Health and Human Services.

NRC (National Research Council) (2000a). *New Horizons in Health: An Integrative Approach.* B.H. Singer and C.D. Ryff (Eds.). Washington DC: National Academy Press.

NRC (National Research Council) (2000b). *From Neurons to Neighborhoods, The Science of Early Childhood Development.* J.P. Shonkoff and D.A. Phillips (Eds.). Washington, DC: National Academy Press.

NRC (National Research Council) (2000c). *The Aging Mind, Opportunities in Cognitive Research.* P.C. Stern and L.L. Carstensen (Eds.). Washington, DC: National Academy Press.

Patrick, D. and Erikson, P. (1993). *Health Status and Health Policy: Quality of Life in Evaluation and Resource Allocation.* New York: Oxford University Press.

Patrick, D., Sittanpalam, Y., Somerville, S., Carter, W.B., and Bergner, M. (1985). A cross-cultural comparison of health status values. *American Journal of Public Health, 75,* 1402–1407.

Rowe, J.W. and Kahn, R.L. (1998). *Successful Aging.* New York: Pantheon Books.

Ryff, C.D. and Singer, B. (1998). The contours of positive health. *Psychological Inquiry 9,* 1–28.

Spilker, B. (Ed.) (1996) *Quality of Life and Pharmacoeconomics in Clinical Trials* (pp. 309–322). Philadelphia: Lippincott-Raven Publishers.

Stokols, D. (1992). Establishing and maintaining healthy environments: Toward a social ecology of health promotion. *American Psychologist, 47,* 6–22.

Stokols, D. (1996). Translating social ecological theory into guidelines for community health promotion. *American Journal of Health Promotion, 10,* 282–298.

United States Department of Health, Education, and Welfare. (1979). *Healthy People.* DHEW Publication Number (PHS) 79-55071. Washington, DC: U.S. Government Printing Office.

Wells, K. (1996). *Caring for Depression.* Cambridge, MA: Harvard University Press.

PART ONE

Biological, Behavioral, and Social Factors Affecting Health

I n the early years of scientific medicine, most clinicians and researchers thought only in terms of single causes: specific agents that cause specific disease. For example, an infection was considered to result only from the proliferation of bacteria, while other kinds of ill health might result from viruses, toxins, accidents, or flaws in a person's genetic makeup. More recent research highlights the relationships between health and behavioral, psychological, and social variables.

Acceptance of the fact that stress is linked to cardiovascular disease or to other health problems has become commonplace. However, research also reveals many reciprocal links among the central nervous system, which recognizes and records experiences; the endocrine system, which produces hormones that govern many body functions; and the immune system, which organizes responses to infections and other challenges.

Similarly, it has long been recognized that specific behaviors are associated with increased risk of specific diseases and related conditions. For example, tobacco use, alcohol consumption, inadequate physical activity, some sexual practices, and high-fat or low-fiber diets have all been recognized as unhealthful. Less widely recognized, however, is the association between socioeconomic status and health, or the influence of social networks, current or anticipated employment status, and personal beliefs. Recent research not only documents the importance of these factors, but also describes some of the mechanisms involved.

Part One reviews some of the most important developments on these topics. Chapter 2 addresses the interactions of biobehavioral factors in health, Chapter 3 reviews behavioral risk factors, and Chapter 4 describes the role of social risk factors.

2

Biobehavioral Factors in Health and Disease

Research into the bidirectional and multilevel relationships between behavior and health has been aided by technology and by conceptual advances in the behavioral, biological, and medical sciences. Our understanding of the interactions between brain function and behavior has been enriched by advances in behavioral neurobiology, neuroscience, and neuroendocrinology from molecular mechanisms to psychological systems. Real-time imaging of the living human brain during different behavioral states has promoted our understanding of the links between human behavior and basic neurochemical processes or specific neuroanatomic pathways. Common availability of monoclonal antibodies, routine production of genetically altered animals, and new understanding of the genetic code have contributed to exploration of how genetics interacts with development and early experiences to influence both vulnerability to disease and resistance to age-related decline. Yet much of the research knowledge is highly compartmentalized, and there is a need to integrate isolated pockets of information.

This chapter addresses the interplay among biological, behavioral, and social factors in health and disease, with an emphasis on biologic factors. Subsequent chapters address behavioral and social factors in greater detail.

STRESS, HEALTH, AND DISEASE

The Stress Response

Over the past 60 years or so, the study of stress has provided a major link in explaining the behavioral variables and the biological factors that influence physical health. Stress both causes and modulates a diversity of physiological effects that can enhance resistance to disease or cause damage and thereby promote disease. For example, stress-related hormones, such as cortisol and epinephrine, have protective and adaptive functions as well as damaging effects. This idea, first introduced by Hans Selye (1956), is reemerging in contemporary biobehavioral research (McEwen, 1998). A characteristic set of physiological effects—the "stress response"—has been identified and investigated in humans and animals (Chrousos, 1998). The primary and secondary effects of the stress response constitute the biologic pathways along which a person's experiences, living and working conditions, interpersonal relations, lifestyle, diet, personality traits, and general socioeconomic status can affect the body. Individual behavior is important because it increases or decreases the pathophysiological cost of stress through diet, exercise, and other activities.

The stress response is an important component of the body's regulatory systems. The maintenance of constant and appropriate internal conditions and functioning in the face of changing environmental demands is called *homeostasis*, an idea first developed by Walter Cannon (1936). The stress response, however, primarily involves reaction in an emergency. This function evolved over millions of years and is critical to the survival of most animals, including humans, when external threats and dangers, such as predation, are encountered. The stress response consists of many co-adapted and simultaneous shifts in the physiological functioning of the cardiovascular, respiratory, muscular, metabolic, immune, and central nervous systems. Physiological changes can be accompanied by altered emotional responses, enhanced vigilance, heightened appraisal of risk, enhanced memory storage and retrieval, and changes in motivation. The stress response is a rapid and pervasive adjustment of internal states to prepare an organism to adapt to a threat—to respond to the rigors of "fight or flight" (Chrousos, 1998).

Many aspects of the stress response, however, are inappropriate or maladaptive in the context of modern postindustrial societies. The threats posed here are different from those our evolutionary ancestors faced. We do not commonly confront acute, life-threatening assault. Instead, contemporary humans face ill-defined, diffuse, often chronic threats that cannot be resolved by fight or flight. Nevertheless, the ancient physiologic stress response is triggered when one experiences, for example, a threat to social position, damage to important interpersonal relationships, loss of possessions, or barriers to the achievement of goals. Because many difficulties of contemporary life and their accompanying stress cannot be rapidly resolved—as could many physical stressors—the stress response persists, homeostasis is not restored, and the response becomes dysfunctional rather than adaptive. An increasing body of evidence indicates that stress is a potent contributor to illness (Cohen and Herbert, 1996; Cohen et al., 1991; Hermann et al., 1995; Kiecolt-Glaser et al., 1996; McEwen, 1998). The continued and unproductive activation of the stress response, including the failure to shut off this response when it is not needed, called *allostatic load*, is discussed below.

The stress response is one aspect of an array of biologic and behavioral processes that either protect or cause damage. For example, secretion of stress-related hormones, such as cortisol and the catecholamines (epinephrine and norepinephrine), typically varies in a daily rhythm that is entrained by the light/dark cycle and by sleep/waking patterns that are part of normal daily life. But chronic increase in cortisol throughout the diurnal cycle is associated with negative consequences, such as accelerated bone mineral loss and hyperglycemia. Because the subjective experience of stress does not always correlate with physiological response (Kirschbaum et al., 1999), long-term measurement of hormone concentrations and of the processes that they regulate (for example, blood cholesterol concentration, fat accumulation, immune function, atrophy of brain structures, blood pressure), constitute an important way to connect life experience and the risk of disease.

Allostasis and Allostatic Load

An important new attempt to understand the relationships between environmental and behavioral challenges and stressors, the physiological responses to these events, and disease uses the terms *allostasis* and *allostatic load*. Allostasis is the maintenance of overall stability (homeostasis) through the constant adjustment and balancing of various components in the process of adapting to challenge. Sterling and Eyer (1988) first used the term to describe cardiovascular system adjustments in response to rest and activity states. Later, the idea was generalized to other physiologic mediators, such as adrenal cortisol and the catecholamines. Allostatic load is the wear and tear the body experiences as a result of repeated allostatic response (McEwen, 1998; McEwen and Stellar, 1993).

Allostasis and allostatic load operate in all systems of the body and focus attention on the protective, as well as the damaging, property of the primary mediators of the stress response: cortisol and the catecholamines. The major aspects are summarized in Figure 2-1. First, the brain integrates and coordinates behavioral and physiologic responses (hormonal and autonomic) to challenge. Some challenges can be perceived as stressful; others are related to circadian rhythms and to coordination of the functions of sleep and waking with the environment. Second, individual differences in the capacity to cope with challenges are based on multilevel relationships between genetic, developmental, and experiential influences. Third, intrinsic to the autonomic, neuroendocrine, and behavioral responses to challenge is the capacity to adapt (allostasis); indeed, neuroendocrine responses, such as the release of cortisol, are by nature protective and acute. Problems arise only when they persist, so efficient initiation and cessation of these responses is vital. Negative effects result when allostatic responses to challenge or stress occur inappropriately or are terminated inefficiently. Fourth, allostasis has a price that is related to the degree of inefficiency in the response and to the number of challenges and stressors a person experiences. Allostatic load is more than chronic stress. It can also reflect a genetically or developmentally induced failure to cope efficiently with the daily challenges related to the sleep/waking cycle and other experiences. And it also includes contributions of lifestyle factors, such as diet, alcohol and tobacco use, physical activity, and sleep, through their influences on the production of stress hormones.

Protective and Damaging Effects of Stress Mediators

A behavioral response to challenge or stress can be protective or damaging. The risk of harm or disease can be increased by such patterns of behavior as hostility or aggression, and it can be reduced by cooperation and conciliation. Cigarette-smoking, excessive alcohol consumption, high fat consumption, and exposure to physical hazards increase the risk, as does insufficient physical activity. The link of allostasis and allostatic load can be applied to various behavioral responses: Such behaviors as smoking, high alcohol consumption, and consumption of high-fat foods all have

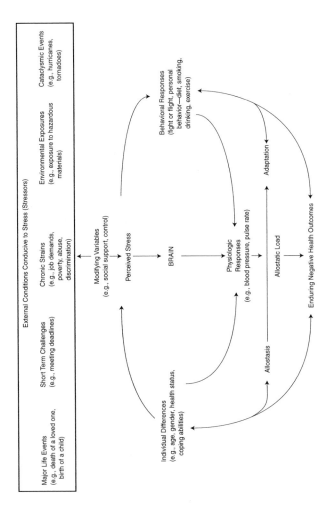

FIGURE 2-1 The Stress Response and Development of Allostatic Load.
Individuals experience objective psychological and environmental conditions that are conducive to stress, referred to as stressors. The perception of stress is influenced by social, psychological, biophysical factors, genetics, and behavior. When the brain perceives an experience as stressful, physiologic and behavioral responses are initiated, leading to allostasis and adaptation. Over time, allostatic load can accumulate, and the overexposure to mediators of neural, endocrine, and immune stress can have adverse effects on various organ systems, leading to enduring negative health outcomes (physiological, e.g., cardiovascular disease; psychological, e.g., depression; behavioral, e.g., alcoholism). Adapted from McEwen, 1998; Israel and Schurman, 1990. Reprinted with permission from Massachusetts Medical Society. Copyright 1998. All rights reserved. Reprinted by permission of Jossey-Bass, Inc., a subsidiary of John Wiley & Sons, Inc.

some perceived adaptive effects in the short-term but damaging effects if they persist. Behavior can attenuate some of the damaging effects of physiologic responses. For example, even a brief period of exercise can enhance glucose uptake by reducing the insulin resistance of muscle tissue (Perseghin et al.,1996).

The mediators of protective and damaging effects of allostatic responses are mainly adrenal steroids and catecholamines. Other hormones—such as dehydroepiandrosterone, prolactin, growth hormones, and the cytokines—also mediate adaptive or maladaptive effects, but their consequences are often specific to an organ or a system. Once the mediators are released, they produce their effects by acting on cellular receptors. The effects can be classified as primary effects; secondary outcomes, which are risk factors for disease; and tertiary outcomes, which are diseases themselves (McEwen and Seeman, 1999). The actions of the mediators adrenal glucocorticoids and catecholamines are shown in Figure 2-2. These substances act via receptors that trigger changes throughout the target cell (including changes in gene expression) that have long-lasting consequences for cell function. It is important to consider the short- and long-term consequences of hormone release for cell function. There are many examples of beneficial and adverse effects of the mediators of allostatic responses. These factors are introduced here and discussed in more detail later.

In the central nervous system, catecholamines and adrenal steroids promote the storage and retrieval of memories of events, pleasant and unpleasant, associated with arousal. However, adrenal steroids acting with excitatory amino acid neurotransmitters are associated with cognitive dysfunction involving various mechanisms that promote atrophy and, in some extreme cases, the death of neurons, particularly in the hippocampal region.

In the cardiovascular system, autonomic responses, in part because of catecholamines, promote allostasis (adaptation) by adjusting heart rate and blood pressure according to the changing demands of sleeping, waking, and physical exertion. Damaging allostatic load occurs as a result of a failure to terminate blood pressure surges efficiently. This accelerates atherosclerosis and synergizes with metabolic hormones to accelerate non-insulin-dependent diabetes.

The immune system is particularly responsive to the mediators of allostatic response. Adrenal steroids and catecholamines promote the movement of immune cells to organs or tissues where they are needed to

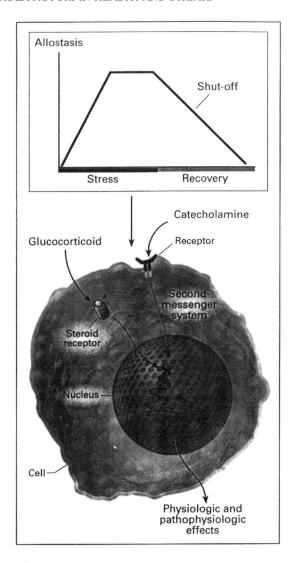

FIGURE 2-2 Allostasis in the Autonomic Nervous System and HPA Axis. Allostatic systems respond to stress (upper panel) by initiating the adaptive response, sustaining it until the stress ceases, and then shutting it off (recovery). Allostatic responses are initiated (lower panel) by an increase in circulating catecholamines from the autonomic nervous system and glucocorticoids from the adrenal cortex. This sets into motion adaptive processes that alter the structure and function of a variety of cellls and tissues. These processes are initiated through intracellular receptors for steroid hormones, plasma-membrane receptors, and second-messenger systems for catecholamines. Cross-talk between catecholamines and glucocorticoid-receptor signaling systems can occur. From McEwen, 1998, by permission of the Massachusetts Medical Society. All rights reserved.

resist infection or other challenge, thereby enhancing the effectiveness of immune responses. But adrenal steroids also can increase allostatic load and suppress immune system response when they are secreted chronically or when their release from the adrenal cortex is not terminated properly.

Allostatic load is associated with at least four patterns of long-term harm to the body. The first is a perception of excessive stress. This can take the form of repeated events of various types that cause recurring increases in the release of stress mediators. For example, the amount and frequency of economic hardship are good predictors of decline in physical and mental functioning and even death (Lynch et al., 1997b). The second pattern involves a failure to adapt to recurrence of the same stressor. This leads to overexposure to stress mediators because of the failure to dampen response to a repeated event. Most people, for example, adapt to repeated public-speaking challenges, but some continue to show elevated cortisol concentrations, which indicate a failure to adapt (Kirschbaum et al., 1995). The third pattern entails the failure to terminate the hormonal stress response or the lack of appearance of the normal trough in the daily cortisol release pattern. Examples are increased blood pressure caused by work-related stress (Gerin and Pickering, 1995), increased evening cortisol and hyperglycemia caused by sleep deprivation (Van Cauter et al., 1997), and the chronically elevated cortisol that often accompanies depressive illness (Michelson et al., 1996). The fourth pattern involves inadequate release of hormones, thus allowing other systems, such as inflammatory cytokines, to become overactive. In the Lewis rats, for example, inadequate release of cortisol is associated with increased susceptibility to inflammatory and autoimmune disturbances (Sternberg, 1997; Sternberg et al., 1996).

Early Development Influences Long-Term Effects of Stress

Developmental influences are implicated in susceptibility to stress-related disorders. Classic work by Levine et al. (1967), Denenberg and Haltmeyer (1967), and Ader (1968), shows that the handling of neonatal rats by experimenters leads to reduced emotionality and stress hormone reactivity throughout life. In contrast, prenatal stress increases emotionality and stress hormone reactivity throughout the life of the animal. Postnatal handling reverses the effects of prenatal stress (Fride et al., 1986; Wakschlak and Weinstock, 1990). Handling is believed to increase maternal licking and grooming of pups, which are associated with reduced reactivity of the hypothalamic/pituitary/adrenal (HPA) axis (Liu et al., 1997). Use of animal models has revealed that age-related brain deterioration is increased by high-stress reactivity and reduced by low-stress reactivity (Dellu et al., 1996; Liu et al., 1997; Meaney et al., 1988). Animals that show high-stress reactivity also show a high propensity for substance abuse (Dellu et al., 1994). Studies in nonhuman primates show that early maternal deprivation alters brain serotonin functioning, increases alcohol preference, increases aggressive behavior, and decreases affiliate behaviors (Higley et al., 1996a, b; Kraemer et al., 1997). In marmosets, altered HPA axis function was found in offspring that experienced negative parenting (Johnson et al., 1996a).

Individual differences in human brain aging are correlated with plasma cortisol concentration (see Lupien et al., 1994, 1998; Seeman et al., 1997), although it is not known whether there are connections to early life events. Some data suggest that extremely low birth weight (Barker, 1997; Wadhwa, 1998) and trauma in early life are risk factors that influence later health in humans (Bremner et al., 1997; Felitti et al., 1998). Studies that link life experience, especially early experience, with stress, allostatic load, and later health risks (Felitti et al., 1998; Bremner et al., 1997; De Bellis et al., 1999a, 1999b) signal the importance of research on the effects of early life experiences on later stress reactivity and health.

Some evidence suggests that even prenatal experiences can have long-term health consequences. In laboratory animals, prenatal stress has been linked to alterations in adrenocortical and central serotonergic and dopaminergic circuits (Nelson and Bloom, 1997). These observations led to the hypothesis (Barker and Sultan, 1995) that disease vulnerabilities in childhood and adult life result from "fetal programming" of homeostatic response set points. This is supported by Eriksson et al. (1999), who report that death from coronary heart disease (CHD) among Finnish men was associated with low birth weight and low ponderal index at birth. In addition, prematurity and low birth weight resulting from maternal behaviors has been seen to increase the life-long risk of CHD (Wadhwa, 1998) and diabetes mellitus (Rich-Edwards et al., 1999).

THE BRAIN AS INTERPRETER, REGULATOR, AND TARGET

The brain is influenced by experiences, including stress, and it is a target of allostatic load, or long-term wear and tear. Since the IOM (1982) report, advances in basic neuroscience and the development of imaging technology have combined to enhance our understanding of how different regions of the brain control behavior. They reveal the plasticity and vulnerability of the brain to effects of life experiences. Advances in the neurobiology of learning and memory have provided important insights into the dynamic nature of brain function throughout life and from the level of the gene to the level of nerve-cell structure and function. Studies of the interplay between brain development and early experience have emphasized their importance in establishing patterns of brain function that persist through life. This section discusses advances in neurobiology that are particularly relevant to the brain as an interpreter of life events, as a regulator of the stress response and daily biological rhythms, and as a target of the protective and the damaging functions of stress mediators. Developmental issues are discussed later in the chapter.

Neurotransmitters, Experience, and Behavior

Changes in balance among neurotransmitters in the brain can influence behavioral responses to potentially stressful situations, can alter the interpretation of stimuli, and might be associated with anxiety and depression. Research that has accelerated rapidly over the past few decades reveals that the human brain has multiple neurotransmitters and neuromodulators. The release of a neurotransmitter sends a message from one neuron to another. Neuromodulators share properties of neurotransmitters and hormones to regulate the general tone of neural systems. Many substances act as neuromodulators, including acetylcholine, histamine, serotonin, the catecholamines, excitatory and inhibitory amino acids, and a host of neuropeptides. In this discussion we emphasize two, serotonin and corticotropin-releasing hormone (CRH)—each with links to the stress response—while recognizing that brain function is a result of the simultaneous interactions of many hormones, neuromodulators, and neurotransmitters.

Serotonin is a neurotransmitter with widespread influences throughout the brain. Most neurons that release serotonin are found in the raphe nuclei in the midbrain. Axons of serotonergic cells have many branches, and they project widely throughout the forebrain, cerebellum, and spinal cord (Cooper et al., 1996). The serotonin system exerts widespread influence over mood and mood disorders, such emotional responses as hostility and aggression, arousal, sensory perception, and higher cognitive functions. For example, low concentrations of brain serotonin are associated with increased incidence of suicide (Brown et al., 1982; Mann, 1998), impulsive aggression (Brown et al., 1982; Higley et al., 1996a, 1996b), and the abuse of alcohol and other substances (Higley et al., 1991).

Experience can alter brain chemistry. One well-studied, common pathway through which the environment effects changes in the brain is the HPA axis. Briefly, to maintain appropriate internal conditions (allostasis) in response to life's stresses, the hypothalamus releases CRH, which travels to the anterior pituitary where it causes the release of adrenocorticotropic hormone. The adrenocorticotropic hormone, in turn, controls the release of other hormones, such as cortisol, from the adrenal cortex (located on top of the kidneys). The HPA axis has been shown to be exquisitely responsive to social environment in rats (Albeck et al, 1997) and in primates (Johnson et al., 1996b; Shively et al., 1997). Social status affects the response of the HPA axis, such that hypothalamic CRH release is deficient in subordinate rats, which also show reduced testosterone concentrations under these conditions (Blanchard et al., 1993; Albeck et al., 1997). CRH involvement in the stress response is complex, with at least one other brain system, involving the amygdala, showing an increase in CRH expression linked to anxiety disorders and depression (Schulkin et al, 1998). Furthermore, behavioral and chemical profiles often depend on the context of the stressful situation (Johnson et al., 1996b).

Arousal and Memory Modulation

Many people report vivid memories of events they associate with intense arousal or strong emotion. Sometimes called "flashbulb memories," these illustrate that memory storage processes are modulated by the degree of arousal associated with an event. The amygdala is a complex collection of nuclei that has several functions, including control of some autonomic responses, elucidation of innate emotional responses, modulation of memory, and control of some aspects of male sexual behavior. The pathway for encoding memories involves the interaction of neural systems in the amygdala and other brain areas, such as the hippocampus, and hormones released by the adrenal cortex (cortisol) and the adrenal medulla (the catecholamines epinephrine and norepinephrine). The amygdala is associated with the modulation of memories of important and arousing life events—events that have strong positive or negative emotional impact (*affect*; Cahill and McGaugh, 1998; LeDoux, 1996). It mediates the effects of the degree of arousal on the storage of memories of all kinds, including those that pertain to spatial information, events, and learning habits.

In relating autonomic and neuroendocrine function to memory processes, it is noteworthy that the encoding of memories is strengthened by glucocorticoids from the adrenal and by norepinephrine released from nerve terminals in the amygdala, hippocampus, and other brain regions. Substances associated with arousal, such as adrenal epinephrine and various peptide hormones, circulating outside the blood-brain barrier act to stimulate receptors in the periphery that then send neural messages to the brain via the vagus nerve (Clark et al., 1995; Williams and Jensen 1991, 1993). Modulated neural messages are then passed via the nucleus of the solitary tract to brain regions where memories are actually encoded (deQuervain et al., 1998; McGaugh et al., 1996; Roozendaal et al., 1996). In support of this mechanism, antagonism of peripheral b-receptors that respond to epinephrine released from the adrenals attenuates the memory-modulated effects of arousal (Cahill et al., 1994; Nielsen and Jensen, 1995). Those findings could be relevant to the biology of post-traumatic stress disorder and depression, which seem to involve overactive functioning of the amygdala (Cahill and McGaugh, 1998; Drevets et al., 1997; Sheline et al., 1998).

Some important advances in animal model studies related to emotional experiences have recently been carried over to human brain function. Human brain-imaging studies have shown that emotionally arousing information (pleasant or unpleasant) activates the amygdala and induces the formation of strong, long-term, episodic memories of that information (Cahill et al., 1996; Hamann et al., 1999). Electric stimulation of the vagus nerve in laboratory rats enhances memory (Clark et al., 1995); this finding was recently expanded to human memory for word recognition (Clark et al., 1999).

Studies of learning and memory have revealed neural plasticity involving structural changes in brain cells and changes in gene expression. It can be seen in the remodeling of neuron structure brought about by training (Greenough and Bailey, 1988). Transcription factors involved in regulating expressions of groups of genes in brain cells also appear essential to the formation of long-term memories in species as varied as fruit flies and mice (Guzowski and McGaugh, 1997; Martin and Kandel, 1996).

Short-term responses of the brain to novel, arousing, or potentially threatening situations are adaptive and result in enhanced learning and in the acquisition of new behavioral strategies for coping. However, repeated stress can increase allostatic load and cause cognitive deficits. The hippocampus is important in declarative, spatial, and contextual memory processes. It also works in processing the contextual associations of strong emotions (Eichenbaum, 1997; Gray, 1982). Atrophy of the hippocampus with age has been reported in animals (Meaney et al., 1988) and humans (Lupien et al., 1998; Lupien et al., 1994) and is accompanied by cognitive impairment. The cumulative effects of life stress, as expressed by the concept of allostatic load, can cause impairment by at least four mechanisms (McEwen, 1997, 1999b): impairing neural excitability, causing atrophy of neurons in the Ammon's horn region of the hippocampus, inhibiting neurogenesis in the dentate gyrus of the hippocampus, and causing permanent loss of neurons in the hippocampus. Each process can occur somewhat independently of the others, and each contributes to some degree to different pathophysiologic conditions associated with traumatic stress, depression, or aging.

Those laboratory findings have been carried over to the human brain by magnetic resonance imaging. Hippocampal atrophy and cognitive impairment have been reported in conditions as diverse as Cushing's syndrome, post-traumatic stress disorder, and recurrent major depression (for reviews, see McEwen et al., 1997; Sapolsky, 1996). The hippocampus is susceptible to those effects and is likely not the only brain region so affected. Atrophy of the amygdala and the prefrontal cortex also has been reported in depressive illness (Drevets et al., 1997; Sheline et al., 1998, 1999). The reversibility or prevention of such atrophy clearly is an important topic for research, as are its implications for cognitive function.

IMMUNE SYSTEM FUNCTION IN HEALTH AND DISEASE

The rebirth of integrative physiology in the context of the growing pool of information about genes and gene regulation has led to the development of new interdisciplinary fields of study, such as neuroendocrine immunology and psychoneuroimmunology—the latter includes psychology and an eclectic mix of other disciplines. At the same time, the more traditional field of immunology has advanced with growing knowledge about the messengers of the immune system, the cytokines and chemokines. Those advances underline the importance of explaining how the immune system functions in the living body, as opposed to examining only its theoretical workings. The immune system is highly integrated with other physiologic systems. It is sensitive to virtually every hormone in the body, and sympathetic, parasympathetic, and sensory nerves innervate the organs of the immune system. These organs also produce hormones that affect cells in the rest of the body. The remarkable capacity to distinguish "self" from "nonself" to protect the body from infectious and malignant challenges is a hallmark of the immune system that has been studied in great detail at the cellular and molecular levels over the past 50 years.

Much progress has been made recently in explaining how the body responds to environmental challenges through immunologic pathways. Research has led to development of the notion of a "danger" hypothesis in which tissue damage (and perhaps a threat to the very survival of the organism) is a signal that activates inflammatory and immune responses (Fuchs and Matzinger, 1996). The response of the immune system to environmental challenge represents a coordinated pattern of gene expression that results in rapid and sustained production of activated cells, secretory products, and effector mechanisms that persist until the challenge is eliminated.

Like many other bodily and behavioral responses to challenge, immune system responses are initially beneficial, but when they are sustained, they can damage healthy host tissue or augment damage produced by pathogens. That potential threat is reduced by the high level of regulation of the immune system and its close integration with the autonomic and endocrine systems. Bidirectional interaction of common chemical messengers and cellular receptors connects the immune system with the nervous system and the endocrine system. In this interactive communication between systems, sensory stimuli to the central nervous system that activates the HPA axis result in the peripheral release of adrenal steroids and catecholamines, both of which can have immunoregulatory effects. Similarly, a challenge that induces an inflammatory response causes the release of cytokines that stimulate the peripheral and central nervous systems (Figure 2-3). This provides an important link through which the neuroendocrine response modulates the development of an inflammatory response at the site of challenge. That is especially important in the lungs, heart, brain, and kidneys, where there are limits to the magnitude an inflammatory response can reach without causing loss of critical function (Hermann et al., 1995).

The movement of immune cells to organs and tissues where they are needed to fight infection or other challenge is highly regulated at multiple levels, including interactions among neural, endocrine, and immune systems (Fauci, 1975; Hermann et al., 1995). Steroid hormones and catecholamines released from the adrenals promote the movement of immune cells. These steroid hormones and catecholamines are immunosuppressive when they are secreted chronically or when their release is not terminated properly—in which case they can actually increase susceptibility to infection and malignancy (Dobbs et al., 1993; Hermann et al., 1993). A deficiency of circulating glucocorticoids and catecholamines, however, allows other immune mediators, such as cytokines, to overreact and thereby increase the risk of autoimmune and inflammatory disorders (Sternberg et al., 1992, 1989; Wilder, 1995).

Neural and Endocrine Effects on the Immune System

The immune system is integrated with the nervous and endocrine systems, which modulate aspects of its function. Many chemical messengers of the nervous and endocrine systems are immunomodulatory, and these substances are important in regulating inflammatory and immune responses (Figure 2.3) (Felten et al., 1987). The presence of receptors—for hormones, neuropeptides, and neurotransmitters—on cells of the immune system suggests some ways by which modulation occurs. The receptors provide a mechanism for other physiologic systems to modulate immune responses. Activation of the HPA axis, which leads to systemic release of potent anti-inflammatory substances, such as cortisol and other glucocorticoids, regulates inflammatory and immune responses (Berczi, 1998). The autonomic system's part in immunoregulation also became clearer once it was demonstrated that primary and secondary lymphoid tissues are highly innervated (Bulloch and Pomerantz, 1984; Felten et al., 1987) and that immune cells in these tissues have receptors for neuromodulators and neurotransmitters.

Effects of Inflammatory and Immune Responses on the Nervous System

Gaining a clear understanding of the bidirectional flow of neuroendocrine and immune interactions had to wait for a revolution in cellular and molecular immunology. Advances in cytokine research provide a context for the study of soluble products produced by activated monocytes and lymphoid cells (circulating and stationary immune cells, respectively).

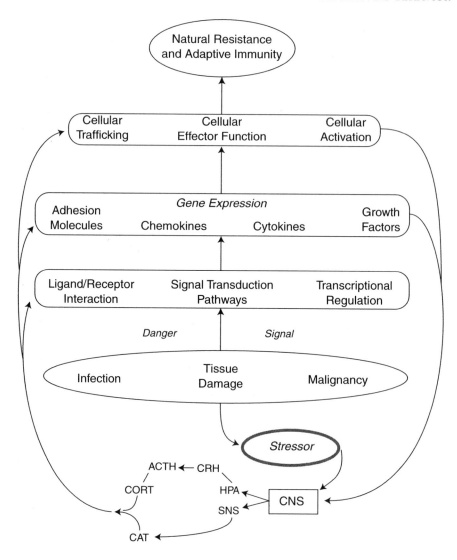

FIGURE 2-3 Neuroendocrine Regulation of Immunity. Tissue damage, infection, and malignancy are hypothesized to generate a danger signal. This signal is transduced at the cellular and molecular levels leading to activation, trafficking and expression of effector functions in the immune system. Products of the immune system, including cytokines, chemokines and growth factors can stimulate the nervous system resulting in the release of steroid hormones, catecholamines, opioids. These products of nervous and endocrine activation modulate molecular and cellular events in an immune response. Adapted from Marucha and Sheridan, 1998. Reprinted with permission from the publisher, Harcourt, Inc. All rights reserved.

These low-molecular-weight products of mononuclear cells are secreted during inflammatory and immune responses. They were shown to be produced by several types of cells; to have several kinds of biologic activity; and to be pleiotropic, affecting cells in many physiologic systems (Arai et al., 1990). The cytokines initiate action by binding to specific receptors on target cell surfaces, and many of them have multiple signaling functions including autocrine (secretion of a substance that stimulates the secretory cell itself), paracrine (the target cell is close to the secretory cell, such as neurotransmitters in the brain), and endocrine (the chemical signal can travel long distances from the secretory cells to the target tissue, via the blood or lymph systems). The pleiotropy of cytokines led to investigations of inflammatory and immune interactions with the nervous system and to the development of the idea that the immune system communicates with the brain through the release of proinflammatory cytokines (Besedovsky et al., 1986). Proinflammatory cytokines released in peripheral tissues function as hormones, and biologically are associated with the development and expression of behaviors associated with illness (Dantzer et al., 1998; Maier et al., 1998) and can induce chronic stress responses (Shanks et al., 1998).

The recognition that cytokines, particularly those that are proinflammatory, communicate with the brain and influence activation of the HPA axis led to investigations of neuroendocrine responses in the etiology of inflammatory (Chrousos, 1995) and autoimmune diseases. Associations between stress responses and autoimmunity have been studied in conditions as diverse as rheumatoid arthritis (Heijnen et al., 1996; Sternberg et al., 1989, 1992), inflammatory bowel disease (Anton and Shanahan, 1998), systemic lupus erythematosus (Utz et al., 1997), and multiple sclerosis (Griffin and Whitacre, 1991). Other studies have examined neuroendocrine responses and immune system reactivity in asthma (Barnes, 1986; Busse et al., 1995; Kang et al., 1998), atopic dermatitis (Buske-Kirschbaum et al., 1998), and allergy (Anderzen et al., 1997).

Stress and Immune System Function

The recognition of the importance of bidirectional communication between neural, endocrine, and immune systems through shared ligands and receptors led to a major research emphasis on immunoregulation by hormones, peptide neuromodulators, and neurotransmitters. The primary function of the immune system is to protect the host from infectious and malignant challenges. Acute stress enhances immune function, and it does so in part by promoting immune cell translocation to sites of immune challenge (Dhabhar et al., 1995, 1996), whereas chronic stress has the opposite effect: it impairs immune function (Dhabhar and McEwen, 1999; Hermann et al., 1995). Various aspects of immune function in states of stress-induced neuroendocrine activation, with a primary emphasis on negative, immunosuppressive outcomes, have been reported (Dobbs et al., 1993; Kiecolt-Glaser et al., 1996).

One important factor in whether a person will develop respiratory infection after challenge with an infectious virus is lack of social support (Cohen, 1995; Cohen et al., 1991). In studies of two-party relationships, marital discord was found to affect general health and immunity significantly (Kiecolt-Glaser et al., 1997).

Because immune system functioning is studied best when the system has been provoked, examinations of stress and immunity have considered the effectiveness and durability of the immune response after the administration of vaccines in humans. The stress of taking a university examination (Glaser et al., 1992) and the chronic stress of being a caregiver (Kiecolt-Glaser et al., 1996; Glaser et al., 1998) were used to characterize responses to vaccination during a stressful period. In each case, the antibody responses to vaccines were poorer in the stressed than in the nonstressed groups.

Similar studies of the mechanisms of neuroendocrine/immune interactions have been performed in animals. Studies of experimental viral infections in mice demonstrate that both the HPA axis and the sympathetic system alter virus-induced pathophysiology under conditions of imposed experimental stress (Hermann et al., 1993). The stress response also can suppress specific components of natural resistance and adaptive immune responses to viral infection, both acute (Dobbs et al., 1993; Sheridan et al., 1991) and latent (Bonneau et al., 1991; Kusnecov et al., 1992). Environmental stress suppresses immunity and enhances the pathogenicity of bacteria, particularly that caused by facultative intracellular parasites, such as mycobacteria (Brown et al., 1993).

Wound healing and other physiologic processes that require substantial proinflammatory responses (including cytokine, chemokine, and growth factor gene expression) are affected by environmental and behavioral stress. The stress of long-term caregiving to dementia patients delays the healing of full-thickness, cutaneous-punch biopsy wounds (Kiecolt-Glaser et al., 1995). Acute stress induced by taking academic examinations delayed the healing of mucosal wounds in the oral cavity; the delay was associated with diminished proinflammatory cytokine responses in the peripheral blood of those who experienced the stress (Marucha et al., 1998). In animal models, restraint stress caused activation of the HPA axis, which was shown to suppress movement of immune cells to wound sites (Padgett et al., 1998).

The effects of disaster-related stress responses on the immune system have been studied (Ironson et al., 1997; Solomon et al., 1997). Major effects of distress of natural disasters include alterations in natural and adaptive immunity, as indicated by lower natural killer-cell cytotoxicity (NKCC) and lower numbers of circulating T lymphocytes. People who were tested after surviving Hurricane Andrew had lower NKCC and fewer suppressor T cells (CD8+) and helper T cells (CD4+) than did comparison subjects (Ironson et al., 1997). Alterations in NKCC were related to psychologic and behavioral factors: Survivors reported greater loss of resources, greater post traumatic disorder symptomology, and more negative intrusive thoughts than did control subjects. Those observations are consistent with conclusions drawn from a growing literature on psychologic stressors and immunity, which has shown NKCC to be diminished by bereavement (Irwin et al., 1987), marital discord (Kiecolt-Glaser et al., 1987), and exposure to earthquakes (Solomon et al., 1997).

The observed reductions in measures of natural and adaptive immunity were statistically significant in a stressed population but did not suggest increased risk for infection or disease in any individual. However, these studies demonstrate that natural disasters, industrial accidents, and psychosocial events are stressors that can affect human immunophysiology and thereby affect both mental and physical well-being.

ADDITIONAL FACTORS INFLUENCE LONG-TERM EFFECTS OF STRESS

Resilience

People differ widely in resilience to and recovery from illness, injury, or surgery and in overcoming adversity. However, relatively little is known about the physiology of resilience and good health. Resilience undoubtedly consists of more than just the absence of allostatic load. It is thought to be the product of cellular processes that protect and build cells and tissues—processes that involve some reserve capacity and resistance to the damaging effects of stressors. Promising research includes how ana-bolic hormones, such as growth hormone and insulin, and neurotrophic factors work in the brain as they are related to voluntary exercise and to recovery from injury and illness. For example, voluntary exercise in rats (running in an activity wheel) increases expression of messenger RNA for a neurotrophin that protects neurons from death and that promotes neuroplasticity and synaptic transmission (Oliff et al., 1998). It is not known, however, what advantages increased neurotrophin concentrations confer on the brains of exercising animals. The animals might be more resilient in the face of severe stress, or their brains might deteriorate more slowly with age. Although the role of neurotrophin regulation in exercise is not known, it has been reported that voluntary exercise increases pro-duction of new neurons in the dentate gyrus of the hippocampus, the brain region that is important in spatial and declarative memory (van Praag et al., 1999).

The study of factors that promote resilience, still poorly defined, is important as a complement to the more traditional approach of studying the damaging effects of stress mediators. Therefore, it will be important for research to relate human life histories, stress, and allostatic load to the production of such substances as the neurotrophins, which are related to tissue growth and repair. It also will be important to identify the influence of social support mechanisms and of individual attitudes that promote beneficial physiologic states associated with the capacity to repair dam-aged tissues and to protect against pathogens and toxic agents, such as free radicals (Epel et al., 1998; Ryff and Singer, 1998; Seeman and McEwen, 1996; Singer et al., 1998; Taylor et al., 1997).

Coping

Coping efforts are important moderators of the impact of stress on health (Baum and Posluszny, 1999). Coping is defined as volitional man-agement of stressful events or conditions and regulation of cognitive, be-havioral, emotional, and physiological responses to stress (Compas et al., 1999; Lazarus and Folkman, 1984). Various classifications of coping re-sponses have been proposed, including coping to solve a problem versus coping to manage emotions, cognitive versus behavioral coping, approach versus avoidance coping, and coping intended to achieve (primary) con-trol over the stressor (the source of stress) versus (secondary) control over response to the stress (emotions).

Coping efforts are important in the process of adaptation to illness. Several consistent findings have emerged from prospective longitudinal studies of breast cancer patients from diagnosis through treatment and recovery (Carver et al., 1993; Epping-Jordan et al., 1999; Stanton and Snider, 1993). Successful coping is facilitated by optimism—the tendency to anticipate positive outcomes. Through the use of strategies including acceptance, positive thinking, and problem solving, optimism is associated with lower psychological distress (reduced symptoms of anxiety and depression). Conversely, pessimistic thinking is associated with coping that involves avoidance and social withdrawal, which are related to higher symptoms of anxiety and depression (Carver et al., 1993; Epping-Jordan et al., 1999). Patients who are more prone to poor coping have histories of social isolation, recent losses, or multiple obligations (Rowland, 1990).

Breast cancer patients who learn to use more direct and confrontational coping strategies are less distressed than are those who use avoidance and denial (Holland and Rowland, 1990). Furthermore, a "fighting spirit" about the illness leads to a probability of longer survival (Green and Berlin, 1987; Greer et al., 1979; Watson et al., 1990). Research suggests that the belief that one has control over the *cause* of the disease leads to poor outcome, whereas belief in control over the *course* of the disease leads to better outcome (Watson et al., 1990). Psychosocial stress has been reported to lead to higher relapse rates in metastatic breast cancer (Ramirez et al., 1989). However, several studies report no significant effect of psychosocial variables on the course of carcinoma (Angell, 1985; Cassileth et al., 1985; Jamison et al., 1987).

Although stress can affect immune function and health, most of the observed effects are relatively small and within the range of normal immune function (Glaser et al., 1999). Therefore, stress-induced immune system changes that are related to disease are likely to be the result of multiple small simultaneous changes in the immune system. Measurement of multiple aspects of the immune system and their interactions is thus necessary to reveal the subtle and complex relationships among stress, immune function, and disease. Study of the effects of coping efforts on stress and immunologic responses is also important because coping might be a crucial mediator of the stress/immune relationship that can be modified through behavioral interventions.

In addition to possible effects on disease onset and etiology, stress also can disrupt the behaviors that normally enhance healthy functioning and protect a person from illness (discussed further in Chapter 3). This can be seen in the association between stress and health risk behaviors, such as smoking (Shiffman et al., 1996), poor diet, and lack of exercise (Greeno and Wing, 1994), and in health-compromising responses to stress that include increased autonomic arousal and elevated blood pressure (Baum and Posluszny, 1999).

Extensive research documents that expression of emotions has beneficial effects on both emotional and physical well-being (Esterling et al., 1999; Pennebaker, 1997). But emotional regulation does not involve the unmodulated ventilation of emotions or the containment or suppression of feelings; rather, successful regulation of emotion appears to involve the controlled and modulated expression and release of feelings in ways that contribute to an increased understanding of those emotions and their meaning. Research by Pennebaker and colleagues (1997) shows that writing about deep feelings is a powerful way to regulate emotional expression. Writing about emotions is associated with improved mood, fewer health problems, and enhanced immune function (Petrie et al., 1995, 1998). The specific mechanisms through which regulation of emotional expression affects health are not fully understood and are the subject of continuing research. However, the regulated expression of emotions through writing is a potentially important component of interventions to change health behavior.

Gender

In animal models and possibly also in humans, there are gender differences in vulnerability to brain damage or brain remodeling as a result of stress (see Galea et al., 1997; Uno et al., 1989). Although the gonadal hormones are important influences in the development of gender differences in early life, hormones and experience also can change brain structure and function in adult life (Greenough and Bailey, 1988; McEwen and Alves, 1999; McEwen, 1999b)—an indication that there is considerable life-long plasticity in the nervous system. And although the role of hormones is a hallmark of sexual differentiation, experience and social factors also are critical, especially in humans and nonhuman primates (Goy, 1970; McEwen, 1999a; Reinisch et al., 1987).

Social Influences

People live in social groups and as members of societies. It is well known that social class or socioeconomic position has a profound effect on health through multiple pathways (Adler et al., 1994; Antonovsky, 1967; Marmot et al., 1991; Syme and Berkman, 1976). Since the 1982 predecessor to this report (IOM, 1982), it has become evident that the degree of a given country's social inequality is related to health in that society (Kaplan et al., 1996; Wilkinson, 1992). And the degree of social integration or connection and the social networks in which people are embedded are related to morbidity and mortality (Berkman, 1995; House et al., 1988). Like economic inequality, social cohesion and social capital are associated with health (Kawachi et al., 1997). Moreover, there are characteristics of the work environment that can produce job stress and significantly influence workers' health (Karasek and Theorell, 1990).

These topics are developed more fully in Chapter 4. Physiologic systems that could mediate the effects of stressful social circumstances on health are discussed here.

CARDIOVASCULAR HEALTH AND DISEASE

Cardiovascular health and disease provide an example of the interactions of behavioral, psychologic, and social factors. This discussion of CHD will be used to point out the biological effects of stress and the psychosocial influences that exist. Despite progress in elucidating the role of genetics in human disease, it is clear that no single cause of CHD can be identified and that these conditions develop as a result of complex interactions among multiple factors.

One example of the effects of disparate factors on the incidence of cardiovascular disease is provided by a recent analysis of changing mortality patterns in Russia (Notzon et al., 1998). Over a 4-year period after the breakup of the former Soviet Union, mean life expectancy declined by 5 years. Most of the decline could be attributed to increased mortality in men aged 25 to 64 because of accidents and cardiovascular disease. Factors implicated in the dramatic change in death rates included economic instability, chronic stress, depression, and the increased use of alcohol and tobacco.

Stress and Cardiovascular Function

Stress clearly is important in cardiovascular health and disease. There is general agreement that acute stress can trigger acute cardiovascular events (Muller and Tofler, 1990), but the more subtle influences of chronic stress and allostatic load are not well understood. The effects of psychosocial stressors are mediated through the central nervous system, so it is relevant to review several pathways through which the brain affects bodily processes related to cardiovascular function. Much new information about function and measurement has contributed to our explanation of the relationships.

The autonomic nervous system regulates internal bodily functions, including all aspects of cardiovascular function. The autonomic system maintains appropriate internal states (homeostasis) and enables the body to respond to external threats perceived as stressors. It has two primary divisions: the sympathetic and parasympathetic. The sympathetic nervous system permits response to extreme conditions: fight or flight. The parasympathetic nervous system modulates functions under resting conditions. Both blood pressure and heart rate are modulated through the autonomic nervous system.

There is strong evidence that increased sympathetic activity is a feature of many cases of hypertension in young adults. Cardiac output increases in the early stages of hypertension and decreases with advancing age. With age, peripheral vascular resistance increases, largely because of remodeling (rerouting) and hypertrophy (overgrowth) of blood vessel walls. Sympathetic activity also can affect the development of atherosclerosis. Mechanisms include increasing insulin resistance, a known risk factor for cardiovascular disease; hemodynamic effects on the arterial wall; and direct metabolic effects, such as increased plasma triglycerides and alteration in the metabolism of low-density lipoproteins (Julius, 1993). Furthermore, increased sympathetic activity can increase the risk of cardiovascular disease through the effects of adrenal epinephrine on platelet aggregation and the development of left ventricular hypertrophy. There is experimental evidence that increased heart rate (Beere et al., 1984) and increased blood pressure variability are both risk factors for atherosclerosis (Sasaki et al., 1994). Decreased heart rate variability itself is associated with the presence of CHD and is a risk factor for cardiovascular morbidity. But it is not known whether this association is causal. For example, reduced heart rate variability might be a consequence of artherosclerotic damage to the carotid sinuses, which could cause impaired baroreceptor reflexes.

Laboratory studies demonstrate that cardiovascular disease can be produced by chronic social stress. Hypertension can be elicited in some strains of mice, but not in others (Henry et al., 1986), and the hypertensive consequences of behavioral stress can be potentiated in genetically normotensive animals by a high-sodium diet (Anderson, 1994). In animals, the combination of emotional stress and high sodium intake has been associated with a greater increase in blood pressure than results from either factor alone (Staesson et al., 1994).

Other studies show that subordinate female cynomolgus monkeys have more atherosclerosis than do dominant females, and the difference appears to be related to suppression of the release of cardioprotective ovarian hormones (Shively and Clarkson, 1994). Atherosclerosis develops faster in dominant male monkeys when they are defending their social position or re-establishing it in an unstable social hierarchy (Manuck et al., 1995). The combination of a high-fat diet with psychosocial stress accelerates the disease process (Brindley and Rolland, 1989).

Studies of chronic stress among people have yielded inconsistent findings: some show activation of the HPA axis and others show its suppression (Ockenfels et al., 1995). Although anticipation or experience of acute stress activates the HPA axis (Smyth et al., 1998), the degree of activation with repeated exposure to stress is greatly variable (Kirschbaum et al., 1995).

The importance of personality, emotion, and social environment in the development of cardiovascular disease is a subject of controversy, but there is evidence that anger, whether expressed openly or repressed, is associated with an increased risk of hypertension (Everson et al., 1998). Job-related stress is also important. The combination of high job demands and low control is associated with hypertension (Schnall et al., 1992). Blood pressure tends to be highest in the workplace, but the increase in blood pressure in people with high-strain jobs is seen at work, at home, and during sleep (Schnall et al., 1992). An imbalance between income and expenditure is associated with high blood pressure (Chin-Hong and McGarvey, 1996; Dressler, 1991).

The prevalence of hypertension in humans varies greatly from one society to another, and it appears to be strongly influenced by society and culture factors. For example, epidemiologic studies indicate that the transition from life in traditional tribal community to urbanized Western society is associated with an increase in blood pressure (Cruz-Coke, 1987; Poulter et al., 1988, 1990), although it is unclear whether this effect is the result of changes in diet or of psychosocial stress.

Behavioral and Psychosocial Factors

Psychosocial factors can influence the course of chronic human disease along several pathways. Behavior that has perceived short-term benefits, such as mood-enhancement induced by cigarette-smoking or excessive alcohol consumption, but that causes long-term injury constitutes one (Chapter 3). Another involves the influence of social and environmental factors, such as socioeconomic status or stress on disease processes (Chapter 4). A third consists of individual psychological factors, such as hostility and depression, that interact with the other two pathways to increase susceptibility to illness. The evidence for a role for these psychological factors in cardiovascular disease is described below.

Hostility

Hostility is the psychosocial variable most often associated with the incidence of CHD (Booth-Kewley and Friedman, 1987). In the context of physical health, hostility is defined usually as a stable attribute characterized by mistrusting cynicism that leads to antagonistic or aggressive behavior and feelings of anger (Miller et al., 1996). The extent to which hostility is a personality trait or a behavioral coping response to environmental stimuli, however, is not known. Most of the research on hostility has been done in men.

Interest in hostility and CHD evolved from earlier research on the type A behavior pattern, an idea originally formulated by Friedman and Rosenman (1974). Type A behavior was characterized by a sense of time urgency, loud and explosive speech, hostility, and competitiveness. Early studies supported an association between type A behavior and the development of CHD (Review Panel, 1981), but later research failed to confirm the association (Case et al., 1985; Shekelle et al., 1985a, 1985b). The original type A behavior data-set was reanalyzed by two teams of investigators to examine inconsistencies and identify variables within the multifaceted type A behavior patterns that were most predictive of CHD (Chesney et al., 1988; Matthews et al., 1977). These analyses revealed that hostility was the best variable for distinguishing men who developed heart disease from men who did not (Hecker et al., 1988; Matthews et al., 1977). Many prospective studies confirmed the relationship between hostility, as assessed by interviews and questionnaires, and CHD incidence (Barefoot et al., 1983; 1989; Dembroski et al., 1989; Houston and Kelly, 1987; Shekelle et al., 1983). Significant associations also have been found between hostility and cardiac mortality (Koskenvuo et al., 1988; Shekelle et al., 1991). Considered together, the cumulative findings constitute substantial evidence of the link between hostility and various aspects of CHD. Although some studies have not found an association (Hearn et al., 1989; Leon et al., 1988; McCranie et al., 1986), the positive reports outnumber negative ones (Scheier and Bridges, 1995). One reason for this inconsistency is that the assessment of hostility often relies on self reports, and people might tend to underreport this socially undesirable trait (Helmers et al., 1995).

There is a hypothesis that people who are hostile have exaggerated cardiovascular reactivity to stress and that this either contributes to the development of atherosclerosis (Matthews et al., 1998) or triggers acute events (Rozanski et al., 1999). However, hostility also is correlated with increased likelihood of smoking, with decreased likelihood of quitting smoking (Lipkus et al., 1994), and with lower socioeconomic status (Barefoot et al., 1991; Carroll et al., 1997). Each of these will increase allostatic load.

Anger

Anger is a psychological state thought to be related to hostility. Expression of anger has been shown to trigger myocardial infarction. In a study of patients undergoing coronary angiography, recall of anger was a potent stimulus that induced vasoconstriction in diseased coronary arteries, but not in healthy arteries (Boltwood et al., 1993). The recall of anger can also produce an acute impairment in ventricular function in patients with CHD (Ironson et al., 1992).

Vital Exhaustion

One common premonitory symptom of myocardial infarction is vital exhaustion, a state of excessive fatigue, increased irritability, and demoralization (Appels et al., 1987). A prospective study of 3877 city employees in Rotterdam, The Netherlands, compared the risk of coronary heart disease among those scoring in the highest third on a measurement scale of exhaustion to those with lower scores. Vital exhaustion predicted myocardial infarction with a relative risk of 2.28—a relatively robust effect for a behavioral predictor (Appels and Mulder, 1989). There appears to be no correlation between the severity of CHD and vital exhaustion score, so it is unlikely that subclinical coronary disease causes the observed fatigue (Kop et al., 1996). Vital exhaustion also has been reported to predict recurrence of arterial blockage after coronary angioplasty (Kop et al., 1994). Job stress is associated with vital exhaustion and is a risk factor for cardiovascular disease (Everson et al., 1997; Keltikangas-Jarvinen et al., 1996a, 1996b; Kop et al., 1998; Lynch et al., 1997a; Raikkonen et al., 1996).

Depression

Depression affects about half of patients who experience myocardial infarction. Depression predicts significantly poorer outcome with heart disease (Denollet et al., 1996; Denollet and Brutsaert, 1998; King, 1997) and roughly doubles the risk of recurrent cardiovascular events (Barefoot et al., 1996; Barefoot and Schroll, 1996; Frasure-Smith et al., 1995). About half of postinfarction patients with depression have a history of depression before the onset of CHD, and there is some evidence suggesting depression as a risk factor for a first infarction (Sesso et al., 1998). The association between depression and mortality seems to be the same in men and women (Frasure-Smith et al., 1999). However, the prevalence of postinfarction depression is about twice as high in women as in men (Carney et al., 1990). It is unlikely that depression is a consequence of CHD, inasmuch as the occurrence of depression often precedes any disease symptoms and there is no relationship between severity of depression and severity of coronary arterial disease (Carney et al., 1995).

Depression is associated with increased sympathetic and decreased parasympathetic tone, as manifested by increased plasma catecholamine concentrations, increased heart rate, and decreased heart rate variability. Myocardial infarctions tend to happen most commonly between 6 A.M. and noon, the time of day that parallels the normal circadian rhythm of sympathetic activity. But the cycles of catecholamines and cortisol are disturbed in people who have depression, peaking earlier in the day than in nondepressed people. Depressed people are more likely than nondepressed people to have myocardial infarction during the night or very early in the morning (Carney et al., 1995).

Twenty years ago it was suggested that the presence of depression predicted a higher subsequent incidence of cancer (Shekelle et al., 1981). Although a large cohort study of employees at Western Electric reported an elevated rate of subsequent cancers among those diagnosed with depression, this finding was not confirmed in a more recent large-scale cohort trial (Zonderman et al., 1989). Zonderman et al. (1989) found no relationship between two measures of depressive symptoms and cancer morbidity or mortality in a large population. The researchers used continuous and not categorical measures of depression, leaving open the possibility that severe clinical depression could be associated with elevated cancer risk. However, this and earlier studies lend little support to the idea that depression increases cancer risk (Fox, 1989). Fox's reanalysis of the original observation suggests that a combination of depression and exposure to toxins could have accounted for the apparent association (Fox, 1989). However, a study by Penninx et al. (1998) did find in a sample of 5000 elderly people that consistent symptoms of depression were predictive of an almost 2-fold elevation in risk of cancer incidence. Thus, depression does not seem to predict cancer incidence, but it is elevated among those who have cancer.

Anxiety, Worry, and Hope

Anxiety and worry have recently received renewed attention as risk factors for cardiovascular disease. Two prospective studies have shown that anxiety predicts the development of CHD (Sloan et al., 1999), and worrying is an important component of anxiety. Men who worry a lot were found to be at increased risk for CHD (Kubzansky et al., 1997).

Hope and optimism, in contrast, have been suggested as important components of psychological well-being and as factors that can contribute to good physical health (Scheier and Carver, 1985; Snyder et al., 1991). A lack of hope is commonly thought to adversely affect health (Scheier and Carver, 1992). However, only recently has there been empirical support for this. One major challenge for researchers and health care providers was to develop ways to measure hope and hopelessness. Hopelessness, as assessed by one question on a four-item questionnaire designed to measure depressed affect, reliably predicted fatal and nonfatal CHD events in a cohort of more than 2800 initially healthy men and women (Anda et al., 1993). Similarly, a two-item hopelessness scale significantly predicted all-cause mortality, the incidence of myocardial infarction and cancer, and death from violence and injury in a sample of 2428 men in the Kuopio ischemic heart disease study in Finland (Everson et al., 1996). Those and similar findings support the general idea that psychosocial factors are important determinants of physical health and disease.

DEVELOPMENTAL TRAJECTORIES

Development is important in the biological and behavioral processes that preserve health or lead to human disease throughout life. Cumulative experience, adaptive plasticity, physical and social exchange with surrounding environments, and genetic predisposition interact to influence development. The unique physiology of each person, partly encoded in the genome and partly determined by prior physical exposures and social experiences, generates the individual behaviors that influence morbidity and mortality.

Although developmental status is a continuing factor in health outcomes over life, it has heightened salience for immediate and long-term health responses during infancy, early childhood, and adolescence. These periods are characterized by extremely rapid biological and psychosocial change. The resolution of the developmental challenges faced at these times determine set points for homeostatic systems, as well as for adopting crucial health-related attitudes and behaviors. These outcomes, in turn, determine trajectories for subsequent biobehavioral functioning that can have long-term effects on health. Therefore, the periods of infancy, early childhood, and adolescence are highlighted here.

Early childhood, infancy, and even prenatal experiences appear to have long-term consequences for health because they influence the biological mechanisms that underlie stress reactivity. There are sociocultural consequences of these experiences as well (NRC, 2000). A secure attachment with a parenting person provides a protective modulator of the environmental influences on an infant. The mother/child attachment is affected by the infant's temperament, which is characterized by reactions to stimuli, the tone of the emotional expression (positive or negative), activity level, and sociability. There is increasing evidence that temperament has a biological base (Boyce et al., 1992), including a genetic component that is heavily influenced by experience (van der Boom, 1994). The minority of infants who have difficult temperaments can experience attachment problems and high levels of stress, with consequences for their stress responses as adults. Unresponsive, insensitive, or abusive parenting also can lead to atypical emotional development. Research with infants of depressed mothers, for example, has shown that diminished parental responsiveness is associated with changes in infant emotional regulation and the balance of left vs. right frontal cortical activation (Dawson et al., 1997). A disproportionate number of severely deprived infants raised in Romanian orphanages exhibited abnormalities in cognitive, emotional, and linguistic development (Fisher et al., 1997). They also showed retarded growth and higher rates of infectious diseases (Albers et al., 1997; Hostetter et al, 1991).

Stress in young children can influence future health. Although currently limited to retrospective analyses, studies of physical and sexual abuse in childhood suggest variable but elevated risk for later depression, somatization, excessive rates of health care use, homelessness, and other indicators of behavioral maladaptation (Cheatsy et al., 1998; Herman et al., 1997; Salmon and Calderbank, 1996; Styron and Janoff-Bulman, 1997). A recent prospective controlled study (Heim et al., 2000) found that, during a relatively mild stress task involving public speaking and mental arithmetic, those with a history of sexual abuse showed significantly elevated concentrations of adrenocorticotropic hormone. This was most pronounced in participants who exhibited symptoms of major depression at the time of testing. The results provide support for increased stress vulnerability and altered HPA axis function in adults who were abused as children (Heim et al., 2000). Elevated prolactin response to serotonin challenge has been found among abused children (Kaufman et al., 1998; Pine et al., 1997), suggesting that the experience could be associated with dysregulation of serotonergic neurotransmission. Activation of specific neuroendocrine systems, such as the HPA axis, also has been found in conditions of normative, acute stress, such as that which accompanies the transition to primary school (Boyce et al., 1995), and prolonged extreme neglect and sensory deprivation, such as adverse rearing in a Romanian orphanage (Gunnar, 1998). Furthermore, chronic stressors in early childhood could impair the emergence of higher cognitive processes such as memory (Nelson and Carver, 1998). The potential for "recovery" from prolonged, severe early adverse experiences through later enrichment is still unknown. All are important areas for research.

Behavioral factors, such as physical activity and diet, are significant in setting health trajectories in children. Nearly half of American children are not regularly physically active, and physical activity declines dramatically among older children (U.S. Department of Health and Human Services, 1996). In the United States, children currently are 20–30% less active than is recommended by the World Health Organization (Salbe et al., 1997). Childhood activity is associated with relative weight, parental obesity, and the proportion of time spent outdoors (Klesges et al., 1990). These statistics are important because the prevalence of overweight children between the ages of 6 and 11 in the National Health and Nutrition

Examination Study increased from 5% to 22% between 1976–1980 and 1988–1991 (Troiano et al., 1995). In the Bogalusa Heart Study, the prevalence of overweight 5- to 24-year-olds doubled between 1973 and 1994 (Freedman et al., 1997). Evidence is growing that obesity in childhood has psychosocial consequences and portends greater risk of disease in adulthood (for reviews, see Dietz, 1998; Must and Strauss, 1999).

Adolescence provides another important period for promoting healthy behaviors. Many of the behaviors associated with adult morbidities and even mortality, such as cigarette smoking, alcohol and drug abuse, unsafe sexual practices, and violent or aggressive responses to stress often begin in adolescence. But because adolescents, in general, are curious about and interested in their bodies, that time of life also provides opportunities to promote good health and to involve young people in decision making about themselves. Effective early intervention can prevent the onset of health-compromising behaviors and can work to prevent their becoming less firmly established as life-long patterns (Millstein et al., 1993).

REFERENCES

Ader R. (1968). Effects of early experiences on emotional and physiological reactivity in the rat. *Journal of Comparative Physiology and Psychology, 66,* 264–268.

Adler, N.E., Boyce, T., Chesney, M.A., Cohen, S., Folkman, S., Kahn, R.L., and Syme, L.S. (1994). Socioeconomic status and health: The challenge of the gradient. *American Psychologist, 49,* 15–24.

Albeck, D.S., McKittrick, C.R., Blanchard, D.C., Blanchard, R.J., Nikulina, J., McEwen, B.S., and Sakai, R.R. (1997). Chronic social stress alters levels of corticotropin-releasing factor and arginine vasopressin mRNA in rat brain. *Journal of Neuroscience, 17,* 4895–4903.

Albers, L., Johnson, D.E., Hostetter, M., Iverson, S., Georgieff, M., and Miller, L. (1997). Health of children adopted from the former Soviet Union and Eastern Europe: Comparison with pre-adoptive medical records. *Journal of the American Medical Association, 278,* 922–924.

Anda, R., Williamson, D., Jones, D., Macera, C., Eaker, E., and Glassman, A. (1993). Depressed affect, hopelessness, and the risk of ischemic heart disease in a cohort of U.S. adults. *Epidemiology, 4,* 285–294.

Anderson, D.E. (1994). Behavior analysis and the search for the origins of hypertension. *Journal of the Experimental Analysis of Behavior, 61,* 255–261.

Anderzen, I., Arnetz, B.B., Soderstrom, T., and Soderman, E. (1997). Stress and sensitization in children: a controlled prospective psychophysiological study of children exposed to international relocation. *Journal of Psychosomatic Research, 43,* 259–269.

Angell, M. (1985). Disease as a reflection of the psyche. *New England Journal of Medicine, 312,* 1570–1572.

Anton, P.A. and Shanahan, F. (1998). Neuroimmunomodulation in inflammatory bowel disease. How far from "bench" to "bedside"? *Annals of the New York Academy of Sciences, 840*, 723–734.

Antonovsky, A. (1967). Social class, life expectancy, and overall mortality. *Milbank Memorial Fund Quarterly, 45*, 31–73.

Appels, A. and Mulder, P. (1989). Fatigue and heart disease. The association between 'vital exhaustion' and past, present and future coronary heart disease. *Journal of Psychosomatic Research, 33*, 727–738.

Appels, A., Hoppener, P., and Mulder, P. (1987). A questionnaire to assess premonitory symptoms of myocardial infarction. *International Journal of Cardiology, 17*, 15–24.

Arai, K., Lee, F., Miyajima, A., Miyatake, S., Arai, N., and Yokota, T. (1990). Cytokines: Coordinators of immune and inflammatory responses. *Annual Review of Biochemistry, 59*, 783–836.

Barefoot, J.C. and Schroll, M. (1996). Symptoms of depression, acute myocardial infarction, and total mortality in a community sample. *Circulation, 93*, 1976–1980.

Barefoot, J.C., Dahlstrom, W.G., and Williams, R.B.J. (1983). Hostility, CHD incidence, and total mortality: a 25-year follow-up study of 255 physicians. *Psychosomatic Medicine, 45*, 59–63.

Barefoot, J.C., Helms, M.J., Mark, D.B., Blumenthal, J.A., Califf, R.M., Haney, T.L., O'Connor, C.M., Siegler, I.C., and Williams, R.B. (1996). Depression and long-term mortality risk in patients with coronary artery disease. *American Journal of Cardiology, 78*, 613–617.

Barefoot, J.C., Peterson, B.L., Dahlstrom, W.G, Siegler, I.C., Anderson, N.B., and Williams, R.B. (1991). Hostility patterns and health implications: Correlates of Cook–Medley Hostility Scale scores in a national survey. *Health Psychology, 10*, 18–24.

Barefoot, J.C., Peterson, B.L., Harrell, F.E.J., Hlatky, M.A., Pryor, D.B., Haney, T.L., Blumenthal, J.A., Siegler, I.C., and Williams, R.B.J. (1989). Type A behavior and survival: A follow-up study of 1,467 patients with coronary artery disease. *American Journal of Cardiology, 64*, 427–432.

Barker, D.J.P. (1997). The fetal origins of coronary heart disease. *Acta Paediatrica Supplement, 422*, 78–82.

Barker, D.J.P. and Sultan, H.Y. (1995). Fetal programming of human disease. In M. A. Hanson, J.A.D. Spencer, and J. H. Rodeck (Eds.) *Growth*, Cambridge, UK: Cambridge University Press.

Barnes, P.J. (1986). Asthma as an axon reflex. *Lancet, 1(8475)*, 242–245.

Baum, A. and Posluszny, D.M. (1999). Health psychology: Mapping biobehavioral contributions to health and illness. *Annual Review of Psychology, 50*, 137–164.

Beere, P.A., Glagov, S., and Zarins, C.K. (1984). Retarding effect of lowered heart rate on coronary atherosclerosis. *Science, 226*, 180–182.

Berczi, I. (1998). The stress concept and neuroimmunoregulation in modern biology. *Annals of the New York Academy of Sciences, 851*, 3–12.

Berkman, L.F. (1995). The role of social relations in health promotion. *Psychosomatic Medicine, 57*, 245–254.

Besedovsky, H., del Rey, A., Sorkin, E., and Dinarello, C.A. (1986). Immunoregulatory feedback between interleukin-1 and glucocorticoid hormones. *Science, 233*, 652–654.

Blanchard, D.C., Sakai, R.R., McEwen, B.S., Weiss, S.M., and Blanchard, R.J. (1993). Subordination stress: Behavioral, brain and neuroendocrine correlates. *Behavioral Brain Research, 58*, 113–121.

Boltwood, M.D., Taylor, C.B., Burke, M.B., Grogin, H., and Giacomini, J. (1993). Anger report predicts coronary artery vasomotor response to mental stress in atherosclerotic segments. *American Journal of Cardiology, 72*, 1361–1365.

Bonneau, R.H., Sheridan, J.F., Feng, N., and Glaser, R. (1991). Stress-induced effects on cell-mediated innate and adaptive memory components of the murine immune response to herpes simplex virus infection. *Brain Behavior and Immunity 5*, 274–295.

Booth-Kewley, S. and Friedman, H.S. (1987). Psychological predictors of heart disease: A quantitative review. *Psychological Bulletin, 101*, 343–362.

Boyce, W. T., Adams, S., Tschann, J. M., Cohen, F., Wara, D., and Gunnar, M. R. (1995). Adrenocortical and behavioral predictors of immune responses to starting school. *Pediatric Research, 38*, 1009–1017.

Boyce, W. T., Barr, R. G., and Zeltzer, L. K. (1992). Temperament and the psychobiology of childhood stress. *Pediatrics, 90*, 483–486.

Bremner, J.D., Randall, P., Vermetten, E., Staib, L., Bronen, R.A., Mazure, C., Capelli, S., McCarthy, G., Innis, R.B., and Charney, D.S. (1997). Magnetic resonance imaging-based measurement of hippocampal volume in posttraumatic stress disorder related to childhood physical and sexual abuse—a preliminary report. *Biological Psychiatry, 41*, 23–32.

Brindley, D. and Rolland, Y. (1989). Possible connections between stress, diabetes, obesity, hypertension and altered lipoprotein metabolism that may result in atherosclerosis. *Clinical Science, 77*, 453–461.

Brown, D.H., Sheridan, J.F., Pearl, D., and Zwilling, B.S. (1993). Regulation of Mycobacterial growth by the hypothalamus-pituitary-adrenal axis: Differential responses of *Mycobacterium bovis* BCG-resistant and susceptible mice. *Infection and Immunity, 61*, 4793–4800.

Brown, G.L., Ebert, M.H., and Goyer, D.C. (1982). Aggression, suicide and serotonin: relationships to CSF amine metabolites. *American Journal of Psychiatry, 139*, 741–746.

Bulloch, K. and Pomerantz, W. (1984). Autonomic nervous system innervation of thymic related lymphoid tissue in wild-type and nude mice. *Journal of Comparative Neurology, 228*, 57–68.

Buske-Kirschbaum, A., Jobst, S., and Hellhammer, D.H. (1998). Altered reactivity of the hypothalamus-pituitary-adrenal axis in patients with atopic dermatitis: Pathologic factor or symptom? *Annals of the New York Academy of Sciences, 840*, 747–754.

Busse, W.W., Kiecolt-Glaser, J.K., Coe, C., Martin, R.J., Weiss, S.T., and Parker, S.R. (1995). NHLBI workshop summary: Stress and asthma. *American Journal of Respiratory and Critical Care Medicine, 151*, 249–252.

Cahill, L. and McGaugh, J.L. (1998). Mechanisms of emotional arousal and lasting declarative memory. *Trends in Neurosciences, 21*, 294–299.

Cahill, L., Haier, R.J., Fallon, J., Alkire, M.T., Tang, C., Keator, D., Wu, J., McGaugh, J.L. (1996). Amygdala activity at encoding correlated with long-term, free recall of emotional information. *Proceedings of the National Academy of Science, 93*, 8016–8021.

Cahill, L., Prins, B., Weber, M., and McGaugh, J.L. (1994). Beta-adrenergic activation and memory for emotional events. *Nature, 371*, 702–704.

Cannon, W.B. (1936). The role of emotions in disease. *Annals of Internal Medicine, 11,* 1453-1465.

Carney, R.M., Freedland, K.E., and Jaffe, A.S. (1990). Insomnia and depression prior to myocardial infarction. *Psychosomatic Medicine, 52,* 603–609.

Carney, R.M., Freedland, K.E., Riggs, B., and Jaffe, A.S. (1995). Depression as a risk factor for cardiac events in established coronary heart disease: a review of possible mechanisms. *Annals of Behavioral Medicine, 17,* 142–149.

Carroll, D., Smith, G.D., Sheffield, D., Shipley, M.J., and Marmot, M.G. (1997). The relationship between socioeconomic status, hostility, and blood pressure reactions to mental stress in men: Data from the Whitehall II study. *Health-Psychology, 16,* 131–136.

Carver, C.S., Pozo, C., Harris, S.D., Noriega, V., Scheier, M.F., Robinson, D.S., Ketcham, A.S., Moffat, F.L., Jr., and Clark, K.C. (1993). How coping mediates the effect of optimism on distress: A study of women with early stage breast cancer. *Journal of Personality and Social Psychology 65,* 375–390.

Case, R.B., Heller, S.S., Case, N.B., Moss, A.J., and the Multicenter Post-Infarction Research Group (1985). Type A behavior and survival after acute myocardial infarction. *The New England Journal of Medicine, 312,* 737–741.

Cassileth, B.R., Lusk, E.J., Miller, D.S., Brown, L.L., and Miller, C. (1985) Psychosocial correlates of survival in advanced malignant disease? *New England Journal of Medicine, 312,* 1551–1555.

Cheasty, M., Clare, A.W., and Collins, C. (1998). Relation between sexual abuse in childhood and adult depression: Case-control study. *British Medical Journal, 6,* 198–201.

Chesney, M.A., Hecker, M.H.L., and Black, G.W. (1988). Coronary-prone components of Type A behavior in the WCGS: A new methodology. In B.K. Houston and C.R. Snyder (Eds.) *Type A Behavior Pattern: Research, Theory, and Intervention* (pp. 168–188). New York: Wiley.

Chin-Hong, P.V. and McGarvey, S.T. (1996). Lifestyle incongruity and adult blood pressure in Western Samoa. *Psychosomatic Medicine, 58,* 131–137.

Chrousos, G.P. (1995). The hypothalamic-pituitary-adrenal axis and immune-mediated inflammation. *New England Journal of Medicine, 332,* 1351–1362.

Chrousos, G.P. (1998) Stressors, stress and neuroendocrine integration of the adaptive response. *Annals of the New York Academy of Science, 851,* 311–335.

Clark, K.B., Krahl, S.E., Smith, D.C., and Jensen, R.A. (1995). Post-training unilateral vagal stimulation enhances retention performance in the rat. *Neurobiology of Learning and Memory, 63,* 213–216.

Clark, K.B., Naritoku, D.K., Smith, D.C., Browning, R.A., and Jensen, R.A. (1999). Enhanced recognition memory following vagus nerve stimulation in humans. *Nature Neuroscience, 2,* 94–98.

Cohen, S. (1995). Psychological stress and susceptibility to upper respiratory infections. *American Journal of Respiratory and Critical Care Medicine, 152,* S53–S58.

Cohen, S. and Herbert, T.B. (1996). Health psychology: Psychological factors and physical disease from the perspective of human psychoneuroimmunology. *Annual Review of Psychology, 47,* 113–142.

Cohen, S., Tyrrell, D., and Smith, A. (1991). Psychological stress and susceptibility to the common cold. *New England Journal of Medicine, 325,* 606–612.

Compas, B.E., Connor, J.K., Saltzman, H., Thomsen, A.H., and Wadsworth, M. (1999). Getting specific about coping: Effortful and involuntary responses to stress in development. In M. Lewis and D. Ramsay (Eds.) *Soothing and Stress* (pp. 229–256). Mahwah, NJ: Lawrence Erlbaum Associates.

Cooper, J.R., Bloom, F.E, and Roth, R.H. (1996). *The Biochemical Basis of Neuropharmacology.* New York: Oxford University Press.

Cruz-Coke, R. (1987). Correlation between prevalence of hypertension and degree of acculturation. *Journal of Hypertension, 5,* 47–50.

Dantzer, R., Bluthe, R.M., Laye, S., Bret-Dibat, J.L., Parnet, P., and Kelley, K.W. (1998). Cytokines and sickness behavior. *Annals of the New York Academy of Sciences, 840,* 586–590.

Dawson, G., Frey, K., Panagiotides, H., Osterling, J., and Hessl, D. (1997). Infants of depressed mothers exhibit atypical frontal brain activity: A replication and extension of previous findings. *Journal of Child Psychology and Psychiatry, 38,* 179–186.

De Bellis, M.D., Baum, A.S., Birmaher, B., Keshavan, M.S., Eccard, C.H., Boring, A.M., Jenkins, F.J., and Ryan, N.D. (1999a). A.E. Bennett research award. Developmental traumatology. Part I: Biological stress systems. *Biological Psychiatry, 45,* 1259–1270.

De Bellis, M.D., Keshavan, M.S., Clark, D.B., Casey, B.J., Giedd, J.N., Boring, A.M., Frustaci, K., and Ryan, N.D. (1999b). A.E. Bennett research award. Developmental traumatology. Part II: Brain development. *Biological Psychiatry, 45,* 1271–1284.

de Quervain, D.J., Roozendaal, B., and McGaugh, J.L. (1998). Stress and glucocorticoids impair retrieval of long-term spatial memory. *Nature, 394,* 787–790.

Dellu, F., Mayo, W., Vallee, M., LeMoal, M., and Simon, H. (1994). Reactivity to novelty during youth as a predictive factor of cognitive impairment in the elderly: a longitudinal study in rats. *Brain Research, 653,* 51–56.

Dellu, F., Mayo, W., Vallee, M., Maccari, S., Piazza, P.V., Le Moal, M., and Simon, H. (1996). Behavioral reactivity to novelty during youth as a predictive factor of stress-induced corticosterone secretion in the elderly—a life-span study in rats. *Psychoneuroendocrinology, 21,* 441–453

Dembroski, T.M., MacDougall, J.M., Costa, P.T., Jr., and Grandits, G.A. (1989). Components of hostility as predictors of sudden death and myocardial infarction in the Multiple Risk Factor Intervention Trial. *Psychosomatic Medicine, 51,* 514–522.

Denenberg, V.H. and Haltmeyer, G.C. (1967). Test of the monotonicity hypothesis concerning infantile stimulation and emotional reactivity. *Journal of Comparative and Physiological Psychology, 63,* 394–396

Denollet, J. and Brutsaert, D.L. (1998). Personality, disease severity, and the risk of long-term cardiac events in patients with a decreased ejection fraction after myocardial infarction. *Circulation 97,* 167–173.

Denollet, J., Sys, S.U., Stroobant, N., Rombouts, H., Gillebert, T.C., Brutsaert, D.L. (1996) Personality as independent predictor of long-term mortality in patients with coronary heart disease. *Lancet, 347,* 417–421.

Dhabhar, F. and McEwen, B. (1999). Enhancing versus suppressive effects of stress hormones on skin immune function. *Proceedings of the National Academy of Sciences, 96,* 1059–1064.

Dhabhar, F.S., Miller, A.H., McEwen, B.S., and Spencer, R.L. (1995). Effects of stress on immune cell distribution. Dynamics and hormonal mechanisms. *Journal of Immunology, 154,* 5511–5527.

Dhabhar, F.S., Miller, A.H., McEwen, B.S., and Spencer, R.L. (1996). Stress-induced changes in blood leukocyte distribution: Role of adrenal steroid hormones. *Journal of Immunology, 157*, 1638–1644.

Dietz, W.H. (1998). Childhood weight affects adult morbidity and mortality. *Journal of Nutrition, 128 (2 Suppl.)*, 411S–414S.

Dobbs, C.M., Vasquez, M., Glaser, R., and Sheridan, J.F. (1993). Mechanisms of stress-induced modulation of viral pathogenesis and immunity. *Journal of Neuroimmunology, 48*, 151–160.

Dressler, W.W. (1991). Social support, lifestyle incongruity, and arterial blood pressure in a southern black community. *Psychosomatic Medicine, 53*, 608–620.

Drevets, W.C., Price, J.L., Simpson, Jr., J.R., Todd, R.D., Reich, T., Vannier, M., and Ralchle, M.E. (1997). Subgenual prefrontal cortex abnormalities in mood disorders. *Nature, 386*, 824–827.

Eichenbaum, H. (1997). How does the brain organize memories? *Science, 277*, 330–332.

Epel, N., McEwen, B., and Ickovics, J. (1998). Embodying psychological thriving: Physical thriving in response to stress. *Journal of Social Issues, 54*, 301–322.

Epping-Jordan, J.E., Compas, B.E., Osowiecki, D.M., Oppedisano, G., Gerhardt, C., Primo, K., and Krag, D.N. (1999). Psychological adjustment to breast cancer: Processes of emotional distress. *Health Psychology, 18*, 1–12.

Eriksson, J.G., Forsén, T., Tuomilehto, J., Winter, P.D., Osmond, C., and Barker, D.J.P. (1999). Catch-up growth in childhood and death from coronary heart disease: Longitudinal study. *British Medical Journal, 318*, 427–431.

Esterling, B.A., L'Abate, L., Murray, E.J., and Pennebaker, J.W. (1999). Empirical foundations for writing in prevention and psychotherapy: Mental and physical health outcomes. *Clinical Psychology Review, 19*, 79–96.

Everson, S.A., Goldberg, D.E., Kaplan, G.A., Cohen, R.D., Pukkala, E. Tuomilehto, J., and Salonen, J.T. (1996). Hopelessness and risk of mortality and incidence of myocardial infarction and cancer. *Psychosomatic Medicine, 58*, 113–121.

Everson, S.A., Goldberg, D.E., Kaplan, G.A., Julkunen, J., and Salonen, J.T. (1998). Anger expression and incident hypertension. *Psychosomatic.Medicine, 60*, 730–735.

Everson, S.A., Lynch, J.W., Chesney, M.A., Kaplan, G.A., Goldberg, D.E., Shade, S.B., Cohen, R.D., Salonen, R., and Salonen, J.T. (1997). Interaction of workplace demands and cardiovascular reactivity in progression of carotid atherosclerosis: Population based study. *British Medical Journal, 314*, 553–558.

Fauci, A.S. (1975). Mechanisms of corticosteroid action on lymphocyte subpopulations. I. Redistribution of circulating T and B lymphocytes to the bone marrow. *Immunology, 28*, 669–680.

Felitti, V.J., Anda, R.F., Nordenberg, D., Williamson, D.F., Spitz, A.M., Edwards, V., Koss, M.P., and Marks, J.S. (1998). Relationship of childhood abuse and household dysfunction to many of the leading causes of death in adults. The adverse childhood experiences (ACE) study. *American Journal of Preventive Medicine, 14*, 245–258.

Felten, D.L., Felten, S., Bellinger, D.L., Carlson, S.L., Ackerman, K.D., Madden, K.S., Olschowki, J.A., and Livnat, S. (1987). Noradrenergic sympathetic neural interactions with the immune system: Structure and function. *Immunological Reviews, 100*, 225–260.

Fisher, L., Ames, E.W., Chisholm, K., and Savoie, L. (1997). Problems reported by parents of Romanian orphans adopted to British Columbia. *International Journal Behavioral Development, 20,* 67–82.

Fox, B.H. (1989) Depressive symptoms and risk of cancer. *Journal of the American Medical Association, 262,* 1231.

Frasure-Smith, N., Lesperance, F., and Talajic, M. (1995). Depression and 18-month prognosis after myocardial infarction. *Circulation, 91,* 999–1005.

Frasure-Smith, N., Lesperance, F., Juneau, M., Talajic, M., and Bourassa, M.G. (1999). Gender, depression, and one-year prognosis after myocardial infarction. *Psychosomatic Medicine, 61,* 26–37.

Freedman, D.S., Srinivasan, S.R., Valdez, R.A., Williamson, D.F., and Berenson, G.S. (1997). Secular increases in relative weight and adiposity among children over two decades: The Bogalusa Heart Study. *Pediatrics, 99,* 420–426.

Fride, E., Dan, Y., Feldon, J., Halevy, G., and Weinstock, M. (1986). Effects of prenatal stress on vulnerability to stress in prepubertal and adult rats. *Physiology and Behavior, 37,* 681–687.

Friedman, M. and Rosenman, R.H. (1974). *Type A Behavior and Your Heart.* New York: Knopf.

Fuchs, E.J. and Matzinger, P. (1996). Is cancer dangerous to the immune system? *Seminars in Immunology, 8,* 271–280.

Galea, L.A.M., McEwen, B.S., Tanapat, P., Deak, T., Spencer, R.L., and Dhabhar, F.S. (1997). Sex differences in dendritic atrophy of CA3 pyramidal neurons in response to chronic restraint stress. *Neuroscience, 81,* 689–697.

Gerin, W. and Pickering, T.G. (1995). Association between delayed recovery of blood pressure after acute mental stress and parental history of hypertension. *Journal of Hypertension, 13,* 603–610.

Glaser, R., Kiecolt-Glaser, J.K., Bonneau, R.H., Malarkey, W., Kennedy, S., and Hughes, J. (1992). Stress-induced modulation of the immune response to recombinant hepatitis B vaccine. *Psychosomatic Medicine, 54,* 22–29.

Glaser, R., Kiecolt-Glaser, J.K., Malarkey, W., and Sheridan, J.F. (1998). The influence of psychological stress on the immune response to vaccines. *Annals of the New York Academy of Sciences, 840,* 649–655.

Glaser, R., Rabin, B., Chesney, M., Cohen, S., and Natelson, B. (1999). Stress-induced immunomodulation: Implications for infectious diseases? *Journal of the American Medical Association, 281,* 2268–2270.

Goy, R.W. (1970). Early hormonal influences on the development of sexual and sex-related behavior. In F.O. Schmitt (Ed.) *The Neurosciences: Second Study Program* (pp. 196–206). New York: Rockefeller University Press.

Gray, J.A. (1982). Precis of the neuropsychology of anxiety: An enquiry into the functions of the septo-hippocamal system. *The Behavioral and Brain Sciences, 5,* 469–534.

Green, M.A. and Berlin, M.A. (1987). Five psychosocial variables related to the existence of post-traumatic stress disorder symptoms. *Journal of Clinical Psychology, 43,* 643-649.

Greeno, C.G. and Wing, R.R. (1994). Stress-induced eating. *Psychological Bulletin, 115,* 444–464.

Greenough, W.T. and Bailey, C.H. (1988). The anatomy of a memory: Convergence of results across a diversity of tests. *Trends in Neurosciences, 11,* 142–147.

Greer, S., Morris, T., and Pettingale, K.W. (1979). Psychological response to breast cancer: Effect on outcome. *Lancet, 2(8146)*, 785–787.

Griffin, A.C. and Whitacre, C.C. (1991). Sex and strain differences in the circadian rhythm fluctuation of endocrine and immune function in the rat: Implications for rodent models of autoimmune disease. *Journal of Neuroimmunology, 35*, 53–64.

Gunnar, M.R. (1998). Neuroendocrine activity in children adopted from Romania: Relations with cognitive and social functioning. *Minneapolis: Institute of Child Development*, University of Minnesota.

Guzowski, J.F. and McGaugh, J.L. (1997). Antisense oligodeoxynucleotide-mediated disruption of hippocampal cAMP response element binding protein levels impairs consolidation of memory for water maze training. *Proceedings of the National Academy of Sciences, 94*, 2693–2698.

Hamann, S.B., Ely, T.D., Grafton, S.T., and Kilts, C.D. (1999). Amygdala activity related to enhanced memory for pleasant and aversive stimuli. *Nature Neuroscience, 3*, 289–293.

Hearn, M.D., Murray, D.M., and Luepker, R.V. (1989). Hostility, coronary heart disease, and total mortality: A 33-year follow-up study of university students. *Journal of Behavioral Medicine, 12*, 105–121.

Hecker, M.H., Chesney, M.A., Black, G.W., and Frautschi, N. (1988). Coronary-prone behaviors in the Western Collaborative Group Study. *Psychosomatic Medicine, 50*, 153–164

Heijnen, C.J., Rouppe van der Voort, C., Wulffraat, N., van der Net, J., Kuis, W., and Kavelaars, A. (1996). Functional alpha-1 adrenergic receptors on leukocytes of patients with polyarticular juvenile rheumatoid arthritis. *Journal of Neuroimmunology, 71*, 223–226.

Heim, C., Newport, D.J., Heit, S., Graham, Y.P., Wilcox, M., Bonsall, R., Miller, A.H., and Nemeroff, C.B. (2000) Pituitary-adrenal and autonomic responses to stress in women after sexual and physical abuse in childhood. *Journal of the American Medical Association, 284*, 592–597.

Helmers, K.F., Krantz, D.S., Merz, C.N., Klein, J., Kop, W.J., Gottdiener, J.S., and Rozanski, A. (1995). Defensive hostility: Relationship to multiple markers of cardiac ischemia in patients with coronary disease. *Health Psychology, 14*, 202–209.

Henry, J.P., Stephens, P.M., and Ely, D.L. (1986). Psychosocial hypertension and the defence and defeat reactions. *Journal of Hypertension, 4*, 687–697.

Herman, D.B., Susser, E.S., Struening, E.L., and Link, B.L. (1997). Adverse childhood experiences: Are they risk factors for adult homelessness? *American Journal of Public Health, 87*, 249–255.

Hermann, G., Beck, F.M., and Sheridan, J.F. (1995). Stress-induced glucocorticoid response modulates mononuclear cell trafficking during an experimental influenza viral infection. *Journal of Neuroimmunology, 56*, 179–186.

Hermann, G., Tovar, C.A., Beck, F.M., Allen, C., and Sheridan, J.F. (1993). Restraint stress differentially affects the pathogenesis of an experimental influenza viral infection in three inbred strains of mice. *Journal of Neuroimmunology, 47*, 83–94.

Higley, J.D., Hasert, M.F., Suomi, S.J., and Linnoila, M. (1991). Nonhuman primate model of alcohol abuse: Effects of early experience, personality, and stress on alcohol consumption. *Proceedings of the National Academy of Science, 88*, 7261–7265.

Higley, J.D., Mehlman, P.T., Higley, S.B., Fernald, B., Vickers, J., Lindell, S.G., Taub, D.M., Suomi, S.J., and Linnoila, M. (1996a). Excessive mortality in young free-ranging male nonhuman primates with low cerebrospinal fluid 5-hydroxyindoleacetic acid concentrations. *Archives of General Psychiatry, 53*, 537–543.

Higley, J.D., Mehlman, P.T., Poland, R.E., Taub, D.M., Vickers, J., Suomi, S.J., and Linnoila, M. (1996b). CSF testosterone and 5-HIAA correlate with different types of aggressive behaviors. *Biological Psychiatry, 40*, 1067–1082.

Holland, J.C. and Rowland, J.H. (Eds.) (1990). *Handbook of Psychooncology: Psychological Care of the Patient with Cancer.* New York: Oxford University Press.

Hostetter, M. K., Iverson, S., Thomas, W., McKenzie, D., Dole, K., and Johnson, D. E. (1991). Prospective medical evaluation of internationally adopted children. *New England Journal of Medicine, 325*, 479–485.

House, J.S., Landis, K.R., and Umberson, R. (1988). Social relationships and health. *Science, 241*, 540–545.

Houston, B.K. and Kelly, K.E. (1987). Type A behavior in housewives: Relation to work, marital adjustment, stress, tension, health, fear-of-failure and self esteem. *Journal of Psychosomatic Research, 31*, 55–61.

Ironson, G., Taylor, C.B., Boltwood, M., Bartzokis, T., Dennis, C., Chesney, M., Spitzer, S., and Segall, G.M. (1992). Effects of anger on left ventricular ejection fraction in coronary artery disease. *American Journal of Cardiology, 70*, 281–285.

Ironson, G., Wynings, C., Schneiderman, N., Baum, A., Rodriguez, M., Greenwood, D., Benight, C., Antoni, M., LaPerriere, A., Huang, H.S., Klimas, N., and Fletcher, M.A. (1997). Posttraumatic stress symptoms, intrusive thoughts, loss, and immune function after Hurricane Andrew. *Psychosomatic Medicine, 59*, 128–141.

Irwin, M., Daniels, M., Smith, T.L., Bloom, E., and Weiner, H. (1987). Impaired natural killer cell activity during bereavement. *Brain, Behavior and Immunity, 1*, 98–104.

Israel, B.A. and Schurman, S.J. (1990) Social support, control and the stress process. In K. Glanz, F.M. Lewis and B.K. Rimer (Eds.) *Health, Behavior and Health Education: Theory, Research, and Practice* (pp. 179–205) San Francisco: Jossey-Bass.

Jamison, R.N., Burish, T.G.; and Wallston, K.A. (1987). Psychogenic factors in predicting survival of breast cancer patients. *Journal of Clinical Oncology, 5*, 768–772.

Johnson, E.O., Kamilaris T.C., Calogero, A.E., Gold, P.W., and Chrousos, G.P. (1996a). Effects of early parenting on growth and development in a small primate. *Pediatric Research, 39*, 999–1005.

Johnson, E.O., Kamilaris, T.C., Carter, C.S., Calogero, A.E., Gold, P.W., and Chrousos, G.P. (1996b) The biobehavioral consequences of psychogenic stress in a small, social primate (*Callithrix jacchus jacchus*). *Biological Psychiatry, 40*, 317–337.

Julius, S. (1993). Corcoran Lecture. Sympathetic hyperactivity and coronary risk in hypertension. *Hypertension, 21*, 886–893.

Kang, D.H., Coe, C.L., Karaszewski, J., and McCarthy, D.O. (1998). Relationship of social support to stress responses and immune function in healthy and asthmatic adolescents. *Research in Nursing and Health, 21*, 117–128.

Kaplan, G.A., Pamuk, E., Lynch, J.W., Cohen, R.D., and Balfour, J.L. (1996). Income inequality and mortality in the United States: Analysis of mortality and potential pathways. *British Medical Journal, 312*, 999–1003.

Karasek, R. and Theorell, T. (1990). *Healthy Work.* New York: Basic Books.

Kaufman J., Birmaher, B., Perel, J., Dahl, R.E., Stull, S., Brent, D., Trubnick, L., al-Shabbout, M., and Ryan, N.D. (1998). Serotonergic functioning in depressed abused children: Clinical and familial correlates. *Biological Psychiatry, 44,* 973–981.

Kawachi, I., Kennedy, B., Lochner, K., and Prothrow-Stith, D. (1997). Social capital, income inequality, and mortality. *American Journal of Public Health, 87,* 1491–1498.

Keltikangas-Jarvinen, L., Raikkonen, K., and Hautanen, A. (1996a). Type A behavior and vital exhaustion as related to the metabolic hormonal variables of the hypothalamic-pituitary-adrenal axis. *Behavioral Medicine, 22,* 15–22.

Keltikangas-Jarvinen, L., Raikkonen, K., Hautanen, A., and Adlercreutz, H. (1996b). Vital exhaustion, anger expression, and pituitary and adrenocortical hormones: Implications for the insulin resistance syndrome. *Arteriosclerosis, Thrombosis, and Vascular Biology, 16,* 275–280.

Kiecolt-Glaser, J.K., Fisher, L.D., Ogrocki, P., Stout, J.C., Speicher, C.E., and Glaser, R. (1987). Marital quality, marital disruption, and immune function. *Psychosomatic Medicine, 49,* 13–34.

Kiecolt-Glaser, J.K., Glaser, R., and Cacioppo, J.T. (1997). Marital conflict in older adults: endocrinological and immunological correlates. *Psychosomatic Medicine, 59,* 339–349.

Kiecolt-Glaser, J.K., Glaser, R., Gravenstein, S., Malarkey, W.B., and Sheridan, J.F. (1996). Chronic stress alters the immune response to influenza virus vaccine in older adults. *Proceedings of the National Academy of Sciences, 93,* 3043–3047.

Kiecolt-Glaser, J.K., Marucha, P.T., Malarkey, W.B., Mercado, A.M., and Glaser, R. (1995). Slowing of wound healing by psychological stress. *Lancet, 346,* 1194–1196.

King, K.B. (1997). Psychologic and social aspects of cardiovascular disease. *Annals of Behavioral Medicine, 19,* 264–270.

Kirschbaum, C., Kudielka, B.M., Gaab, J., Schommer, N.C., and Hellhammer, D.H. (1999). Impact of gender, menstrual cycle phase and oral contraceptive use on the activity of the hypothalamo-pituitary-adrenal axis. *Psychosomatic Medicine, 61,* 154–162.

Kirschbaum, C., Prussner, J.C., Stone, A.A., Federenko, I., Gaab, J., Lintz, D., Schommer, N., and Hellhammer, D.H. (1995). Persistent high cortisol responses to repeated psychological stress in a subpopulation of healthy men. *Psychosomatic Medicine, 57,* 468–474.

Klesges, R.C., Eck, L.H., Hanson, C.L., Haddock, C.K., and Klesges, L.M. (1990). Effects of obesity, social interactions, and physical environment on physical activity in preschoolers. *Health Psychology, 9,* 435–449.

Kop, W.J., Appels, A.P., Mendes, D.L.C., and Bar, F.W. (1996). The relationship between severity of coronary artery disease and vital exhaustion. *Journal of Psychosomatic Research, 40,* 397–405.

Kop, W.J., Appels, A.P., Mendes, d.L.C., de Swart, H.B., and Bar, F.W. (1994). Vital exhaustion predicts new cardiac events after successful coronary angioplasty. *Psychosomatic Medicine, 56,* 281–287.

Kop, W.J., Hamulyak, K., Pernot, C., and Appels, A. (1998). Relationship of blood coagulation and fibrinolysis to vital exhaustion. *Psychosomatic Medicine, 60,* 352–358.

Koskenvuo, M., Kaprio, J., Rose, R.J., Kesaniemi, A., Sarna, S., Heikkila, K., and Langinvainio, H. (1988). Hostility as a risk factor for mortality and ischemic heart disease in men. *Psychosomatic Medicine, 50,* 330–340.

Kraemer, G.W., Schmidt, D.E. and Ebert, M.H. (1997) The behavioral neurobiology of self-injurious behavior in rhesus monkeys, in *The Neurobiology of Suicide: From the Bench to the Clinic*. In D.M. Stoff and J.J. Mann (Eds.) *Annals of the New York Academy of Sciences*, 836, 12–38.

Kubzansky, L.D., Kawachi, I., Spiro, A., Weiss, S.T., Vokonas, P.S., and Sparrow, D. (1997). Is worrying bad for your heart? A prospective study of worry and coronary heart disease in the Normative Aging Study. *Circulation*, 95, 818–824.

Kusnecov, A.V., Grota, L.J., Schmidt, S.G., Bonneau, R.H., Sheridan, J.F., Glaser, R., and Moynihan, J.A. (1992). Decreased herpes simplex viral immunity and enhanced pathogenesis following stressor administration in mice. *Journal of Neuroimmunology*, 38, 129–137.

Lazarus, R.S. and Folkman, S. (1984). *Stress, Appraisal, and Coping*. New York: Springer-Verlag.

LeDoux, J.E. (1996). *The Emotional Brain*. New York: Simon and Schuster.

Leon, G.R., Finn, S.E., Murray, D., and Bailey, J.M. (1988). Inability to predict cardiovascular disease from hostility scores or MMPI items related to type A behavior. *Journal of Consulting and Clinical Psychology*, 56, 597–600.

Levine, S., Glick, D., and Nakane, P.K. (1967). Adrenal and plasma corticosterone and vitamin A in rat adrenal glands during postnatal development. *Endocrinology*, 80, 910–914.

Lipkus, I.M., Barefoot, J.C., Williams, R.B., and Siegler, I.C. (1994). Personality measures as predictors of smoking initiation and cessation in the UNC Alumni Heart Study. *Health Psychology*, 13, 149–155.

Liu, D., Diorio, J., Tannenbaum, B., Caldji, C., Francis, D., Freedman, A., Sharma, S., Pearson, D., Plotsky, P.M., and Meaney, M.J. (1997). Maternal care, hippocampal glucocorticoid receptors, and hypothalamic-pituitary-adrenal responses to stress. *Science*, 277, 1659–1662.

Lupien, S., Lecours, A.R., Lussier, I., Schwartz, G., Nair, N.P.V., and Meaney, M.J. (1994). Basal cortisol levels and cognitive deficits in human aging. *Journal of Neuroscience*, 14, 2893–2903.

Lupien, S.J., DeLeon, M.J., De Santi, S., Convit, A., Tarshish, C., Nair, N.P.V., Thakur, M., McEwen, B.S., Hauger, R.L., and Meaney, M.J. (1998). Cortisol levels during human aging predict hippocampal atrophy and memory deficits. *Nature Neuroscience*, 1, 69–73.

Lynch, J., Krause, N., Kaplan, G.A., Tuomilehto, J., and Salonen, J.T. (1997a). Workplace conditions, socioeconomic status, and the risk of mortality and acute myocardial infarction: The kuopio ischemic heart disease risk factor study. *American Journal of Public Health*, 87, 617–622.

Lynch, J.W., Kaplan, G.A., and Shema, S.J. (1997b). Cumulative impact of sustained economic hardship on physical, cognitive, psychological, and social functioning. *New England Journal of Medicine*, 337, 1889–1895.

Maier, S., Goehler, L.E., Fleshner, M., and Watkins, L.R. (1998). The role of the vagus in cytokine to brain communication. *Annals of the New York Academy of Sciences*, 840, 289–300.

Mann, J.J. (1998). The neurobiology of suicide. *Nature Medicine*, 4, 25–30.

Manuck, S.B., Kaplan, J.R., Adams, M.R., and Clarkson, T.B. (1995). Studies of psychosocial influences on coronary artery atherosclerosis in cynomolgus monkeys. *Health Psychology*, 7, 113–124.

Marmot, M.G., Davey Smith, G., Stansfeld, S., Patel, C., North, F., Head, J., White, I., Brunner, E., and Feeney, A. (1991). Health inequalities among British civil servants: The Whitehall II study. *Lancet*, 337, 1387–1393.

Martin, K.C. and Kandel, E.R. (1996). Cell adhesion molecules, CREB, and the formation of new synaptic connections. *Neuron*, 17, 567–570.

Marucha, P.T., Kiecolt-Glaser, J.K., and Favagehi, M. (1998). Mucosal wound healing is impaired by examination stress. *Psychosomatic Medicine*, 60, 362–365.

Matthews, K.A., Glass, D.C., Rosenman, R.H., and Bortner, R.W. (1977). Competitive drive, pattern A, and coronary heart disease: A further analysis of some data from the Western Collaborative Group Study. *Journal of Chronic Diseases*, 30, 489–498.

Matthews, K.A., Owens, J.F., Kuller, L.H., Sutton-Tyrrell, K., and Jansen-McWilliams, L. (1998). Are hostility and anxiety associated with carotid atherosclerosis in healthy postmenopausal women? *Psychosomatic.Medicine*, 60, 633–638.

McCranie, E.W., Watkins, L.O., Brandsma, J.M., and Sisson, B.D. (1986). Hostility, coronary heart disease (CHD) incidence, and total mortality: Lack of association in a 25-year follow-up study of 478 physicians. *Journal of Behavioral Medicine*, 9, 119–125.

McEwen, B., Biron, C., Brunson, K., Bulloch, K., Chambers, W.H., Dhabhar, F.S., Goldfarb, R.H., Kitson, R.P., Miller, A.H., Spencer, R.L., and Weiss, J.M. (1997). The role of adrenocorticoids as modulators of immune function in health and disease: Neural, endocrine, and immune interactions. *Brain Research Reviews*, 23, 79–133.

McEwen, B.S. (1997). Possible mechanisms for atrophy of the human hippocampus. *Molecular Psychiatry*, 2, 255–262.

McEwen, B.S. (1998). Protective and damaging effects of stress mediators. *New England Journal of Medicine*, 338, 171–179.

McEwen, B.S. (1999a). Permanence of brain sex differences and structural plasticity of the adult brain. *Proceedings of the National Academy of Sciences*, 96, 7128–7130.

McEwen, B.S. (1999b). Stress and hippocampal plasticity. *Annual Review of Neuroscience*, 22, 105–122.

McEwen, B.S. and Alves, S.H. (1999). Estrogen actions in the central nervous system. *Endocrine Reviews*, 20, 279–307.

McEwen, B.S. and Seeman, T. (1999). Protective and damaging effects of mediators of stress: Elaborating and testing the concepts of allostasis and allostatic load. *Annals of the New York Academy of Sciences*, 896, 30–47.

McEwen, B.S. and Stellar, E. (1993), Stress and the individual: Mechanisms leading to disease. *Archives of Internal Medicine*, 153, 2093–2101.

McGaugh, J.L., Cahill, L., and Roozendaal, B. (1996). Involvement of the amygdala in memory storage: Interaction with other brain systems. *Proceedings of the National Academy of Sciences*, 93, 13508–13514.

Meaney, M., Aitken, D., Berkel, H., Bhatnager, S., and Sapolsky, R. (1988). Effect of neonatal handling on age-related impairments associated with the hippocampus. *Science*, 239, 766–768.

Michelson, D., Stratakis, C., Hill, L., Reynolds, J., Galliven, E., Chrousos, G., and Gold, P. (1996). Bone mineral density in women with depression. *New England Journal of Medicine*, 335, 1176–1181.

Miller, T.Q., Smith, T.W., Turner, C.W., Guijarro, M.L., and Hallet, A.J. (1996). A meta-analytic review of research on hostility and physical health. *Psychological Bulletin, 119*, 322–348.

Millstein, S.G., Petersen, A.C., and Nightingale, E.O. (Eds.) (1993). *Promoting the Health of Adolescents: New Directions for the Twenty-first Century.* New York: Oxford University Press.

Muller, J.E. and Tofler, G.H. (1990). A symposium: triggering and circadian variation of onset of acute cardiovascular disease. *American Journal of Cardiology, 66*, 1–70.

Must, A. and Strauss, R.S. (1999). Risks and consequences of childhood and adolescent obesity. *International Journal of Obesity and Related Metabolic Disorders, 23 suppl. 2*, S2–S11.

National Research Council (NRC). (2000). *From Neurons to Neighborhoods: The Science of Early Childhood Development.* Washington, DC: National Academy Press.

Nelson, C., and Bloom, F. (1997). Child development and neuroscience. *Child Development, 68*, 970-987.

Nelson, C.A. and Carver, L.J. (1998). The effects of stress and trauma on brain and memory: A view from developmental cognitive neuroscience. *Development and Psychopathology, 10*, 793–809.

Nielsen, K.A. and Jensen, R.A. (1995). Beta-adrenergic receptor antagonist anti-hypertensive medications impair arousal-induced modulation of working memory in elderly humans. *Behavioral and Neural Biology, 62*, 190–200.

Notzon, F.C., Komarov, Y.M., Ermakov, S.P., Sempos, C.T., Marks, J.S., and Sempos, E.V. (1998). Causes of declining life expectancy in Russia. *Journal of the American Medical Association, 279*, 793–800.

Ockenfels, M.C., Porter, L., Smyth, J., Kirschbaum, C., Hellhammer, D.H., and Stone, A.A. (1995). Effect of chronic stress associated with unemployment on salivary cortisol: Overall cortisol levels, diurnal rhythm, and acute stress reactivity. *Psychosomatic Medicine, 57*, 460–467.

Oliff, H.S., Berchtold, N.C., Isackson, P., and Cotman, C.W. (1998). Exercise-induced regulation of brain-derived neurotrophic factor (BDNF) transcripts in the rat hippocampus. *Brain Research Molecular Brain Research, 61*, 147–153.

Padgett, D.A., Marucha, P.T., and Sheridan, J.F. (1998). Restraint stress slow cutaneous wound healing in mice. *Brain, Behavior and Immunity, 12*, 64–73.

Pennebaker, J.W. (1997). Writing about emotional experiences as a therapeutic process. *Psychological Science, 8*, 162–166.

Penninx, B.W., Guralnik, J.M., Pahor, M., Ferrucci, L., Cerhan, J.R., Wallace, R.B., and Havlik, R.J. (1998). Chronically depressed mood and cancer risk in older persons. *Journal of the National Cancer Institute, 90*, 1888–1893.

Perseghin, G., Price, T.B., Petersen, K.F., Roden, M., Cline, G.W., Gerow, K., Rothman, D.L., and Shulman, G.I. (1996). Increased glucose transport-phosphorylation and muscle glycogen synthesis after exercise training in insulin-resistant subjects. *New England Journal of Medicine, 335*, 1357–1362.

Petrie, K.J., Booth, R.J., and Pennebaker, J.W. (1998). The immunological effects of thought suppression. *Journal of Personality and Social Psychology, 75*, 1264–1272.

Petrie, K.J., Booth, R.J., Pennebaker, J.W., Davison, K.P, and Thomas, M.G. (1995). Disclosure of trauma and immune response to a hepatitis B vaccination program. *Journal of Consulting and Clinical Psychology, 63*, 787–792.

Pine, D.S., Coplan, J.D., Wasserman, G.A., Miller, L.S. Fried, J.E., Davies, M., Cooper, T.B., Greenhill, L., Shaffer, D., and Parsons, B. (1997). Neuroendocrine response to fenfluramine challenge in boys. Associations with aggressive behavior and adverse rearing. *Archives of General Psychiatry, 54,* 839–846.

Poulter, N.R., Khaw, K.T., and Sever, P.S. (1988). Higher blood pressures of urban migrants from an African low-blood pressure population are not due to selective migration. *American Journal of Hypertension, 1,* 143S–145S.

Poulter, N.R., Khaw, K.T., Hopwood, B.E., Mugambi, M., Peart, W.S., Rose, G., and Sever, P.S. (1990). The Kenyan Luo migration study: Observations on the initiation of a rise in blood pressure. *British Medical Journal, 300,* 967–972

Raikkonen, K., Hautanen, A., and Keltikangas-Jarvinen, L. (1996). Feelings of exhaustion, emotional distress, and pituitary and adrenocortical hormones in borderline hypertension. *Journal of Hypertension, 14,* 713–718.

Ramirez, A.J.; Craig, T.K.; Watson, J.P.; Fentiman, I.S.; North, W.R.; and Rubens, R.D. (1989). Stress and relapse of breast cancer. *Biomedical Journal, 298,* 291-293.

Reinisch, J.M., Rosenblum, L.A., and Sanders, S.A. (Eds.) (1987). *Masculinity/Femininity.* New York: Oxford University Press.

Review Panel. (1981). Coronary-prone behavior and coronary heart disease: A critical review. *Circulation, 63,* 1199–1215.

Rich-Edwards, J.W., Colditz, G.A., Stampfer, M.J., Willett, W.C., Gillman, M.W., Hennekens, C.H., Speizer, F.E., and Manson, J.E. (1999). Birthweight and the risk of type 2 diabetes mellitus in adult women. *Annals of Internal Medicine, 130,* 278–284.

Roozendaal, B., Portillo-Marquez, G., and McGaugh, J.L. (1996). Basolateral amygdala lesions block glucocorticoid-induced modulation of memory for spatial learning. *Behavioral Neuroscience, 110,* 1074–1083.

Rowland, J. (1990). Interpersonal resources: Coping. In J.C. Holland and J.R. Holland (Eds.) *Psychooncology: Psychological Care of the Patient with Cancer.* New York: Oxford University Press. pp. 44-57.

Rozanski, A., Blumenthal, J.A., and Kaplan, J. (1999). Impact of psychological factors on the pathogenesis of cardiovascular disease and implications for therapy. *Circulation, 99,* 2192–2217.

Ryff, C.D. and Singer, B. (1998). The contours of positive health. *Psychological Inquiry, 9,* 1–28.

Salbe, A.D., Fontvieille, A.M., Harper, I.T., and Ravussin, E. (1997). Low levels of physical activity in 5-year-old children. *Journal of Pediatrics, 131,* 423–429.

Salmon, P. and Calderbank, S. (1996). The relationship of childhood physical and sexual abuse to adult illness behavior. *Journal of Psychosomotic Research, 40,* 329-336.

Sapolsky, R.M. (1996). Why stress is bad for your brain. *Science, 273,* 749–750.

Sasaki, S., Yoneda, Y., Fujita, H., Uchida, A., Takenaka, K., Takesako, T., Itoh, H., Nakata, T., Takeda, K., and Nakagawa, M. (1994). Association of blood pressure variability with induction of atherosclerosis in cholesterol-fed rats. *American Journal of Hypertension, 7,* 453–459.

Scheier, M.F. and Bridges, M.W. (1995). Person variables and health: Personality predispositions and acute psychological states as shared determinants for disease. *Psychosomatic Medicine, 57,* 255–268.

Scheier, M.F. and Carver, C.S. (1985). Optimism, coping, and health: Assessment and implications of generalized outcome expectancies. *Health Psychology, 4,* 219–247.

Scheier, M.F. and Carver, C.S. (1992). Effects of optimism on psychological and physical well-being: Theoretical overview and empirical update. *Cognitive Therapy and Research, 16,* 201–228.

Schnall, P.L., Schwartz, J.E., Landsbergis, P.A., Warren, K., and Pickering, T.G. (1992). Relation between job strain, alcohol, and ambulatory blood pressure. *Hypertension, 19,* 488–494.

Schulkin, J., Gold, P.W., and McEwen, B.S. (1998). Induction of corticotropin-releasing hormone gene expression by glucocorticoids: Implication for understanding the states of fear and anxiety and allostatic load. *Psychoneuroendocrinology, 23,* 219–243.

Seeman, T.E. and McEwen, B.S. (1996). The impact of social environment characteristics on neuroendocrine regulation. *Psychosomatic Medicine, 58,* 459–471.

Seeman, T.E., McEwen, B.S., Singer, B.H., Albert, M.S., and Rowe, J.W. (1997). Increase in urinary cortisol excretion and memory declines: MacArthur studies of successful aging. *Journal of Clinical Endocrinology and Metabolism, 82,* 2458–2465.

Selye, H. (1956). *The Stress of Life.* New York: McGraw-Hill.

Sesso, H.D., Kawachi, I., Vokonas, P.S., and Sparrow, D. (1998). Depression and the risk of coronary heart disease in the Normative Aging Study. *American Journal of Cardiology, 82,* 851–856.

Shanks, N., Harbuz, M.S., Jessop, D.S., Perks, P., Moore, P.M., and Lightman, S.L. (1998). Inflammatory disease as chronic stress. *Annals of the New York Academy of Sciences, 840,* 599–607.

Shekelle, R.B., Raynor, W.J., Jr., Ostfeld, A.M., Garron, D.C., Bieliauskas, L.A., Liu, S.C., Maliza, C., and Paul, O. (1981). Psychological depression and 17-year risk of death from cancer. *Psychosomatic Medicine, 43,* 117–125.

Shekelle, R.B., Gale, M., and Norusis, M. (1985a). Type A score (Jenkins Activity Survey) and risk of recurrent coronary heart disease in the Aspirin Myocardial Infarction Study. *American Journal of Cardiology, 56,* 221–225.

Shekelle, R.B., Gale, M., Ostfeld, A.M., and Paul, O. (1983). Hostility, risk of coronary heart disease, and mortality. *Psychosomatic Medicine, 45,* 109–114.

Shekelle, R.B., Hulley, S.B., Neaton, J.D., Billings, J.H., Borhani, N.O., Gerace, T.A., Jacobs, D.R., Lasser, N.L., Mittlemark, M.B., and Stamler, J., for the Multiple Risk Factor Intervention Trial Research Group (1985b). The MRFIT behavior pattern study, Type A behavior and the incidence of coronary heart disease. *American Journal of Epidemiology, 122,* 559–570.

Shekelle, R.B., Vernon, S.W., and Ostfeld, A.M. (1991). Personality and coronary heart disease. *Psychosomatic Medicine, 53,* 176–184

Sheline, Y.I., Gado, M.H., and Price, J.L. (1998). Amygdala core nuclei volumes are decreased in recurrent major depression. *NeuroReport, 9,* 2023–2028.

Sheline, Y.I., Sanghavi, M., Mintun, M.A., and Gado, M.H. (1999). Depression duration but not age predicts hippocampal volume loss in medically healthy women with recurrent major depression. *Journal of Neuroscience, 19 ,* 5034–5043.

Sheridan, J.F., Feng, N.G., Bonneau, R.H., Allen, C.M., Huneycutt, B.S., and Glaser, R. (1991). Restraint stress differentially affects anti-viral cellular and humoral immune responses in mice. *Journal of Neuroimmunology, 31,* 245–255.

Shiffman, S., Hickcox, M., Paty, J.A., Gnys, M., Kassel, J.D., and Richards, T.J. (1996). Progression from a smoking lapse to relapse: Prediction from abstinence violation effects, nicotine dependence, and lapse characteristics. *Journal of Consulting and Clinical Psychology, 64,* 993–1002.

Shively, C.A. and Clarkson, T.B. (1994). Social status and coronary artery atherosclerosis in female monkeys. *Arteriosclerosis and Thrombosis, 14*, 721–726.

Shively, C.A., Laber-Laird, K, and Anton, R.F. (1997) Behavior and physiology of social stress and depression in female cynomolgus monkeys. *Biological Psychiatry, 41*, 871–882.

Singer, B., Ryff, C.D., Carr, D., and Magee, W.J. (1998). Linking life histories and mental health: A person-centered strategy. *Sociological Methodology, 28*, 1–51.

Sloan, R.P., Shapiro, P.A., Bagiella, E., Myers, M., and Gorman, J.M. (1999). Cardiac autonomic control buffers blood pressure variability responses to challenge: A psychophysiologic model of coronary artery disease. *Psychosomatic.Medicine, 61*, 58–68.

Smyth, J., Ockenfels, M.C., Porter, L., Kirschbaum, C., Hellhammer, D.H., and Stone, A.A. (1998). Stressors and mood measured on a momentary basis are associated with salivary cortisol secretion. *Psychoneuroendocrinology, 23*, 353–370.

Snyder, C.R., Harris, C., Anderson, J.R., Holleran, S.A., Irving, L.M., Sigmon, S.T., Yoshinobu, L., Gibb, J., Langelle, C., and Harney, P. (1991). The will and the ways: Development and validation of an individual-differences measure of hope. *Journal of Personality and Social Psychology, 60*, 570–585.

Solomon, G.F., Segerstrom, S.C., Grohr, P., Kemeny, M., and Fahey, J. (1997). Shaking up immunity: Psychological and immunologic changes after a natural disaster. *Psychosomatic Medicine, 59*, 114–127.

Staessen, J.A., Poulter, N.R., Fletcher, A.E., Markowe, H.L., Marmot, M.G., Shipley, M.J., and Bulpitt, C.J. (1994). Psycho-emotional stress and salt intake may interact to raise blood pressure. *Journal of Cardiovascular Risk, 1*, 45–51.

Stanton, A.L. and Snider, P.R. (1993). Coping with a breast cancer diagnosis: A prospective study. *Health Psychology, 12*, 16–23.

Sterling, P. and Eyer, J. (1988). Allostasis: A new paradigm to explain arousal pathology. In S. Fisher and J. Reason (Eds.) *Handbook of Life Stress, Cognition and Health* (pp. 629–649). New York: John Wiley and Sons.

Sternberg, E.M. (1997). Neural-immune interactions in health and disease. *Journal of Clinical Investigation, 100*, 2641–2647.

Sternberg, E.M., Chrousos, G.P., Wilder, R.I., and Gold, P.W. (1992). The stress response and the regulation of inflammatory disease. *Annals of Internal Medicine, 117*, 854–866.

Sternberg, E.M., Hill, J.M., and Chrousos, G.P. (1996). Inflammatory mediator-induced hypothalamic-pituitary-adrenal axis activation is defective in streptococcal cell wall arthritis susceptible Lewis rats. *Proceedings of the National Academy of Sciences, 86*, 2374–2378.

Sternberg, E.M., Hill, J.M., Chrousos, G.P., Kamilaris, T., Listwak, S.J., Gold, P.W., and Wilder, R.I. (1989). Inflammatory mediator-induced hypothalamic-pituitary-adrenal axis activation is defective in streptococcal cell wall arthritis susceptible Lewis rats. *Proceedings of the National Academy of Sciences, 86*, 2374–2378.

Styron, T. and Janoff-Bulman, R. (1997). Childhood attachment and abuse: Long-term effects on adult attachment, depression, and conflict resolution. *Child Abuse and Neglect, 21*, 1015–1023.

Syme, S. and Berkman, L. (1976). Social class, susceptibility and sickness. *American Journal of Epidemiology, 104*, 1–8.

Taylor, S.E., Repetti, R.L., and Seeman, T. (1997). Health Psychology: What is an unhealthy environment and how does it get under the skin? *Annual Review of Psychology*, 48, 411–447.

Troiano, R.P., Flegal, K.M., Kuczmarski, R.J., Campbell, S.M., and Johnson, C.L. (1995). Overweight prevalence and trends for children and adolescents. *Archives of Pediatrics and Adolescent Medicine*, 149, 1085–1091.

U.S. Department of Health and Human Services. (1996). *Physical Activity and Health: A Report of the Surgeon General*. Washington, DC: Centers for Disease Control and Prevention National Center for Chronic Disease Prevention and Health Promotion. The President's Council on Physical Fitness and Sports.

Uno, H., Ross, T., Else, J., Suleman, M., and Sapolsky, R. (1989). Hippocampal damage associated with prolonged and fatal stress in primates. *Journal of Neuroscience*, 9, 1705–1711.

Utz, P.J., Hottelet, M., Schur, P.H., and Anderson, P. (1997). Proteins phosphorylated during stress-induced apoptosis are common targets for autoantibody production in patients with systemic lupus erythematous. *Journal of Experimental Medicine*, 185, 843–854.

van Cauter, E., Polonsky, K.S., and Scheen, A.J. (1997). Roles of circadian rhythmicity and sleep in human glucose regulation. *Endocrine Reviews*, 18, 716–738.

van den Boom, D.C. (1994) The influence of temperament and mothering on attachment and exploration: An experimental manipulation of sensitive responsiveness among lower-class mothers with irritable infants. *Child Development*, 65, 1457–1477.

van Praag, H., Kempermann, G., and Gage, F. H. (1999). Running increases cell proliferation and neurogenesis in the adult mouse dentate gyrus. *Nature Neuroscience*, 2, 266–270.

Wadhwa, P.D. (1998). Prenatal stress and life-span development. In *Encyclopedia of Mental Health*. San Diego: Academic Press.

Wakschlak, A. and Weinstock, M. (1990). Neonatal handling reverses behavioral abnormalities induced in rats by prenatal stress. *Physiology and Behavior*, 48, 289–92.

Watson, M., Pruyn, J., Greer, S., and van den Borne, B. (1990). Locus of control and adjustment to cancer. *Psychology Representative*, 66, 39–48.

Wilder, R.L. (1995). Neuroendocrine-immune system interactions and autoimmunity. *Annual Review of Immunology*, 13, 307–338.

Wilkinson, R.G. (1992). Income distribution and life expectancy. *British Medical Journal*. 304, 165–168.

Williams C.L. and Jensen R.A. (1993). Effects of vagotomy on Leu-enkephalin-induced changes in memory storage processes. *Physiology and Behavior*, 54, 659–663.

Williams, C.L. and Jensen, R.A. (1991). Vagal afferents: A possible mechanism for the modulation of memory by peripherally acting agents. In R.C.A. Frederickson, J.L. McGaugh, and D.L. Felten (Eds.) *Peripheral Signaling of the Brain: Role in Neural-Immune Interactions, Learning and Memory* (pp. 467–472). Lewiston, NY: Hogrefe and Huber.

Zonderman, A.B., Costa, P.T., Jr., and McCrae, R.R. (1989). Depression as a risk for cancer morbidity and mortality in a nationally representative sample. *Journal of the American Medical Association*, 262, 1191–1195.

3

Behavioral Risk Factors

S everal behaviors that exert a strong influence on health are reviewed in this section: tobacco use, alcohol consumption, physical
activity and diet, sexual practices, and disease screening. Although
epidemiologic data on the relationships between these behaviors and various health outcomes were available in the early 1980s, many refinements
in knowledge have occurred since then. Causal conclusions have been
strengthened by more sophisticated research designs, dose/response relationships have been clarified, the influence of many of these behaviors on
overall public health has been quantified, and scientific guidelines have
been formulated. This chapter summarizes the important recent epidemiologic evidence on the health effects of these behaviors.

TOBACCO USE

Since the release in 1964 of the surgeon general's first report on smoking, there has been a tremendous increase in scientific knowledge about
the health consequences of tobacco use (U.S. Department of Health and
Human Services [USDHHS], 1989, 1990, 2000). Cigarette-smoking is the
major cause of *preventable* mortality and morbidity in the United States
(National Center for Health Statistics [NCHS], 1998a; USDHHS, 2000).
Not only does smoking lead to an increased risk of the two leading causes
of death in the United States—heart disease and cancer (NCHS, 1998b;

USDHHS, 2000)—but smoking during pregnancy has been linked to adverse pregnancy outcomes (DiFranza and Lew, 1995; Hebel et al., 1988; LeClere and Wilson, 1997; Li et al., 1993; Shu et al., 1995; USDHHS, 2000; Ventura et al., 1997; Walsh, 1994). Nonsmoking people are not immune to tobacco's health hazards, inasmuch as exposure to second-hand smoke has serious health consequences for adults and children (USDHHS, 1986, 2000; U.S. Environmental Protection Agency [USEPA], 1992).

Although cigarette-smoking among adults leveled off in the 1990s, tobacco use among adolescents increased in that period (USDHHS, 2000). That cigarette-smoking among younger people has increased is particularly alarming for several reasons. Evidence shows not only that tobacco is addictive (USDHHS, 2000) and that only a relatively small percentage of smokers can stop smoking permanently each year (Centers for Disease Control and Prevention [CDC], 1993, 1996b; USDHHS, 2000), but also that nicotine addiction develops in most smokers during adolescence (Institute of Medicine [IOM], 1994; USDHHS, 1988a, 1994, 2000). Curbing or eradicating tobacco use might remain a daunting task. Prevention is the primary objective, but many benefits are associated with smoking cessation, and such efforts should not be ignored.

Measuring the Public Health Burden of Cigarette-Smoking

There is widespread agreement in the public health and medical communities that cigarette-smoking is the biggest external (nongenetic) contributor to death in the United States. Tobacco-related diseases account for more than 400,000 deaths among adults in the United States each year (CDC, 1993; NCHS, 1998b; USDHHS, 2000). Deaths attributable to tobacco use have been found to exceed deaths from acquired immunodeficiency syndrome (AIDS), traffic accidents, alcohol use, suicide, homicide, fire, and use of illegal drugs combined (IOM, 1994). One World Health Organization report showed that the burden of disease and death attributable to tobacco in developed countries was substantially higher than that attributable to any other risk factor, including alcohol use, unsafe sex, hypertension, and physical inactivity (Murray and Lopez, 1996).

Because there is a long delay between the onset of persistent smoking and the full development of its adverse health consequences, current tobacco-attributable mortality and morbidity are consequences of smoking that began decades ago. If current U.S. tobacco use patterns persist, it is estimated that 5 million persons who were under the age of 18 in 1995 will die from a smoking-related disease (CDC, 1996a; USDHHS, 2000).

Major Smoking-Related Diseases

Cigarette-smoking leads to an increased risk of heart disease, the leading cause of death in the United States (USDHHS, 2000); and the surgeon general's 1983 report (USDHHS, 1983) concluded that cigarette-smoking is the most important modifiable risk factor for coronary heart disease. Cigarette-smoking is also linked with cancer, the second-leading cause of death in the United States (NCHS, 1998b). Smoking causes cancers of the lung, larynx, esophagus, pharynx, mouth, and bladder, and contributes to cancer of the pancreas, kidney, and cervix (USDHHS, 2000). Tobacco use is the leading contributor to lung cancer incidence, and refraining from smoking could prevent most lung cancer cases (National Cancer Institute, 1986; NCHS, 1998b). In 1996, lung cancer accounted for about 28% of all cancer deaths (NCHS, 1998b; Ries et al., 1996; Ventura et al., 1997). An estimated 172,000 new cases are diagnosed each year, and lung cancer causes an estimated 153,000 deaths each year (NCHS, 1998b). Smoking also causes other lung diseases, such as chronic bronchitis and chronic obstructive pulmonary disease (USDHHS, 2000).

According to the Surgeon General's 1990 report (USDHHS, 1990), smoking is the most important modifiable cause of poor pregnancy outcome in the United States. It is estimated that 15–30% of all pregnant women smoke (Chandra, 1995; Ventura et al., 1997). Pregnancy complications associated with maternal smoking include premature detachment of the placenta, development of the placenta in the lower uterine segment, which can cause hemorrhaging in the last trimester; bleeding during pregnancy; premature membrane rupture; and premature delivery. Maternal smoking also has been associated with spontaneous abortions and low birthweight (DiFranza and Lew, 1995; Hebel et al., 1988; LeClere and Wilson, 1997; Li et al., 1993; Shu et al., 1995; USDHHS, 2000; Ventura et al., 1997; Walsh, 1994). Evidence indicates that in some groups of pregnant women smoking one to six cigarettes a day increases by about two-thirds the risk of giving birth to a low birthweight infant (LeClere and Wilson, 1997; Ventura et al., 1997). Smoking in the last few weeks of pregnancy has the biggest impact on fetal weight gain. Women who stop smoking before becoming pregnant or who quit in the first 3–4 months of pregnancy have infants of the same birthweight as those born to women who never smoked. Women who stop smoking later in pregnancy have higher birthweight infants than do women who smoke throughout pregnancy.

The complex issues associated with the real and perceived risk of tobacco and tobacco harm-reduction products are explored in an IOM report (2001).

Consequences of Second-Hand Smoke

Exposure to second-hand smoke has serious health consequences (USDHHS, 1986, 2000; USEPA, 1992). At least 43 of the roughly 4000 chemicals identified in tobacco smoke have been shown to cause cancer in humans and animals (USDHHS, 2000; USEPA, 1992). About 3000 nonsmoking Americans die of lung cancer and 150,000–300,000 children suffer from lower respiratory tract infections each year because of exposure to second-hand smoke (USDHHS, 2000; USEPA, 1992). Second-hand smoke exposure exacerbates asthma and leads to 500,000 child visits to physicians each year (DiFranza and Lew, 1996; USDHHS, 2000). Second-hand smoke exposure also has been linked to increased risk of heart disease among adults (Glantz and Parmely, 1995; Howard et al., 1998; USDHHS, 2000). Data gathered in a study of the U.S. population over the age of 3 showed that almost 88% of nonusers of tobacco had detectable serum cotinine, a biological marker of exposure to second-hand smoke (Pirkle et al., 1996; USDHHS, 2000). Another study showed that almost 22% of Americans under the age of 18 (about 15 million people) were exposed to second-hand smoke in their homes (CDC, 1997b; USDHHS, 2000). A 1996 study showed that home and workplace environments contribute significantly to the widespread exposure to second-hand smoke in the United States (Pirkle et al., 1996; USDHHS, 2000).

Socioeconomic Characteristics of Smokers

Although smoking among adults declined steadily from the middle 1960s through the 1980s, it leveled off in the 1990s (USDHHS, 2000). In 1995, the prevalence of smoking among adults was almost 25% (CDC, 1997a; NCHS, 1998b; USDHHS, 2000). Men are more likely to smoke than are women—27% and 22%, respectively (CDC, 1997a; USDHHS, 2000)—although those rates could change because cigarette use among high school senior girls almost equals that among boys (NCHS, 1998a; USDHHS, 2000). American Indians and Alaska Natives are more likely (34%), and Hispanics, Asians, and Pacific islanders are less likely (16%), to smoke than are other racial and ethnic groups (African American, 26%; White, 25%) (USDHHS, 2000). Cigarette-smoking was about twice as common among poor men and women as among more affluent persons in 1995 (NCHS, 1998a). One study showed that non-Hispanic White and African Americans living in poverty were more likely to smoke than were people with middle and high incomes in 1995 (NCHS, 1998a).

Among adolescents, tobacco use increased in the 1990s, after decreasing in the 1970s and 1980s (USDHHS, 2000). Several factors place young people at an increased risk of initiating tobacco use (USDHHS, 2000). Sociodemographic risk factors include low socioeconomic status of one's family. Environmental risk factors include accessibility and availability of tobacco products, cigarette advertising and promotion, the price of tobacco products, perceptions that tobacco use is normative, use and approval of tobacco use by peers and siblings, and lack of parental involvement. Personal risk factors include poor self-image and low self-esteem relative to peers, the belief that tobacco use is functional (useful or providing a benefit), and lack of confidence in one's ability to refuse an offer to use tobacco (USDHHS, 1994, 2000).

Primary Prevention of Cigarette-Smoking

When the surgeon general's first report on smoking was released in 1964, 42% of American adults smoked tobacco; in 1995, use had declined to 24.7% (47 million) of American adults (CDC, 1997a). Among adults, the number of former smokers (43 million) is now almost the same as current smokers (46 million) (IOM, 1994). Given the progress since 1964, it is possible to envision a smoke-free society; however, maintaining the current rate of progress will be challenging. There is overwhelming evidence that the nicotine in tobacco is addictive (USDHHS, 1988a, 2000). Almost 70% of current smokers want to quit smoking, and about 45% quit smoking for at least a day (Howard et al., 1998). However, only 2.5% of smokers stop smoking permanently each year (CDC, 1996b, 1993; USDHHS, 2000).

Nearly all first-time use of tobacco occurs before high school graduation. That is important because nicotine addiction occurs in most smokers during adolescence (IOM, 1994; USDHHS, 1988a, 1994, 2000).

Smoking patterns among American youth and the short- and long-term health consequences of initiating smoking in adolescence were described in the Surgeon General's 1994 report *Preventing Tobacco Use Among Young People* (USDHHS, 1994). The same report provides a summary of efforts to prevent tobacco use among young people; such prevention emerged as a major focus of tobacco control efforts (IOM, 1994; USDHHS, 2000).

Benefits of Smoking Cessation

Given the addictive nature of nicotine and the cumulative nature of health damage due to smoking, strategies to reduce tobacco use should emphasize primary prevention rather than smoking cessation. However, smoking's prevalence in the U.S. population points to the need to continue cessation efforts.

Scientific data on the benefits of smoking cessation were reviewed in the surgeon general's 1990 report (USDHHS, 1990). In the 25 years between 1965 and 1990, half of all living Americans who had ever smoked had stopped. The 1990 report concluded that smoking cessation has major and immediate health benefits for men and women of all ages. Former smokers live longer than continuing smokers. For example, on the average, people who quit smoking before reaching the age of 50 have half the risk of dying before the age of 65 than those who do not quit before the age of 50 (USDHHS, 2000, 1990).

OBESITY: PHYSICAL ACTIVITY AND DIET

Recent years have seen an epidemic in obesity in the United States (Mokdad et al., 1999). Obesity is a major health risk for diabetes (Must et al., 1999), and the relationship of weight to the disease has been extensively reviewed in the literature (Kopelman, 2000; Leong and Wilding 1999; National Task Force on the Prevention and Treatment of Obesity, 2000; Scheen, 2000; USDHHS, 1980). Overweight adults also are at an increased risk for hypertension, coronary heart disease, and some forms of cancer (NCHS, 1998a; Pi-Sunyer, 1993). They also run the risk of developing gallbladder disease, osteoarthritis, sleep apnea, respiratory problems (USDHHS, 2000), and a variety of musculoskeletal problems (Foreyt et al., 1996). There is some disagreement about whether the principal threat to health is from an increase in body fat per se, or from a lack of physical activity, but there is no disagreement that major behavioral change is needed to correct this increase in obesity (Hill and Peters, 1998; Taubes, 1998).

Although genetic factors are important, physical activity and diet contribute significantly to maintenance of appropriate body weight. The combination of inactivity and detrimental dietary patterns has been ranked as the second leading factor contributing to mortality in the United States, after tobacco use (McGinnis and Foege, 1993). In addition, both diet and physical activity, in and of themselves, influence health. Studies show that men and women who are physically active have, on the average, lower mortality than people who are inactive (Kaplan et al., 1987, 1996; Kujala et al., 1998; Kushi et al., 1997; Leon et al., 1987; Lindsted et al., 1991; Paffenbarger et al., 1993; Sherman et al., 1994; Slattery et al., 1989). A sedentary lifestyle has been linked to 23% of deaths from major chronic diseases (Hahn et al., 1990). Furthermore, studies show that dietary factors are associated with 4 of the 10 leading causes of death, including coronary heart disease, stroke, some forms of cancer, and non-insulin-dependent diabetes mellitus (CDC, 1997c; USDHHS, 2000).

This section will review some of the factors that influence obesity, with a particular emphasis on physical activity and diet, and describe the relevance of body weight, physical activity, and diet to cardiovascular disease, cancer, and musculoskeletal problems. It is not meant to be a comprehensive review but rather a sampling of the influences these behaviors can have on health and disease.

Prevalence and Trends

Obesity and overweight are increasing in the United States. Currently, "overweight" is defined as a body mass index (BMI)[1] of 25–30 while "obesity" is defined as a BMI greater than 30 (National Heart Lung Blood Institute Obesity Task Force, 1998).[2] For most of the 1960s and 1970s the

---

[1]BMI is used in all these guidelines as a measure of adiposity. It is calculated as weight (in kilograms) divided by height (in meters) squared. Growing evidence suggests that BMI reflects adiposity well through middle age, but might be less clearly related to adiposity at older ages when lean muscle mass can decrease and mass is redistributed to the abdomen.

[2]The correlation between BMI and body fat is both age and sex dependent, and it is valid for comparison across ethnic groups (Gallagher et al., 1996; USDHHS, 2000). A limitation of the BMI measure is that it does not provide information about body fat distribution, which has been identified as an independent predictor of health risk (National Institute of Health, 1993; USDHHS, 2000). However, until a better measure of body fat is developed, BMI will be used as a proxy to screen for overweight and obesity.

prevalence of overweight adults (25–74 years of age) was nearly constant at about 25%. However, by 1988–1994, that rose to approximately 35% (NCHS, 1998a), and the prevalence continues to increase. Obesity increased from 12% in 1991 to almost 18% in 1998 and 19% in 1999 (Mokdad et al., 1999; 2000). Obesity in children over the age of 6 and in adolescents also is increasing (Troiano and Flegal, 1998; USDHHS, 2000). Because overweight and obesity that develop in childhood or adolescence can persist into adulthood, this trend increases the risk for chronic disease later in life (USDHHS, 2000).

Relatively few Americans participate in regular physical activity. Only 11% of the U.S. adult population reported regular, vigorous physical activity for 20 minutes or longer more than twice each week (USDHHS, 2000). Furthermore, physical activity tends to decline during adolescence (CDC, 1998; Pate et al., 1994), and a major decrease in vigorous physical activity (much more for girls than for boys) occurs in grades 9–12 (USDHHS, 2000). A consensus is emerging that physical activity does not need to be vigorous to be beneficial to health.[3] For people who are inactive, even small increases have been associated with measurable health benefits (USDHHS, 2000).

In 1994–1996, the proportion of Americans who ate away from home was approximately 57%, or an increase of about one-third from the late 1970s (USDA, 1997; USDHHS, 2000). Recent data indicate that 40% of the family food budget is spent at restaurants and carry-outs (USDA, 1996; USDHHS, 2000). Food purchased from restaurants, fast-food outlets, school cafeterias, and vending machines generally is higher in saturated fat, cholesterol, and sodium and lower in fiber and calcium than is food prepared and eaten at home (Lin and Frazao, 1997; USDHHS, 2000). And people tend to eat larger portions of higher calorie foods when they eat out. The larger food portions in restaurants further exacerbate this

---

[3]Generally terms used to define the intensity of physical activity are *light*, *moderate*, *hard* or *vigorous*, and *very hard* or *strenuous*. A common classification is to use MET (metabolic equivalent task) values. One MET is the number of kilocalories expended in 1 hour of resting. Often, activities with a MET value below 3.0 are considered light activities; easy walking and regular housework are examples. Activities with MET values of at least 3.0 but less than 6.0 are often classified as moderate; examples are brisk walking, heavy gardening, and calisthenics. Activities with MET values of at least 6.0 but less than 12.0 are often called vigorous, and include jogging, running, swimming, aerobics, and bicycling. Strenuous or very hard activities—such as bicycle or foot racing, speed skating, and competitive cross-country skiing—have MET values of 12.0 or higher.

problem (McCrory et al., 2000). One study pointed to an association between the frequency of eating restaurant food and elevated BMI (McCrory et al., 1999). A 1995 survey found that school meals and snacks had the highest saturated-fat density of all foods people eat away from home, including food from restaurants, fast-food outlets, and vending machines (Lin and Frazao, 1997; USDHHS, 2000). Although schools are required to plan menus that comply with U.S. dietary guidelines, these standards do not apply to a la carte foods or to foods sold in snack bars, school stores, or vending machines (USDHHS, 2000). Because many dietary habits are established during childhood (CDC, 1996c; Kelder et al., 1994; USDHHS, 2000), educating school-aged children about nutrition can help them establish healthy eating habits early in life. Implementation of curricula that encourage healthy eating and that provide students with the skills they need to adopt and maintain healthy eating habits has led to positive changes in student dietary behaviors and to reductions in cardiovascular disease risk factors (CDC, 1996c; Contento et al., 1995; Lytle and Achterberg, 1995; USDHHS, 2000).

Similar increases in the incidence of overweight and obesity are evident throughout the world, although rates differ (Flegal, 1999). In Europe obesity is especially prevalent in Southern and Eastern countries, particularly among women (Seidell, 1995). In Sweden, between 1980 and 1996 the prevalence of obesity rose from 9% to 12% in women and from 6.6% to 10% in men (Lissner et al., 2000). Between 1982 and 1994, the percentage of overweight people in New Zealand increased from about 53% to 64% for men and 36.5% to 45% for women (Simmons et al., 1996). In many countries, as in the United States, obesity is an increasing concern in children (for example, Great Britain: Chinn and Rona, 2001; Germany: Kromeyer-Hauschild et al., 1999; Singapore: Ho et al., 1983). Even in the developing world, the rates of obesity are showing increases (Shetty, 1997). As reviewed above for the United States, these international trends are attributed to high fat, energy dense diets and reduced physical activity (Shetty, 1997; Seidell, 1995) .

Socioeconomic Characteristics

Although overweight and obesity are increasing among all sociodemographic groups, the prevalence is influenced by specific sociocultural variables, including gender, ethnicity, socioeconomic status, and education. From 1988 to 1994, about one-third of U.S. adults were overweight, with a higher prevalence among poor women (46%) (NCHS, 1998a). A clear gradient with family income exists for the prevalence of overweight in women (but not in men). Poor women are 1.4 times more likely to be overweight than are middle-income women and 1.6 times more likely to be overweight than are women with high incomes (NCHS, 1998a). Obesity is particularly common among Hispanic, African American, Native American, and Pacific Islander women (USDHHS, 2000).

Populations also differ in amount of physical activity. The proportion of the population reporting no leisure-time physical activity is higher among women than men, among Hispanics than among Whites, among older than younger adults, and among the less affluent than the wealthier (USDHHS, 1996, 2000). A sedentary lifestyle is less likely with increasing income. African American men living in poverty are 3 times more likely to be sedentary than were those with high family incomes. For Hispanic and non-Hispanic White men, a sedentary lifestyle was about 2.5 times more prevalent among the poor than among those with a higher family income. Women had similar income-related gradients in sedentary lifestyle, with higher income groups experiencing a lower prevalence of sedentary lifestyle (NCHS, 1998a).

Adult Weight Gain

Adult weight gain is observed in many industrialized societies. Because full adult height generally is attained by age 18, weight gain in adulthood is almost exclusively through the addition of adipose tissue. Lack of weight gain, particularly among men over 50, does not imply an absence of gain in fat. Above this age, muscle mass is, to varying degrees, redistributed to fat, much of it within the abdomen (Rimm et al., 1995).

Avoiding weight gain as an adult is a high priority because treatment of obesity has poor long-term success, and lost weight often is regained (Chapter 5). Several studies show that greater leisure-time physical activity is associated with lower weight gain (Ravussin et al., 1988; Rissanen et al., 1991), and it reduces the weight gain often observed after cessation of cigarette-smoking (Kawachi et al., 1996). Although many people try to lose weight, most regain the weight within 5 years (NIH, 1993; USDHHS, 2000). In order to maintain weight loss, permanent lifestyle changes that combine good dietary habits, decreased sedentary behavior, and increased physical activity are essential. Changes in the physical and social environment can help people maintain the necessary long-term lifestyle changes both for diet and for physical activity (USDHHS, 2000). Preventing weight gain in the first place also substantially reduces the likelihood that conditions such as hypertension and diabetes will develop (Colditz et al., 1995). A reduction of even 10–15% of body weight in substantially overweight people has been shown to ameliorate hyperglycemia, hyperlipidemia, and hypertension (see Mertens and Van Gaal, 2000; Oster et al., 1999; de Leiva, 1998; Goldstein, 1992).

Weight and Disease

Several authors have pointed out the consequences of overweight and obesity for morbidity and mortality (Allison et al., 1999; Calle et al., 1999; Must et al., 1999). A linear relationship exists between adiposity and most health conditions. The shape of the curve for mortality has been debated, in part because of excess mortality among the leanest people. The positive relationship between leanness and mortality is confounded by cigarette-smoking (smokers tend to be leaner but also are at higher risk of disease), and by reverse causation—the major illnesses that predispose to death lead first to weight loss. The effect of disease on weight might result in the leaner segment of the population being overrepresented among those at a higher risk of death.

Observed statistical associations between weight and mortality have driven recommendations for weight guidelines, but setting the guidelines has been problematic because of the U-shaped relationship described above, and recommendations have varied over time. The Dietary Guidelines Advisory Committee (USDA and USDHHS, 1995a) concluded that mortality risk increased significantly among persons with a BMI of 25 or higher (Lee and Paffenbarger, 1992; Rimm et al., 1995; Willett et al., 1995), whereas a linear increase in risk of diabetes, hypertension, and coronary heart disease begins well below that value (Chan et al., 1994; Colditz et al., 1995; Willett et al., 1995). A 2- to 4-fold increase in risk of these diseases is observed among those with BMI 24–25, compared with those whose BMI is 21. The lower cut-point for the healthy weight range is set at a BMI of 19, below which a person is considered excessively thin and at risk of other health complications (USDHHS, 2000; USDA, 1995a, b; USDA and USDHHS, 1995a, b).

Diet and physical activity are behaviors that have a direct influence on weight. However, they may also have direct effects on diseases. These direct and indirect actions are explored below in examples of diseases.

Cardiovascular Diseases

Several cohort studies have documented the adverse cardiovascular health effects experienced by overweight adults. In part, cardiac failure develops as a consequence of the increased demands on the heart to supply blood to the increased body fat (Kopelman, 2000). The Nurses Cohort Study (Willet et al., 1995) demonstrated a 2-fold increase in coronary heart disease in overweight women and a 3.6-fold increase with obesity. Similarly, the Framingham Heart Study showed increased incidence in heart disease proportionate to excess weight (Hubert et al., 1983). Adult weight gain is an additional risk (Hubert et al., 1983). For example, compared with men and women who maintained weight to within 2 kg of their weight at age 18–20, those who gained 5–9.9 kg experienced a 1.5- to 2-fold higher risk of coronary heart disease (Rimm et al., 1995; Willett et al., 1995) and hypertension (Ascherio et al., 1992; Huang, 1998).

Many studies show that physically active people have a substantially lower risk of coronary heart disease than do the inactive (Berlin and Colditz, 1990; Kaplan et al., 1987; Kushi et al., 1997; Leon et al., 1987; Lindsted et al., 1991; Slattery et al., 1989). Prospective data from a cohort study of 72,000 female nurses (40–65 years old in 1986) indicated that walking and vigorous physical activity reduce the incidence of coronary events (Manson et al., 1999). Brisk walking for 3 hours or more each week reduced the risk of coronary disease by 30–40%, and increasing the time or intensity of the physical activity produced even greater reductions in risk (Manson et al., 1999). Several clinical trials suggest that moderate physical activity can produce a similar, or even larger, reduction in blood pressure than vigorous activity does (Hagberg et al., 1989; Marceau et al., 1993; Matsusaki et al., 1992). Although vigorous physical activity rarely is associated with myocardial infarction or sudden cardiac death (USDHHS, 1996), some risks exist. Even persons who exercise regularly have a transient increase in the risk of sudden cardiac death during and immediately after vigorous physical activity (Kohl et al., 1992).

More than 20 prospective studies have addressed components of diet and risk of coronary heart disease (Willett, 1998). Research in humans and laboratory animals shows that diets low in saturated fatty acids and cholesterol are associated with low risks and rates of coronary heart disease (USDHHS, 2000). Although consumption of trans-fatty acids increases the risk of coronary heart disease (Ascherio et al., 1994; Expert Panel on Trans Fatty Acids and Coronary Heart Disease, 1995; Hu et al., 1997; Willett et al., 1993, Willett and Ascherio, 1994), eating foods higher in polyunsaturated fat and monounsaturated fat decreases the risk of coronary heart disease. In addition, fiber intake is strongly protective against coronary heart disease (Willett, 1998). Emerging evidence suggests that low folate and high circulating concentrations of homocysteine are major contributors to risk of coronary heart disease and stroke (Boushey et al., 1995; Chasan-Taber et al., 1996; Rimm et al., 1996; Selhub et al., 1995). Vitamin E appears to reduce the risk of coronary heart disease (Rimm et al., 1993; Stampfer et al., 1993).

Cancer

Obesity has been associated with an increased risk for some forms of cancer. The data have been most consistent for postmenopausal breast cancer (Barnes-Josiah et al., 1995; Huang et al., 1997) and endometrial cancer (Le Marchand et al., 1991). A prospective study by Sonnenschein et al. (1999) reported a relative risk for breast cancer of 2.36 in postmenopausal women in the fourth quartile of BMI. Women in this weight range also showed a 4-fold greater risk for endometrial cancer (Goodman et al., 1997). The mechanisms of these effects are not known, but they could be related to levels of sex hormones.

Physical inactivity has been examined as a contributing factor in a variety of cancers. Many studies conducted in men show an inverse relationship between physical activity and risk of colon cancer (Giovannucci et al., 1995; Lee et al., 1991; Severson et al., 1989; Slattery et al., 1988; Whittemore et al., 1990; Wu et al., 1987). A large prospective cohort study in women found a similarly strong inverse association between physical activity and colon cancer (Martinez et al., 1997). Physical activity not only increases intestinal motility (Thor et al., 1985) and aids in the suppression of colon cell proliferation (Lee, 1994; Shephard et al., 1991), but it is hypothesized to decrease gastrointestinal transit time (Lee, 1994; Shephard, 1993) and thus the duration of contact between the colon mucosa and potential carcinogens.

Increased physical activity has been hypothesized to prevent breast cancer by reducing cumulative lifetime exposure to circulating ovarian hormones (Kramer and Wells, 1996). However, the epidemiologic findings are inconsistent. Several studies report reductions in breast cancer risk with more physical activity (Bernstein et al., 1994; D'Avanzo et al., 1996; Mittendorf et al., 1995; Thune et al., 1997); others found a modest association at best (Albanes et al., 1989; Chen et al., 1997; Friedenreich and Rohan, 1995; Gammon et al., 1998; McTiernan et al., 1996; Rockhill et al., 1998) or even increased risk (Albanes et al., 1989; Dorgan et al., 1994). Similarly, findings from studies on the relationship between physical activity and prostate cancer are inconsistent (USDHHS, 1996).

Diet also could be an etiologic factor in cancer. For instance, evidence indicates that low folate intake works a role in the development of colon cancer (Freudenheim et al., 1991; Giovannucci et al., 1998; Mason and Levesque, 1996). A consistent relationship between intake of fruit and vegetables and lower risk of many malignancies supports an anticancer effect of some component of these foods (Steinmetz and Potter, 1991). Yet, despite epidemiologic evidence that fruits and vegetables that contain carotenoids reduce the risk of lung cancer (Ziegler et al., 1996), randomized trials of the specific carotenoid, β-carotene, fail to show any benefit (Albanes et al., 1996; Hennekens et al., 1996). In fact, the β-Carotene and Retinol Efficacy Trial (Omenn et al., 1996) found an increase in mortality in patients taking supplements of β-carotene and vitamin A. Evidence linking high-fatty-acid diets with cancer are inconclusive, and there is continuing debate about the relationship between colorectal, prostate, and breast cancers and total fat content or type of fat in the diet (NRC 1989; Ip and Carroll, 1997; USDHHS, 2000). Randomized clinical trials are attempting to clarify the relationship between dietary total fat and the risk of cancer (Freeman et al., 1993; Schatzkin et al., 1996; USDHHS, 2000).

Musculoskeletal Health

Physical activity contributes to the development of bone mass during childhood and adolescence and to the maintenance of skeletal mass during adulthood (USDHHS, 1996). Increased bone mineral density is positively associated with aerobic exercise (Snow-Harter et al., 1996; USDHHS, 2000). Through its load-bearing effect on the skeleton, physical activity influences bone density and bone architecture—the higher the load, the greater the bone mass (Lanyon, 1987, 1993). Conversely, if the skeleton is unloaded, because of inactivity or immobility, bone mass declines.

Calcium intake is essential for the formation and maintenance of bones (USDHHS, 1988b; USDHHS, 2000). Higher calcium intake has been linked to increased bone density in short-term studies, but high protein intake and high dairy calcium intake are both related to increased risk of fractures in long-term prospective studies of men and women (Feskanich et al., 1996, 1997; Owusu et al., 1997, 1998). Because ideal calcium intake for development of peak bone mass has not been determined, it has not been established to what extent increased calcium intake will prevent osteoporosis.

Although most young children meet the dietary requirements for calcium, the intake of calcium declines precipitously with age (USDHHS, 2000). In part as a consequence of inadequate calcium in the diet, osteoporosis is prevalent, affecting more than 25 million people in the United States alone. It is the principal underlying cause of bone fractures in postmenopausal women and the elderly (NIH, 1994; USDHHS, 2000). Physical activity can help. Strength training has been shown to help postmenopausal women preserve bone density (Nelson et al., 1994; USDHHS, 2000).

In addition to strengthening bone, physical activity reduces the risk of fractures in the elderly by increasing muscle strength and balance, thus reducing the risk of falling. Muscle strength has been shown to decline with age, and studies have documented a relationship between muscle strength and physical function (Brown et al., 1995; USDHHS, 2000). However, age-related loss of strength can be attenuated with strengthening exercises and this can help the older population maintain a threshold of strength necessary to perform basic weight-bearing activities, such as walking (Evans, 1995; Tseng et al., 1995; USDHHS, 2000). Thus, regular physical activity can help to maintain the functional independence of the elderly population (Buchner, 1997; LaCroix et al., 1993; Nelson et al., 1994).

Osteoarthritis, the most common form of arthritis, increases with age, and it is the leading cause of activity limitation among older persons (USDHHS, 1996). Although some competitive athletic activities (such as running, soccer, football, and weight-lifting) are associated with increased risk of osteoarthritis in specific joints (USDHHS, 1996), regular noncompetitive physical activity is not harmful to joints (Lane, 1995; Panush and Lane, 1994) and might actually relieve symptoms and improve functioning among persons who already have osteoarthritis or rheumatoid arthritis (Ettinger et al., 1997; Ettinger and Afable, 1994; Fisher and Pendergast, 1994; Minor, 1991).

Physical activity poses some potential risks. Musculoskeletal injury is the most common. Increased risks of roadway accidents also could be associated with running or bicycling on roads, and various sports are associated with specific hazards, such as downhill skiing at high velocities and collisions with other players in football and hockey.

ALCOHOL CONSUMPTION

Alcohol has been identified as a top contributor to death in the United States (McGinnis and Foege, 1993), after tobacco use and diet and activity patterns. Compared with other threats to human health, alcohol causes the widest variety of injuries (Rose, 1992). Approximately 100,000 deaths are related to alcohol consumption in the United States each year (McGinnis and Foege, 1993; Rose, 1992), which translates into 15% of potential years of life lost before the age of 65 (Rose, 1992).

A significant proportion of the U.S. population drinks alcohol. Among current drinkers, 46% report having been intoxicated at least once in the past year, and almost 4% report having been intoxicated weekly (USDHHS, 2000). Almost 10% of current drinkers (approximately 8 million people) meet diagnostic criteria for alcohol dependence, and an additional 7% (more than 5.6 million people) meet diagnostic criteria for alcohol abuse (National Institute on Alcohol Abuse and Alcoholism [NIAAA], 1993; USDHHS, 2000). In 1995, the cost of alcohol abuse and alcoholism was estimated at $167 billion in the United States, of which more than two-thirds was due to lost productivity (Harwood et al., 1998; USDHHS, 2000).

Alcohol use and alcohol-related problems are common among adolescents (O'Malley et al., 1998; USDHHS, 2000). Research shows that the age at which a person starts drinking strongly predicts development of alcohol dependence over a lifetime. Approximately 40% of people who begin drinking before the age of 15 develop alcohol dependence at some stage in their lives. About 10% of people who begin drinking at age 21 or older develop alcohol dependence at some stage in life (Grant and Dawson, 1997; USDHHS, 2000). People with a family history of alcoholism have a higher prevalence of lifetime alcohol dependence than do those with no such history (Grant, 1998; USDHHS, 2000).

Socioeconomic Factors

Studies conducted in 1994–1996 showed that people of both sexes and all races and ethnic groups—with the exception of Hispanic women—displayed a strong inverse relationship between education and heavy alcohol consumption (NCHS, 1998a). Generally, heavy drinking tends to decrease with education, and moderate alcohol use increases with education (NCHS, 1998a; Substance Abuse and Mental Health Services Administration, 1993). In 1994–1996, African American men and women with less than a high school education were almost twice as likely to report heavy alcohol use as were those who had more than a high school education (NCHS, 1998a). White men with high school diplomas were 20% more likely to report heavy alcohol use than were those with more education. White women with less than a high school diploma were 40% more likely to report heavy drinking than were women with more education.

Negative Health Effects

As early as 1926, a U-shaped relationship was described between mortality and consumption of alcohol (Pearl, 1926). The wide range of alcohol-induced illnesses and injuries is primarily attributable to differences in the amount, duration, and patterns of alcohol consumption as well as to differences in genetic vulnerability to particular alcohol-related consequences (USDHHS, 1997a; 2000). Long-term excessive drinking increases risk for high blood pressure, irregularities of heart rhythm (i.e., arrhythmias), disorders of the heart muscle (i.e., cardiomyopathy), and stroke (USDHHS, 2000). Long-term, heavy drinking also increases the risk of developing cancer of the esophagus, mouth, throat, and voice box and of the colon and rectum (NIAAA, 1993; USDHHS, 2000). Alcohol consumption appears to increase the risk of breast cancer in women (Smith-Warner et al., 1998); consumption of two or more drinks per day has been shown to slightly increase women's risk of developing breast cancer (Reichman, 1994; USDHHS, 2000).[4] The *Dietary Guidelines for Americans* (USDA, 1995a) advises women to consume no more than 1 drink per day; while men are advised to consume no more than two per day. Because men and women have less body water as they age, older persons can lower their risk of alcohol problems by drinking no more than one drink per day (Dufour et al., 1992; USDHHS, 2000). Heavy and chronic alcohol use is a cause of poor pregnancy outcomes (NCHS, 1998a; USDHHS, 1993), including fetal alcohol syndrome, a major nongenetic

---

[4]A drink is defined as 0.54 ounces of ethanol, which is the approximately the amount of alcohol in 12 ounces of regular beer, 5 ounces of wine, or 1.5 ounces of 80-proof distilled spirits.

cause of mental retardation (American Academy of Pediatrics, 1993; Bagheri et al., 1998; IOM, 1996). Sustained heavy alcohol consumption worsens the outcome for patients with hepatitis C (NIH, 1997a; USDHHS, 2000) and increases the risk for cirrhosis and other liver disorders (Saadatamand et al., 1997; USDHHS, 2000). Cirrhosis, primarily attributable to heavy drinking, is one of the 10 leading causes of death in the United States (Bureau of the Census, 1997; Hasin et al., 1990; Popham et al., 1984; Saadatamand et al., 1997; Schmidt, 1980).

Progress has been made in reducing the rate of alcohol-related driving fatalities, but it is still a serious problem. Overall, the rate of alcohol-related driving fatalities declined from 9.8 deaths per 100,000 people in 1987 to 6.5 per 100,000 in 1996 (USDHHS, 2000). It is estimated that even at current rates, 3 out of every 10 Americans will be involved in an alcohol-related crash sometime during their lives. The populations of greatest concern for alcohol-related driving fatalities include Native Americans and those between the ages of 15 and 24. In 1994, the alcohol involvement rate in fatal traffic crashes for American Indian and Alaska Native males was 4 times higher (28 per 100,000 population) than for the general population, and, for 15- to 24-year olds, the rate was almost 13 per 100,000 population (USDHHS, 2000).

The consequences of excessive alcohol consumption extend beyond death rates. Alcohol consumption also contributes to risk of injury. In addition to injuries and deaths from traffic accidents, a significant proportion of injuries and deaths from falls, fires, and drowning has been linked with use of alcohol (Saadatamand et al., 1997; USDHHS, 2000). Alcohol consumption contributes to destruction of personal and social relationships (Brookoff et al., 1997); it is a factor in homicide, suicide, marital violence, and child abuse (Roizen, 1993; USDHHS, 2000); and it contributes to high-risk sexual behavior (Strunin and Hingson, 1992, 1993; USDHHS, 2000).

Positive Health Effects

In contrast with those harmful effects, however, evidence is overwhelming of a beneficial effect of moderate consumption of alcohol (1-2 drinks per day) on reducing risk of coronary heart disease and thrombotic stroke. Light-to-moderate drinking can have beneficial effects on the heart, especially among people at greatest risk for heart attacks, including men over age 45 and women after menopause (USDHHS, 2000; Zakhari,

1997). Moderate alcohol-drinking reduces the risk of death from those cardiovascular causes, on the average, by approximately 20–40% (Doll, 1997; Thun et al., 1997). A reduction in cardiovascular disease mortality will translate into a reduction in total mortality in many populations because cardiovascular disease is by far the leading cause of death in middle and old age. The inverse association between alcohol consumption and cardiovascular disease risk is causal: ethanol has been shown in short-term experimental studies to increase the serum concentration of high-density lipoprotein cholesterol (Rimm et al., 1999), and it also appears to affect platelet function and other components of clotting and fibrinolysis (Hendriks et al., 1994; Meade et al., 1987; Renaud et al., 1992).

Quantifying Net Public Health Benefit

The positive and negative effects of alcohol on mortality raise the question, "Is alcohol consumption good for health?" The answer is conditional. The net benefit of alcohol consumption in a population depends on age distribution of the population, because the ratio of mortality from conditions that are prevented by alcohol to mortality from conditions that are made more common by it varies greatly with age. The net benefit also will vary with the population prevalence of factors that predispose to (or protect from) cardiovascular disease, and they might differ in men and women.

Optimal public health guidelines on alcohol consumption are not the same across or even within populations, because the importance of cardiovascular disease and injuries or trauma varies significantly with age and sex as well as from one society to another. For instance, in Sub-Saharan and Latin American countries, the ratio of deaths from coronary heart disease to deaths from violence is close to 1.0, and sometimes even less than 1.0 among men (Murray and Lopez, 1996). Groups inherently at high risk from the detrimental effects of alcohol (such as adolescents and young adults, binge drinkers, and those with lower socioeconomic status) in which deaths from injuries (including motor vehicle injuries), violence, and other external causes are high, have not been included in epidemiologic studies that analyze the alcohol/mortality relationship. For example, among U.S. men aged 15–29, deaths from injuries and other external causes account for 75% of all deaths, compared with 4% from cardiovascular diseases (Schoenborn and Marano, 1988). In another study involving Swedish military recruits in the same age range, a linear increase in risk of death from all causes was found with increasing alcohol consumption (Andreasson et al., 1988).

Although alcohol consumption is unlikely to reduce total mortality in people under 45 (Doll, 1997), the optimal duration of moderate alcohol consumption is not known in terms of reducing risk of cardiovascular disease mortality in older people. Furthermore, even though some of the benefits of alcohol are the result of long-term, habitual consumption (Jackson et al., 1992), many of the important effects of ethanol on high-density lipoproteins and clotting components are acute; thus, it is likely that alcohol consumption beginning in middle age would suffice while avoiding much of the risk of injuries and other external causes of death (although not necessarily of cancers or cirrhosis of the liver).

Optimal alcohol consumption differs for men and women for several reasons. Women metabolize alcohol less efficiently than men do (making women more prone to some health problems than are men who drink the same amount), and because women have less body water than men (making them more prone to intoxication than men after drinking the same amount of alcohol) (USDHHS, 2000). Women also have lower age-specific risks of cardiovascular disease and greater susceptibility to liver damage than men, and women are prone to a relatively high risk of breast cancer, which appears to increase with consumption of any amount of alcohol (Smith-Warner et al., 1998). Although men might be at risk for alcohol-related problems if they consume more than 14 drinks per week or more than 4 drinks per occasion, women could be at risk if they consume more than 7 drinks per week or more than 3 per occasion (USDHHS, 1995, 2000).

The problem of alcohol consumption is frequently one of maldistribution, with many abstaining and many consuming at a hazardous level (Holman and English, 1996). There seems to be no precedent for a public health campaign that simultaneously seeks to "pull in" both tails of a risk factor distribution, in this case reduction of both the prevalence of abstention and of heavy drinking (Holman and English, 1996). There are risks in promoting a population wide alcohol policy that discourages abstention, even if the policy encourages only light-to-moderate regular consumption. First, there is no evidence that moderate drinking is harmless. Second, a public health recommendation that encourages even light drinking over abstention could increase the number of heavy drinkers in a population since it has been noted that population distributions of risk factors tend to shift, either downward or upward, as an entity (Rose, 1992).

Researchers have noted that it is unethical for governments and other public institutions to promote low alcohol intake as a disease prevention measure because of the potential adverse risks at the population level, but they also note that it is similarly unethical to promote abstinence (Holman and English, 1996). In an editorial accompanying publication of a large study by the American Cancer Society, a question was raised about whether alcohol consumption is the method of choice for preventing cardiovascular disease. One important consideration is whether physical activity and diet would be as effective as moderate alcohol consumption—with lower risk of harm—in lowering cardiovascular disease mortality (Potter, 1997). The data on physical activity and some dietary factors would seem to suggest that they *are* equally effective, and they have the additional benefit of reducing risks of many other diseases.

SEXUAL PRACTICES

Sexual relationships and practices are complex to investigate, but their study is important because infectious disease has always been a possible outcome of sexual relationships, as has unwanted pregnancy. Both are crucial public health issues of our time. Recently released figures show that the United States is among the highest in incidence and prevalence of sexually transmitted infection (also called sexually transmitted disease) in the industrialized world (USDHHS, 2000).

Concern about AIDS has been an important motivation for recent studies of sexual behaviors, including a large national survey of sexual behaviors and attitudes (Laumann, 1994). Most of the issues that arise in relating sexual behavior to risk of infection with the human immunodeficiency virus (HIV) pertain to many other, far more common, sexually transmitted infections. But HIV has made unsafe sex a matter of life and death. In 1995, there were more than 43,000 deaths from AIDS in the United States, making it the eighth-leading cause of death in that year, and the leading cause of death among Americans 25–44 years old (Anderson et al., 1997). It is now the second-leading cause of death among all Americans aged 25–44, but it is the leading cause of death for African Americans in this age group (USDHHS, 2000). Other, more common sexually transmitted infections—human papilloma virus, gonorrhea, chlamydia, and genital herpes—vary in the severity of their consequences; but if left untreated, these diseases can compromise health and even become life threatening.

Prevalence of Sexually Transmitted Infections

In 1996, the United States had 15.3 million new cases of sexually transmitted infection. This was higher than the 12 million annual new cases estimated by the Centers for Disease Control and Prevention a decade before (Tanne, 1998). The increase is partly real and partly the result of more sensitive tests that can now identify asymptomatic infection.

More than 68 million Americans now have an incurable sexually transmitted infection (Tanne, 1998); for instance, 1 out of every 5 Americans has genital herpes (Tanne, 1998). Every year, 15 million people are infected with a sexually transmitted disease, almost 4 million of them teenagers (American Social Health Association, 1998; USDHHS, 2000). Sexually transmitted infections are more prevalent in teenagers and young adults than in older persons, partly because of the greater propensity of younger persons to engage in unprotected sex and to switch sexual partners relatively frequently (Laumann, 1994). Despite its prominence in the media, AIDS represents only a tiny proportion of sexually transmitted infections, basically less than half of one percent of all the new cases of sexually transmitted infection (Laumann, 1994). The most commonly reported sexually transmitted infection in the United States is chlamydia, with 3 million new cases each year (Tanne, 1998). The direct and indirect costs of the primary sexually transmitted diseases and their complications, including sexually transmitted HIV infection, are estimated at $17 billion each year (St. Louis et al., 1997; USDHHS, 2000).

Data from a University of Chicago national survey on sexual behaviors (Laumann, 1994) indicate that 16.9% of U.S. adults aged 18–59 years old have had a sexually transmitted infection (15.9% of men, 17.8% of women). The risk of sexually transmitted infection rises monotonically and dramatically with the number of sex partners. Lifetime occurrence of any sexually transmitted infection rises from 4% for those with only one partner after the age of 18 years to 40.4% for those with more than 20 partners. The number of sex partners is the most succinct measure of the extent of exposure to infection. Another important aspect of extent of exposure is type of sexual practice: anal intercourse is an especially efficient way of transmitting infections, especially HIV, because it often leads to small breaks in the skin.

Contributing Factors That Affect Transmission

Although sexually transmitted infections are behavior-linked diseases that result from unprotected sex (IOM, 1997; USDHHS, 2000), other factors contribute to their rapid spread in a population. Because most sexually transmitted infections are asymptomatic, or produce very mild symptoms, they often are disregarded, so infected persons do not seek immediate medical care. About 85% of women and about 50% of men with chlamydia have no symptoms (Fish et al., 1989; Handsfield et al., 1986; Stamm and Holmes, 1990; USDHHS, 2000). There is also a long interval between the acquisition of a sexually transmitted infection and the eventual recognition of a clinically significant health problem; it is sometimes several years before an infection manifests itself. Thus, because the original infection is often asymptomatic, there is frequently no perceived connection between the original sexually acquired infection and the health problem associated with it.

Another contributing biological factor is that women are at higher risk than men for most sexually transmitted diseases, and for some of these infections, young women are more susceptible than older women. This is especially alarming because analyses of adolescent females' sexual activity not only demonstrate the frequency of those behaviors, but also reveal that not all sexually experienced young females willingly enter into a sexual relationship (Abma et al., 1998; USDHHS, 2000). In 1995, more than 16% of females who experienced their first sexual intercourse when they were aged 15 or younger indicated that it was not voluntary (Abma et al., 1997; USDHHS, 2000). Sexual violence against women contributes both directly and indirectly to the transmission of disease. Directly, women who experience this type of violence are less able to protect themselves from sexually transmitted infections or pregnancy (USDHHS, 2000). Indirectly, studies show that sexually abused girls engage in high-risk sexual behaviors such as voluntary intercourse at earlier ages and multiple partners, which are risk factors for sexually transmitted diseases (Miller et al., 1995; Stock et al., 1997).

There is an association between sexually transmitted infections and substance abuse, particularly the abuse of alcohol and other drugs. The introduction of new, illicit substances into communities, for instance, often drastically alters sexual behavior in high-risk sexual networks, thereby causing an epidemic of sexually transmitted diseases (Marx et al., 1991; USDHHS, 2000). The epidemic in crack cocaine use intensified the U.S. syphilis epidemic in the late 1980s (Gunn et al., 1995; USDHHS, 2000).

One social factor that contributes to the spread of sexually transmitted infections in the United States is the stigma connected with them. Another is the overall discomfort many people have with discussing intimate aspects of life, particularly those related to sex (Brandt, 1985;

USDHHS, 2000). This is what most significantly separates the United States from industrialized countries that have low rates of sexually transmitted infection. (USDHHS, 2000). Even in the most intimate relationships, talking openly and comfortably about sex and sexuality is difficult for many Americans. A recent survey indicated that approximately one-fourth of married women and one-fifth of married men had no knowledge about their partner's sexual history (EDK Associates, 1995; USDHHS, 2000). The secrecy surrounding sexuality hampers sexuality education programs for adolescents, and it discourages open discussion between parents and their children and between sex partners regarding sexually transmitted diseases. It also impedes balanced messages from mass media, health care professionals' education and counseling activities, and community activism (IOM, 1997; USDHHS, 2000).

Sexually Transmitted Infections and Cancer

Several sexually transmitted viral infections are known or strongly suspected to cause cancer. The most important of these are the sexually transmitted types of human papilloma virus. At least 90% of the approximately 16,000 cases of cervical cancer diagnosed each year are estimated to be attributable to infection with the human papilloma virus (Morrison et al., 1997).

A strong link between hepatitis B and hepatitis C viruses and hepatocellular carcinoma (liver cancer) became evident during the 1980s. Hepatitis B infection occurs more frequently among persons who have multiple sex partners and who also have a history of sexually transmitted infection. An estimated 53,000 cases of hepatitis B virus (out of a total of 200,000–300,000 cases) were sexually transmitted in the United States in 1994 (IOM, 1997).

Disproportionate Affliction of Sexually Transmitted Infections

Although people in all communities—including all racial, cultural, economic, and religious groups—and sexual networks are at risk for sexually transmitted infections, some are disproportionately affected by these diseases and their associated complications. For instance, not only do sexually transmitted diseases occur more frequently in women than in men, but women also suffer more serious complications (USDHHS, 2000), including pelvic inflammatory disease, ectopic pregnancy, infertility, and chronic pelvic pain (Chandra and Stephen, 1998; USDHHS, 2000). In addition, women are biologically more susceptible to infection when exposed to a sexually transmitted disease agent, and sexually transmitted diseases are more difficult to diagnose in women because of female physiology and the anatomy of the reproductive tract (USDHHS, 2000).

Sexually transmitted diseases pose a risk to unborn children. The diseases not only cause serious health problems in pregnant women, but they can result in the death of the fetus or newborn (Brunham et al., 1990; USDHHS, 2000). Sexually transmitted disease in a mother also can result in congenital or perinatal infections that permanently damage the child's brain, spinal cord, eyes, auditory nerves, or immune system. Sexually transmitted infection can complicate a pregnancy even without directly reaching the fetus or newborn, causing spontaneous abortion, stillbirth, premature membrane rupture, or premature delivery (Goldenberg et al., 1997; USDHHS, 2000). Women with bacterial vaginosis, for instance, are 40% more likely than women without this condition to deliver a preterm, low-birthweight baby (Hillier et al., 1995; Meis et al., 1995; USDHHS, 2000).

Sexually transmitted infections disproportionately affect adolescents and young adults for several reasons, including behavioral, social, and biological (Alan Guttmacher Institute, 1994; USDHHS, 2000). In 1996, 15-to 19-year-olds had the highest reported rates of chlamydia and gonorrhea (USDHHS, 1997b; USDHHS, 2000), and the herpes infection rate of white adolescents between the ages of 12 and 19 was shown to have increased almost 5-fold over just 10 years (Fleming et al., 1997; USDHHS, 2000). Several factors contribute these incidences. Because many teenagers are sexually active, they are at risk for sexually transmitted infections; in 1995, just over 50% of females aged 15–19 indicated they had already had sexual intercourse, and more than 51% of high school males reported having experienced sexual intercourse by age 16. Teenagers are more likely than older persons to have serial sex partners who are active in a sexual network that already is infected with untreated sexually transmitted diseases (USDHHS, 2000).

Rates of sexually transmitted diseases are higher for minority and ethnic groups (primarily African American and Hispanic populations) than for whites. For example, although chlamydia is a widely distributed sexually transmitted infection in all racial and ethnic groups, the prevalence is higher in minorities. In 1996, African Americans accounted for approximately 78% of the total number of gonorrhea cases reported—32 times the rate for whites. These high rates also apply to African American adolescents and young adults, with the average about 24 times higher than that for 15- to 19-year-old white adolescents and 30 times higher than for 20- to 24 year-old whites in 1996. In 1996, the gonorrhea rate for Hispanics was 3 times the rate for whites. Since 1990, syphilis rates have declined in all racial and ethnic groups, except for American Indians and Alaska Natives, but the rates for African Americans and Hispanics continue to be greater than those for non-Hispanic whites. In 1996, African Americans accounted for approximately 84% of all reported cases of syphilis (USDHHS, 2000).

Young, heterosexual women, especially minorities, are increasingly acquiring HIV infection and developing AIDS. In 1996, 39% of the reported AIDS cases occurred in 13- to 24-year-olds and, of the AIDS cases reported in women, almost 4 of every 5 occurred in the minority population, consisting primarily of African Americans or Hispanics (USDHHS, 2000).

Prevention of Sexually Transmitted Infections

Behavioral means for prevention of sexually transmitted infections include delaying the onset of sexual activity, limiting the number of partners, abstaining from sex with people not known to be infection free, and using effective barrier contraception.

Community-focused interventions also are useful in reducing sexually transmitted infections. Such interventions generally aim to change behavioral norms. Research conducted in the past decade has shown that sexual behavior and sexual preference exhibit persistent social regularities, which implies that social forces are important in shaping sexual expression (Laumann, 1994). Thus, changing norms that encourage safe sexual behaviors holds great potential for reducing the population burden of sexually transmitted infections. Mass media campaigns, for example, have used reinforcing messages to increase knowledge about HIV infection and ways to prevent it. Because only a small percentage of adolescents receive any prevention information from parents, and because for most teenagers schools are the main source of information about sexually transmitted infections, school-based interventions can be significant in motivating young people to modify their behaviors (American Social Health Association, 1996; USDHHS, 2000). In fact, most states and school districts now require teaching about prevention of sexually transmitted infections (IOM, 1997). Curricula including information about both abstinence and contraceptive use appear to be effective in delaying the onset of sexual intercourse and in encouraging contraceptive use once intercourse has begun (IOM, 1997). Currently available contraceptives differentially affect risk of pregnancy and sexually transmitted infections. There is a contraceptive trade-off dilemma with currently existing methods: the contraceptives with the best record of preventing pregnancy have the worst record for preventing sexually transmitted infections (Cates, 1996). For instance, oral contraceptives are highly effective at preventing pregnancy, but offer no protection against sexually transmitted infections. Furthermore, they appear to increase risk of cervical chlamydial infection (Cottingham and Hunter, 1992). Intrauterine devices, also effective in preventing pregnancy, are associated with pelvic inflammatory disease, especially in the first month after insertion (Farley et al., 1992). The condom is effective at preventing sexually transmitted diseases, but it is less effective than are other contraceptive methods for preventing pregnancy (USDHHS, 2000). For such reasons, use of dual methods of contraception could help prevent unwanted pregnancies and transmission of infections (Cates and Stone, 1992; USDHHS, 2000).

DISEASE SCREENING PRACTICES

Screening asymptomatic persons to detect preclinical disease has become an important part of public health. But preclinical screening makes sense only if treatment initiated earlier in the disease process will reduce morbidity and mortality from the disease: there is no benefit in living with a diagnosis if a person's life or quality of life is not extended. Although some screening tests can be highly effective in reducing morbidity and mortality, others are of unproven benefit. Poor specificity can produce a large number of false-positives, which in turn can lead to unnecessary and potentially harmful follow-up with diagnostic testing and treatment and needless psychological distress.

The selection of appropriate tests for a given individual depends primarily on that person's age and sex. In addition, consideration of individual risk factors, such as lifestyle or family history, often is used to determine which tests are appropriate tests and how often testing should be done.

In 1984, the U.S. Public Health Service commissioned the U.S. Preventive Services Task Force. This panel was charged with developing recommendations for clinicians on the appropriate use of preventive interventions, including screening for preclinical disease and screening for disease risk, based on a systematic review of evidence of clinical effectiveness. In 1989, the first *Guide to Clinical Preventive Services* (U.S. Preventive Services Task Force, 1989) was published. In 1990, the task force was reconvened to continue and update the scientific review process through examination of new and emerging evidence on preventive interventions. The second edition of the *Guide to Clinical Preventive Services* (U.S. Preventive Services Task Force, 1996) was published in 1996. Much of the discussion below concerning screening tests for the major chronic diseases of middle and older age derives from that Guide.

According to the task force, screening must satisfy two major requirements to be considered effective for use in a population. First, the test must be able to detect the target condition earlier than would be possible without screening and with enough accuracy to preclude large numbers of false-positive and false-negative results. Second, screening for and treating persons with early disease should improve the likelihood of favorable health outcomes (e.g., reduced disease-specific morbidity or mortality) as compared with what would happen in treating patients who present on their own with signs or symptoms of the disease. In addition, the tests must be cost-effective and acceptable to the target population (fear of or distaste for colorectal screening and tests involving drawing of blood, for example, could prevent some people from participating). Documented effectiveness should be the most basic requirement for providing a health care service (U.S. Preventive Services Task Force, 1996).

Primary versus Secondary Prevention

Primary prevention aims to reduce the incidence of disease; *secondary prevention* attempts to prevent the prevalence of disease, usually by shortening the course of the disease through early and effective intervention. Screening, as a component of early detection of extant disease, is one aspect of secondary prevention. However, some forms of screening, such as high-blood-cholesterol or high-blood-pressure screening, can be thought of as primary prevention for cardiovascular disease—they are in essence screening for risk of disease. As the tests have become better able to detect very early stages of such diseases as cancer (for example, in situ breast cancer and very small colon polyps), the boundary between primary and secondary prevention has blurred.

The following is a summary of general guidelines for screening for the major chronic diseases of middle and older ages. For people with unusual family histories of disease, or other medical concerns, screening procedures can vary at the discretion of the physician.

Screening for Hypertension and High Blood Cholesterol

The U.S. Preventive Services Task Force recommends screening for hypertension for all children and adults (U.S. Preventive Services Task Force, 1996). The prevalence of hypertension increases with age, and it is more common in African Americans than whites. It is estimated that 40–50 million Americans have hypertension (Burt et al., 1995). Office sphygmomanometry (use of the blood pressure cuff) is the most appropriate way to screen for hypertension in the general population. However, there are special problems with accuracy when testing children under the age of 3. (The definition of hypertension in childhood is somewhat arbitrary, based on age-specific percentiles.)

There is a positive relationship between the magnitude of blood pressure elevation and the benefits of treatment. In persons with malignant hypertension, the benefits of treatment are most dramatic: treatment increases 5-year survival from near 0 to 75% (Hansson, 1988). The efficacy of treating less severe hypertension has been demonstrated in randomized clinical trials. The greatest benefits are associated with reduction in morbidity and mortality from stroke. Improved detection and treatment of high blood pressure is responsible for a substantial portion of the greater than 50% reduction in age-adjusted stroke mortality that has been observed in this country since 1972 (Joint National Committee on Detection and Treatment of High Blood Pressure, 1993). The Joint National Committee on Detection, Evaluation, and Treatment of High Blood Pressure and the American Heart Association recommend blood pressure measurement at least once every 2 years for adults with a diastolic blood pressure below 85 mm Hg (millimeters of mercury) and a systolic pressure below 130 mm Hg. More frequent testing is recommended for persons with higher measures, with frequency depending on degree of elevation. The American Academy of Pediatrics, the American Medical Association, and the American Heart Association recommend that children and adolescents have their blood pressure monitored every 1 or 2 years during regular office visits to a physician (U.S. Preventive Services Task Force, 1996).

Along with hypertension, elevated blood cholesterol is a major modifiable risk factor for cardiovascular disease. Total cholesterol can be measured in venipuncture or fingerstick specimens from fasting or nonfasting individuals. Because of normal physiologic variation and measurement error, a single cholesterol measurement might not reflect a person's true average concentration. A single measurement of blood cholesterol can vary by as much as 14% from an individual's average value, under normal laboratory circumstances (Cooper et al., 1992). For this reason, some experts advise telling people their "cholesterol range," rather than providing them with a single value (Belsey and Baer, 1990). When a precise estimate of blood cholesterol is needed, an average of two or three measures has been recommended.

Based on evidence from clinical trials showing that lowering serum cholesterol can reduce risk of coronary heart disease, periodic screening for high blood cholesterol (once every 5 years) is recommended for all men aged 35–65 (U.S. Preventive Services Task Force, 1996). Although there are few trial data pertaining to women, the epidemiology and pathophysiology of coronary heart disease is similar in men and women, and it is likely that reduction of high cholesterol will benefit women as well. However, the later onset of coronary heart disease in women, due to protection from estrogen, suggests that routine screening for high cholesterol in women should begin around age 45. Thus, periodic screening is recommended for women aged 45–65 (U.S. Preventive Services Task Force, 1996).

According to the U.S. Preventive Services Task Force, there is insufficient evidence to recommend for or against routine screening of all asymptomatic persons over age 65. Cholesterol appears to plateau by age 65 in women, and earlier in men (U.S. Preventive Services Task Force, 1996). Continued screening, therefore, would be less important in persons who have shown desirable concentrations throughout middle age. However, screening in older persons might be recommended on a case-by-case basis. Older persons with important coronary heart disease risk factors, such as smoking, hypertension, or diabetes, could be more likely to benefit from screening, based on their high risk of coronary heart disease and the proven benefits of lowering cholesterol in older persons with symptomatic coronary heart disease. There is also insufficient evidence to recommend for or against routine screening in children, adolescents, or young adults; again, however, screening could be recommended for people who have a family history of very high cholesterol, premature coronary heart disease in a first-degree relative, or major risk factors for coronary heart disease.

Cervical Cancer Screening

Approximately 16,000 women are diagnosed with cervical cancer each year in the United States, and 4800 women die from the disease annually (NCHS, 1998b). The 5-year survival rate is about 90% for women with localized cervical cancer but is only about 14% for women with advanced disease (NCHS, 1998b). The incidence of invasive cervical cancer has decreased greatly over the past 40 years, due largely to organized screening programs to detect early-stage disease (U.S. Preventive Services Task Force, 1996). Women with a history of multiple sexual partners, early age at onset of sexual intercourse, or both, are at highest risk of cervical cancer. Infection with HIV or some types of the human papilloma virus sharply increases risk.

The Pap smear is the principal screening test for cervical cancer. The U.S. Preventive Services Task Force, American Cancer Society, the National Cancer Institute, the American College of Obstetricians and Gynecologists, and the American Medical Association recommend that all women who are or have been sexually active, or who are 18 years of age or older, should have annual Pap smears. The recommendation permits Pap testing less frequently after 3 or more normal annual smears, at the discretion of individual physicians. There is no consensus on the age at which to discontinue Pap testing.

Colorectal Cancer Screening

Colorectal cancer is the second-most-common form of cancer in the United States, after lung cancer, and is the second-leading cause of cancer death. Each year, about 140,000 new cases are diagnosed, and 55,000 persons die of the disease (NCHS, 1998b). The average patient who dies of colorectal cancer loses 13 years of life, and in addition to the mortality associated with this disease, its treatment can produce significant morbidity. Screening for early-stage colorectal cancer as well as its precursor lesions (adenomatous polyps) thus can significantly reduce morbidity and mortality associated with colorectal cancer.

Colorectal cancer screening can act as both primary and secondary prevention because the tests can detect and (in the case of sigmoidoscopy and colonoscopy) remove precancerous polyps as well as carcinomas. The principal tests for detecting polyps and early malignancy in asymptomatic persons are the fecal occult blood test (FOBT) and flexible sigmoidoscopy. There is a large literature on the accuracy and effectiveness of these tests under varying conditions and in different groups of persons. As reviewed by the Preventive Services Task Force (1996), it is estimated that most positive reactions to FOBT (70–90%) are falsely positive for colorectal cancer. However, despite its low positive predictive value, FOBT is effective in reducing colorectal cancer mortality, especially when done annually (Towler et al., 1998). Unlike FOBT, flexible sigmoidoscopy is both a screening and diagnostic tool; any polyps detected can be biopsied and removed during the procedure. Evidence shows that screening with sigmoidoscopy reduces both incidence of and mortality from colorectal cancer (U.S. Preventive Services Task Force, 1996).

Screening for colorectal cancer is recommended by a variety of groups for all persons aged 50 years and older, although there is no consensus about whether FOBT or sigmoidoscopy, or a combination of the two, produces the greatest benefit. For persons with a family history of colorectal cancer, screening is recommended to begin at an earlier age, particularly if a family member was diagnosed with colorectal cancer at a young age. For persons with a family history of hereditary syndromes associated with very high risk of colorectal cancer, and for those with a previous diagnosis of high-risk adenomatous polyps or colon cancer, regular screening with colonoscopy (at least once a year) is part of routine management. As mentioned above, FOBT screening should be performed annually to achieve maximum benefit. There is insufficient evidence to determine the optimal screening interval for sigmoidoscopy; however, a frequency of 3–5 years has been recommended by some expert groups.

Prostate Cancer Screening

Prostate cancer is the most common non-skin cancer among American men. After lung cancer, it accounts for more cancer deaths in men than any other. Each year about 245,000 men are diagnosed with prostate cancer, and 40,000 die (NCHS, 1998b). The PSA (prostate-specific antigen) test is the principal screening test for prostate cancer. Although this test has adequate sensitivity to detect clinically important cancers at an early stage, it is also likely to detect a large number of cancers of uncertain clinical significance. Because treatment for prostate cancer can cause substantial morbidity as a result of impaired sexual, urinary, and bowel function, and because prostate cancer also carries a nonnegligible mortality risk (estimated 0.7%–2% 30-day mortality risk [Murphy et al., 1994;

Wasson et al., 1993]), the question of which cancers should be treated after detection with PSA testing is critical.

The absence of proof that screening can reduce mortality from prostate cancer, together with the strong potential that screening will increase treatment-related morbidity, argue against a policy of routine screening in asymptomatic men. Thus, the U.S. Preventive Services Task Force (1996) does not recommend routine screening for prostate cancer. However, the American Cancer Society does recommend yearly PSA testing beginning at age 50 for white men and at age 40 for African American men, in whom risk of the disease is higher.

Breast Cancer Screening

Each year, some 180,000 women are diagnosed with breast cancer in the United States (NCHS, 1998b). This accounts for about 30% of all incident cancers among women. Each year, 44,000 women die of breast cancer (NCHS, 1998b), making it the second-leading cause of cancer deaths among American women, after lung cancer. Breast cancer is extremely rare among women younger than 20, and is uncommon among women under the age of 30. Incidence rates increase sharply with age, however, and become substantial before age 50 years. Rates continue to rise, although less quickly, in postmenopausal women.

As reviewed by the U.S. Preventive Services Task Force (1996), several clinical trials conducted among women aged 40 years and older have shown an overall reduction of breast cancer mortality due to screening. The average reduction is 20–30% (over roughly a 10-year period) for women aged 50–69 who are screened periodically for breast cancer (U.S. Preventive Services Task Force, 1996). However, there is no consensus about the optimal screening interval for women in this age group. Although annual screening has been recommended by many groups, an analysis of data from Sweden revealed little evidence that screening every year provides a greater benefit than does screening every 2 years (Tabar et al., 1987).

Based on data from clinical trials, there is disagreement in the scientific community over whether routine mammographic screening should be recommended for women in their forties. This disagreement has at times been strident and strong (Taubes, 1997). Although none of the randomized clinical trials enrolled enough women in their forties to study the benefit of screening in this age group with statistical confidence, a summary analysis of the trials nonetheless suggested a benefit. The magnitude (10–15% reduction in breast cancer mortality risk over roughly a 10-year period) was smaller than the benefit observed in women aged 50 and older (U.S. Preventive Services Task Force, 1996). A consensus conference convened by NIH in 1997 to examine the question of whether regular mammography screening should be recommended for women in their forties. The group concluded that the decision to screen should be made by individual women in consultation with their physicians (NIH, 1997b). The American College of Physicians, the U.S. Preventive Services Task Force, and the National Cancer Institute agree with that conclusion, but other groups (the American Cancer Society, the American College of Obstetricians and Gynecologists, and the American Medical Association) defer, recommending annual routine mammography for women aged 40–49 (U.S. Preventive Services Task Force, 1996). A detailed review of the literature on behavior change and health communication issues associated with mammography is provided in an IOM report (2001b).

Screening for Sexually Transmitted Diseases

Screening and treatment of sexually transmitted diseases affect both transmission and duration. Studies show that screening for sexually transmitted diseases meets criteria for a successful preventive intervention (USDHHS, 2000; U.S. Preventive Services Task Force, 1996). During the 1990s, for example, significant progress was made toward reducing the burden of disease of the common bacterial sexually transmitted diseases in the United States (i.e., gonorrhea and syphilis) (USDHHS, 2000). For those diseases that often are asymptomatic, research indicates that screening and proper treatment even benefit people who are likely to suffer acute complications if infections are not detected and treated early (Hillis et al., 1995; USDHHS, 2000). For instance, data are becoming available indicating that chlamydia screening is reducing disease burden and preventing associated complications (USDHHS, 2000). In a randomized, controlled trial conducted by a managed care organization, screening for chlamydia was demonstrated to reduce the incidence of subsequent pelvic inflammatory disease by 56% in a screened group (Scholes et al., 1996; USDHHS, 2000). Selective chlamydia screening in the Pacific Northwest decreased disease burden by 60% in 5 years in the screened population (Britton et al., 1992; USDHHS, 2000).

Testing has been identified, as has counseling, as an effective tool for assisting HIV-infected individuals both in coping with their infections and in preventing them from infecting other people. The combination of counseling and testing provides the opportunity to guide people with seronegative test results on behaviors and strategies for avoiding infection, in addition to referring them to other needed medical and social services. After the 1994 findings that perinatal HIV transmission rates could be considerably reduced with zidovudine therapy, the Public Health Service issued guidelines suggesting that HIV counseling and voluntary testing be a part of routine prenatal care for pregnant women (USDHHS, 2000). A primary objective of this policy is to ensure that HIV-infected women have access to adequate health care for themselves and have the opportunity to reduce the risk of HIV transmission to their babies.

REFERENCES

Abma, J., Chandra, A., Mosher, W., Peterson, L., and Piccinino, L. (1997). Fertility, family planning, and women's health: New data from the 1995 National Survey of Family Growth. National Center for Health Statistics. *Vital Health Statistics, 23*, 1–114.

Abma, J., Driscoll, A., and Moore, K. (1998). Young women's degree of control over first intercourse: An exploratory analysis. *Family Planning Perspectives, 30*, 12–18.

Alan Guttmacher Institute (1994). *Sex and America's Teenagers.* New York: Alan Guttmacher Institute..

Albanes, D., Blair, A., and Taylor, P.R. (1989). Physical activity and risk of cancer in the NHANES I population. *American Journal of Public Health, 79*, 744–750.

Albanes, D., Heinonen, O.P., Taylor, P.R., Virtamo, J., Edwards, B.K., Rautalahti, M., Hartman, A.M., Palmgren, J., Freedman, L.S., Haapakoski, J., Barrett, M.J., Pietinen, P., Malila, N., Tala, E., Liippo, K., Salomaa, E.R., Tangrea, J.A., Teppo, L., Askin, F.B., Taskinen, E., Erozan, Y., Greenwald, P., and Huttunen, J.K. (1996). Alpha-tocopherol and beta-carotene supplements and lung cancer incidence in the alpha-tocopherol, beta-carotene cancer prevention study: effects of base-line characteristics and study compliance. *Journal of the National Cancer Institute, 88*, 1560–1570.

Allison, D.B., Fontaine, K.R., Manson, J.E., Steverns, J., and VanItallie, T.B. (1999) Annual deaths attributable to obesity in the United States. *Journal of the American Medical Association, 282*, 1530–1538.

American Academy of Pediatrics Committee on Substance Abuse and Committee on Children with Disabilities: Fetal alcohol syndrome and fetal alcohol effects. (1993). *Pediatrics, 91*, 1004–1006.

American Social Health Association. (1996). Teenagers know more than adults about STDs, but knowledge among both groups is low. *STD News, 3*, 1–5.

American Social Health Association. (1998). *Sexually Transmitted Diseases in America: How Many Cases and at What Cost?* Menlo Park, CA: Kaiser Family Foundation.

Anderson, R., Kochanek, K., and Murphy, S. (1997). *Report of Final Mortality Statistics, 1995.* Hyattsville, MD: US Department of Health and Human Services, Centers for Disease Control and Prevention, National Center for Health Statistics.

Andreasson, S., Allebeck, P., and Romelsjo, A. (1988). Alcohol and mortality among young men: Longitudinal study of Swedish conscripts. *The British Medical Journal*, *296*, 1021–1025.

Ascherio, A., Hennekens, C.H., Buring, J.E., Master, C., Stampfer, M.J., and Willett, W.C. (1994). Trans fatty acids intake and risk of myocardial infarction. *Circulation*, *89*, 94–101.

Ascherio, A., Rimm, E.B., Giovannucci, E.L, Colditz, G.A., Rosner, B., Willett, W.C., Sacks, F., and Stampfer, M.J. (1992). A prospective study of nutritional factors and hypertension among US men. *Circulation*, *86*, 1475–1484.

Bagheri, M.M., Burd, L., Martsolf, J.T., and Klug, M.G. (1998). Fetal alcohol syndrome: Maternal and neonatal characteristics. *Journal of Perinatal Medicine*, *26*, 263–269.

Barnes-Josiah, D., Potter, J.D., Sellers, T.A., and Himes, J.H. (1995). Early body size and subsequent weight gain as predictors of breast cancer incidence (Iowa, United States). *Cancer Causes and Control*, *6*, 112–118.

Belsey, R. and Baer, D. (1990). Cardiac risk classification based on lipid screening. *Journal of the American Medical Association*, *263*, 1250–1252.

Berlin, J. and Colditz, G. (1990). A meta-analysis of physical activity in the prevention of coronary heart disease. *American Journal of Epidemiology*, *132*, 612–628.

Bernstein, L., Henderson, B.E., Hanisch, R., Sullivan-Halley, J., and Ross, R.K. (1994). Physical exercise and reduced risk of breast cancer in young women. *Journal of the National Cancer Institute*, *86*, 1403–1408.

Boushey, C.J., Beresford, S.A.A., Omenn, G.S., and Motulsky, A.G. (1995). A quantitative assessment of plasma homocysteine as a risk factor for vascular disease: probable benefits of increasing folic acid intakes. *Journal of the American Medical Association*, *274*, 1049–1057.

Brandt, A. (1985). *No Magic Bullet: A Social History of Venereal Disease in the United States Since 1880*. New York: Oxford University Press.

Britton, T., DeLisle, S., and Fine, D. (1992). STDs and family planning clinics: A regional program for chlamydia control that works. *American Journal of Gynecological Health*, *6*, 80–87.

Brookoff, D., O'Brien, K., Cook, C., Thompson, T., and Williams, C. (1997). Characteristics of participants in domestic violence. Assessment at the scene of domestic assault. *Journal of the American Medical Association*, *277*, 1369–1373.

Brown, M., Sinacore, D.R., and Host, H.H. (1995). The relationship of strength to function in the older adult. *Journal of Gerontology*, *50A*, 55–59.

Brunham, R., Holmes, K., and Embree, J. (1990). Sexually transmitted diseases in pregnancy. In K. Holmes, P. Mardh, P. Sparling, P. Weisner, W. Cates, S. Lemon et al. (Eds.) *Sexually Transmitted Diseases, 2nd edition*. New York: McGraw-Hill.

Buchner, D.M. (1997). Preserving mobility in older adults. *Western Journal of Medicine*, *167*, 258–264.

Bureau of the Census. (1997). *Statistical Abstract of the United States: 1997, 117th edition*. Washington, DC: Department of Commerce.

Burt, V., Whelton, P., Roccella, E., Brown, C., Cutler, J.A., Higgins, M., Horan, M.J., and Labarthe, D. (1995). Prevalence of hypertension in the U.S. adult population: Results from the Third National Health and Nutrition Examination Survey, 1988–1991. *Hypertension*, *25*, 305–313.

Calle, E.E., Thun, M.J., Petrelli, J.M., Rodriguez, C., and Heath, C.W. (1999) Body-mass index and mortality in a prospective cohort of U.S. adults. *The New England Journal of Medicine, 341,* 1097–1105.

Cates, W. and Stone, K. (1992). Family planning, sexually transmitted diseases, and contraceptive choice: A literature update. *Family Planning Perspectives, 24,* 75–84.

Cates, W., Jr. (1996). Contraception, unintended pregnancies, and sexually transmitted diseases: Why isn't a simple solution possible? *American Journal of Epidemiology, 143,* 311–318.

CDC (Centers for Disease Control and Prevention) (1993). Smoking cessation during previous year among adults—United States, 1990 and 1991. *Morbidity and Mortality Weekly Report, 42,* 504–507.

CDC (Centers for Disease Control and Prevention) (1996a). Projected smoking-related deaths among youth—United States. *Morbidity and Mortality Weekly Report, 45,* 971–974.

CDC (Centers for Disease Control and Prevention) (1996b). Cigarette smoking before and after an excise tax increase and an antismoking campaign. *Morbidity and Mortality Weekly Report, 45,* 966-970.

CDC (Centers for Disease Control and Prevention) (1996c). Guidelines for school health programs to promote lifelong healthy eating. *Morbidity and Mortality Weekly Report, 45, (RR-9),* 1–42.

CDC (Centers for Disease Control and Prevention) (1997a). Cigarette smoking among adults—United States, 1995. *Morbidity and Mortality Weekly Report, 46,* 1217–1220.

CDC (Centers for Disease Control and Prevention) (1997b). State-specific prevalence of cigarette smoking among adults, and children's and adolescents' exposure to environmental tobacco smoke—United States. *Morbidity and Mortality Weekly Report, 46,* 1038–1043.

CDC (Centers for Disease Control and Prevention) (1997c). Report of Final Mortality Statistics, 1995. *Monthly Vital Statistics Report, 45, Supplement 2.* Atlanta: National Center for Health Statistics.

CDC (Centers for Disease Control and Prevention) (1998). Youth risk behavior survey, United States, 1997. *Morbidity and Mortality Weekly Report, 47,* 1–31.

Chan, J.M., Rimm, E.B., Colditz, G.A., Stampfer, M.J., and Willett, W.C. (1994). Obesity, fat distribution, and weight gain as risk factors for clinical diabetes in men. *Diabetes Care, 17,* 961–969.

Chandra, A. (1995). Health aspects of pregnancy and childbirth: United States, 1982-88. *Vital Health Statistics, 23,* 1–74.

Chandra, A. and Stephen, E. (1998). Impaired fecundity in the United States: 1982–1995. *Family Planning Perspectives, 30,* 34–42.

Chasan-Taber, L., Selhub, J., Rosenberg, I.H., Malinow, M.R., Terry, P., Tishler, P.V., Willett, W., Hennekens, C.H., and Stampfer, M.J. (1996). A prospective study of folate and vitamin B$_6$ and risk of myocardial infarction in US physicians. *Journal of the American College of Nutrition, 15,* 136–143.

Chen, C.L., White, E., Malone, K.E., and Daling, J.R. (1997). Leisure-time physical activity in relation to breast cancer among young women (Washington, United States). *Cancer Causes and Control, 8,* 77–84.

Chinn, S. and Rona, R.J. (2001) Prevalence and trends in overweight and obesity in three corss sectional studies of British children, 1974–94. *British Medical Journal, 322,* 24–26.

Colditz, G.A., Willett, W.C., Rotnitzky, A., and Manson, J.E. (1995). Weight gain as a risk factor for clinical diabetes mellitus in women. *Annals of Internal Medicine, 122,* 481–486.

Contento, I., Balch, G.I., Bronner, Y.L., et al. (1995). Nutrition education for school-aged children. *Journal of Nutrition Education, 27,* 298–311.

Cooper, G., Myers, G., Smith, S., and Schlant, R. (1992). Blood lipid measurements: Variations and practical utility. *Journal of the American Medical Association, 267,* 3009–3014.

Cottingham, J. and Hunter, D. (1992). Chlamydia trachomatis and oral contraceptive use: A quantitative review. *Genitourinary Medicine, 8,* 209–216.

D'Avanzo, B., Nanni, O., La Vecchia, C., Franceschi, S., Negri, E., Giacosa, A., Conti, E., Montella, M., Talamini, R., and Decarli, A. (1996). Physical activity and breast cancer risk. *Cancer Epidemiology, Biomarkers and Prevention, 5,* 155–160.

de Leiva, A. (1998). What are the benefits of moderate weight loss? *Experimental And Clinical Endocrinology and Diabetes, 106 Suppl. 2,* 10–13.

DiFranza, J.R. and Lew, R.A. (1995). Effect of maternal cigarette smoking on pregnancy complications and sudden infant death syndrome. *Journal of Family Practice, 40,* 385–394.

DiFranza, J.R. and Lew, R.A. (1996). Morbidity and mortality in children associated with the use of tobacco products by other people. *Pediatrics, 97,* 560–568.

Doll, R. (1997). One for the heart. *The British Medical Journal, 315,* 1664–1668.

Dorgan, J.F., Brown, C., Barrett, M., Splansky, G.L., Kreger, B.E., D'Agostino, R.B., Albanes, D., and Schatzkin, A. (1994). Physical activity and risk of breast cancer in the Framingham Heart Study. *American Journal of Epidemiology, 139,* 662–669.

Dufour, M.C., Archer, L., and Gordis, E. (1992). Alcohol and the elderly: Health promotion and disease prevention. *Clinics in Geriatric Medicine, 8,* 127–141.

EDK Associates. (1995). *The ABCs of STDs.* New York: EDK Associates.

Ettinger, W.J. Jr., Burns R., Messier S.P., Applegate, W., Rejeski, W.J., Morgan, T., Shumaker, S., Berry, M.J., O'Toole, M., Monu, J., and Craven, T. (1997) A randomized trial comparing aerobic exercise and resistance exercise with a health education program in older adults with knee osteoarthritis. The Fitness Arthritis and Seniors Trial. *Journal of the American Medical Association, 277,* 25–31

Ettinger, W.H. Jr. and Afable, R. (1994). Physical disability from knee osteoarthritis: The role of exercise as an intervention. *Medicine and Science of Sports and Exercise, 26,* 1435–1440.

Evans, W.J. (1995). Effects of exercise on body composition and functional capacity of the elderly. *Journal of Gerontology, 50A,* 147–150.

Expert Panel on Trans Fatty Acids and Coronary Heart Disease. (1995). *Trans* fatty acids and coronary heart disease risk. *American Journal of Clinical Nutrition, 62,* 655S–708S.

Farley, T., Rosenberg, M., Rowe, P., Chen, J., and Meirik, O. (1992). Intrauterine devices and pelvic inflammatory disease: An international perspective. *Lancet, 339,* 785–788.

Feskanich, D., Willett, W.C., Stampfer, M.J., and Colditz, G.A. (1996). Protein consumption and bone fractures in women. *American Journal of Epidemiology, 143,* 472–479.

Feskanich, D., Willett, W.C., Stampfer, M.J., and Colditz, G.A. (1997). Milk, dietary calcium, bone fractures in women: A 12-year prospective study. *American Journal of Public Health, 87,* 992–997.

Fish, A., Fairweather, D., Oriel, J., and Ridgeway, G. (1989). Chlamydia trachomatis infection in a gynecology clinic population: Identification of high-risk groups and the value of contact tracing. *European Journal of Obstetrics, Gynecology and Reproductive Biology, 31,* 67–74.

Fisher, N. and Pendergast, D. (1994).Effects of a muscle exercise program on exercise capacity in subjects with osteoarthritis. *Archives of Physical Medicine and Rehabilitation, 75,* 792–797.

Flegal, K.M. (1999) The obesity epidemic in children and adults: Current evidence and research issues. *Medical Science in Sports and Exercise 31 (11 Suppl),* S509–S514.

Fleming, D.T., McQuillan, G.M., Johnson, R.E., Nahmias, A.J., Aral, S.O., Lee, F.K., and St. Louis, M.E. (1997). Herpes simplex virus type 2 in the United States, 1976 to 1994. *New England Journal of Medicine, 337,* 1105–1111.

Foreyt, J.P., Poston, W.S.C., II, and Goodrick, G.K. (1996). Future directions in obesity and eating disorders. *Addictive Behavior, 21,* 767–778.

Freeman, L., Prentice, R., Clifford, C., Harlan, W., Henderson, M., and Roussow, J. (1993). Dietary fat and breast cancer: Where we are. *Journal of the National Cancer Institute, 85,* 764–765.

Freudenheim, J. L., Graham, S., Marshall, J.R., Haughey, B.P., Cholewinski, S., and Wilkinson, G. (1991). Folate intake and carcinogenesis of the colon and rectum. *International Journal of Epidemiology, 20,* 368–374.

Friedenreich, C.M. and Rohan, T.E. (1995). Physical activity and risk of breast cancer. *European Journal of Cancer Prevention, 4,* 145–151.

Gallagher, D., Visser, M., Sepulveda, D., Pierson, R.N., Harris, T., and Heymsfield, S.B. (1996). How useful is body mass index for comparison of body fatness across age, sex, and ethnic groups? *American Journal of Epidemiology, 143,* 228-39.

Gammon, M.D., Schoenberg, J.B., Britton, J.A., Kelsey, J.L., Coates, R.J., Brogan, D., Potischman, N., Swanson, C.A., Daling, J.R., Stanford, J.L., and Brinton, L.A. (1998). Recreational physical activity and breast cancer risk among women under age 45 years. *American Journal of Epidemiology, 147,* 273–280.

Giovannucci, E., Ascherio, A., Rimm, E.B., Colditz, G.A., Stampfer, M.J., and Willett, W.C. (1995). Physical activity, obesity, and risk for colon cancer and adenoma in men. *Annals of Internal Medicine, 122,* 327–334.

Giovannucci, E., Stampfer, M., Colditz, G., Hunter, D., Fuchs, C., Rosner, B., Speizer, F.E., and Willett, W.C. (1998). Multivitamin use, folate, and colon cancer in women in the Nurses' Health Study. *Annals of Internal Medicine, 129,* 517–524.

Glantz, S.A. and Parmely, W.W. (1995). Passive smoking and heart disease: Mechanism and risk. *Journal of the American Medical Association, 273,* 1047–1053.

Goldenberg, R.L., Andrews, W.W., Yuan, A.C., MacKay, H.T., and St. Louis, M.E. (1997). Sexually transmitted diseases and adverse outcomes of pregnancy. *Clinics in Perinatology, 24,* 23–41.

Goldstein, D.J. (1992). Beneficial health effects of modest weight loss. *International Journal of Obesity and Related Metabolic Disorders, 16*, 397–415.

Goodman, M.T., Hankin, J.H., Wilkens, L.R., Lyu, L.C., McDuffie, K., Liu, L.Q., and Kolonel, L.N. (1997). Diet, body size, physical activity, and the risk of endometrial cancer. *Cancer Research, 57*, 5077–5085.

Grant, B.F. (1998). The impact of a family history of alcoholism on the relationship between age at onset of alcohol use and DSM-IV alcohol dependence. *Alcohol Health and Research World, 22*, 144–148.

Grant, B.F. and Dawson, D.A. (1997). Age at onset of alcohol use and its association with DSM-IV alcohol abuse and dependence: Results from the National Longitudinal Alcohol Epidemiologic Survey. *Journal of Substance Abuse, 9*, 103–110.

Gunn, R., Montes, J., Toomey, K., Rolfs, R., Greenspan, J., Spitters, C., and Waterman, S.H. (1995). Syphilis in San Diego County 1983–1992: Crack cocaine, prostitution, and the limitations of partner notification. *Sexually Transmitted Diseases, 22*, 60–66.

Hagberg, J., Montain, S., Martin, W.I., and Ehsani, A. (1989). Effect of exercise training in 60–69-year-old persons with essential hypertension. *American Journal of Cardiology, 64*, 348–353.

Hahn, R., Teutsch, S., Rothenberg, R., and Marks, J. (1990). Excess deaths from nine chronic diseases in the United States, 1986. *Journal of the American Medical Association, 264*, 2654–2659.

Handsfield, H., Jasman, L., Roberts, P., Hanson, V.W., Kothenbeutel, R.L., and Stamm, W.E. (1986). Criteria for selective screening for Chlamydia trachomatis infection in women attending family planning clinics. *Journal of the American Medical Association, 255*, 1730–1734.

Hansson, L. (1988). Current and future strategies in the treatment of hypertension. *American Journal of Cardiology, 61*, 2C–7C.

Harwood, H., Fountain, D., and Livermore, G. (1998). *The economic costs of alcohol and drug abuse in the United States 1992* (NIH publication number 98-4327). Washington, DC: U.S. Department of Health and Human Services.

Hasin, D., Grant, B., and Harford, T. (1990). Male and female differences in liver cirrhosis mortality in the United States, 1961–1985. *Journal of Studies on Alcohol, 51*, 123–129.

Hebel, J.R., Fox, N.L., and Sexton, M. (1988). Dose-response of birth weight to various measures of maternal smoking during pregnancy. *Journal of Clinical Epidemiology, 41*, 483-489.

Hendriks, H.F., Veenstra, J., Velthuis-te Wierik, E.J., Schaafsma, G. and Kluft, C. (1994). Effect of moderate dose of alcohol with evening meal on fibrinolytic factors. *British Medical Journal, 308*, 1003-1006.

Hennekens, C.H., Buring, J.E., Manson, J.E., Stampfer, M., Rosner, B., Cook, N.R., Belanger, C., LaMotte, F., Gaziano, J.M., Ridker, P.M., Willett, W., and Peto, R. (1996). Lack of effect of long-term supplementation with beta carotene on the incidence of malignant neoplasms and cardiovascular disease. *New England Journal of Medicine, 334*, 1145–1149.

Hill, J.O. and Peters, J.C. (1998). Environmental contributions to the obesity epidemic. *Science, 280*, 1371–1374.

Hillier, S., Nugent, R., Eschenbach, D., Krohn, M., Gibbs, R., Martin, D., Cotch, M.F., Edelman, R., Pastorek, J.G. 2nd, Rao, A.V., et al. (1995). Association between bacterial vaginosis and preterm delivery of a low birth weight infant. *New England Journal of Medicine, 333,* 1737–1742.

Hillis, S., Nakashima, A., Amsterdam, L., Pfister, J., Vaughn, M., Addiss, D., Marchbanks, P.A., Owens, L.M., and Davis, J.P. (1995). The impact of a comprehensive chlamydia prevention program in Wisconsin. *Family Planning Perspectives, 27,* 108–111.

Ho, T.F., Chay, S.O., Yip, W. C., Tay, J.S., and Wong, H.B. (1983) The prevalence of obesity in Singapore primary school children. *Australian Paediatric Journal, 19,* 248–250.

Holman, C. and English, D. (1996). Ought low alcohol intake to be promoted for health reasons? *Journal of the Royal Society of Medicine, 89,* 123–129.

Howard, G., Wagenknecht, L.E., Burke, G.E., Diez-Roux, A., Evans, G.W., McGovern, P., Nieto, F.J., and Tell, G.S. (1998). Cigarette smoking and progression of atherosclerosis: The Atherosclerosis Risk in Communities (ARIC) Study. *Journal of the American Medical Association, 279,* 119–124.

Hu, F.B., Stampfer, M.J., Manson, J.E., Rimm, E., Colditz, G.A., Rosner, B.A., Hennekens, C.H. and Willett, W.C. (1997). Dietary fat intake and the risk of coronary heart disease in women. *New England Journal of Medicine, 337,* 1491–1499.

Huang, Z., Hankinson, S.E., Colditz, G.A., Stampfer, M.J., Hunter, D.J., Manson, J.E., Hennekens, C.H., Rosner, B., Speizer, F.E., and Willett, W.C. (1997). Dual effects of weight and weight gain on breast cancer risk. *Journal of the American Medical Association, 278,* 1407–1411.

Huang, Z., Willett, W.C., Manson, J.E., Rosner, B., Stampfer, M.J., Speizer, F.E., and Colditz, G.A. (1998). Body weight, weight change, and risk for hypertension in women. *Annals of Internal Medicine, 128,* 81–88.

Hubert, H.B., Feinleib, M., McNamara, P.M., and Castelli, W.P. (1983). Obesity as an independent risk factor for cardiovascular disease: A 26-year follow-up of participants in the Framingham Heart Study. *Circulation, 67,* 968–977.

IOM (Institute of Medicine) (1994). *Growing Up Tobacco Free: Preventing Nicotine Addiction in Children and Youths.* B.S. Lynch and R.J. Bonnie (Eds.) Washington, DC: National Academy Press.

IOM (Institute of Medicine) (1996). *Fetal Alcohol Syndrome: Diagnosis, epidemiology, prevention, and treatment.* K. Stratton, C. Howe, and F. Battaglia (Eds.). Washington, DC: National Academy Press.

IOM (Institute of Medicine) (1997). *The Hidden Epidemic: Confronting Sexually Transmitted Diseases.* T.R. Eng and W.T. Butler (Eds.). Washington, DC: National Academy Press.

IOM (Institute of Medicine) (2001a). *Clearing the Smoke, Assessing the Science Base for Tobacco Harm Reduction.* K. Stratton, P. Shetty, R. Wallace, and S. Bondurant (Eds.). Washington, DC: National Academy Press.

IOM (Institute of Medicine) (2001b). *Speaking of Health: Assessing Health Communication. Strategies for Diverse Populations.* C. Chrvala and S. Scrimshaw (Eds.). Washington, DC: National Academy Press.

Ip, C. and Carroll, K. (Eds.) (1997). Individual fatty acids and cancer. *American Journal of Clinical Nutrition, 65,* 1505S–1586S.

Jackson, R., Scragg, R., and Beaglehole, R . (1992). Does recent alcohol consumption reduce the risk of acute myocardial infarction and coronary death in regular drinkers? *American Journal of Epidemiology, 136*, 819–824.

Joint National Committee on Detection and Treatment of High Blood Pressure. (1993). *The Fifth Report of the Joint National Committee on Detection, Evaluation, and Treatment of High Blood Pressure.* Bethesda, MD: National Institutes of Health.

Kaplan, G., Seeman, T., Cohen, R., Knudsen, L., and Guralnik, J. (1987). Mortality among the elderly in the Alameda County Study: Behavioral and demographic risk factors. *American Journal of Public Health, 77*, 307–312.

Kaplan, G.A., Strawbridge, W.J., Cohen, R.D., and Hungerford, L.R. (1996). Natural history of leisure-time physical activity and its correlates: Associations with mortality from all causes and cardiovascular disease over 28 years. *American Journal of Epidemiology, 144*, 793–797.

Kawachi, I., Troisi, R., Rotnitzky, A., Coakley, E., and Colditz, G. (1996). Can physical activity minimize weight gain in women after smoking cessation? *American Journal of Public Health, 86*, 999–1004.

Kelder, S.H., Perry, C.L., Klepp, K.I., and Lytle, L.L. (1994). Longitudinal tracking of adolescent smoking, physical activity, and food choice behaviors. *American Journal of Public Health, 84*, 1121–1126.

Kohl, H.I., Powell, K., Gordon, N., Blair, S., and Paffenbarger, R.J. (1992). Physical activity, physical fitness, and sudden cardiac death. *Epidemiologic Reviews, 14*, 37–58.

Kopelman, P.G. (2000). Obesity as a medical problem. *Nature, 404*, 635–643.

Kramer, M.M. and Wells, C.L. (1996). Does physical activity reduce risk of estrogen-dependent cancer in women? *Medicine and Science in Sports and Exercise, 28*, 322–334

Kromeyer-Hauschild, K., Zellner, K., Jaeger, U., and Hoyer, H. (1999). Prevalence of overweight and obesity among school children in Jena (Germany). *International Journal of Obesity and Related Metabolic Disorders, 23*, 1143–1150.

Kujala, U.M., Kaprio, J., Sarna, S., and Koskenvuo, M. (1998). Relationship of leisure-time physical activity and mortality: The Finnish twin cohort. *Journal of the American Medical Association, 279*, 440–444.

Kushi, L., Fee, R., Folsom, A., Mink, P., Anderson, K., and Sellers, T. (1997). Physical activity and mortality in postmenopausal women. *Journal of the American Medical Association, 277*, 1287–1292.

LaCroix, A.Z., Guralnik, J.M., Berkman, L.F., Wallace, R.B., and Satterfield, S. (1993). Maintaining mobility in late life. II. Smoking, alcohol consumption, physical activity, and body mass index. *American Journal of Epidemiology, 137*, 858–869.

Lane, N. (1995). Exercise: a cause of osteoarthritis. *Journal of Rheumatology, 22*, 3–6.

Lanyon, L. (1987). Functional strain in bone tissue as an objective and controlling stimulus for adaptive bone remodelling. *Journal of Biomechanics, 20*, 1083–1093.

Lanyon, L. (1993). Osteocytes, strain detection, bone modeling and remodeling. *Calcified Tissue International, 53*, S102–S107.

Laumann, E. (1994). *The Social Organization of Sexuality.* Chicago: University of Chicago Press.

Le Marchand, L., Wilkens, L.R., and Mi, M.-P. (1991). Early-age body size, adult weight gain and endometrial cancer risk. *International Journal of Cancer, 48*, 807–811.

LeClere, F.B. and Wilson, J.B. (1997). Smoking behavior of recent mothers, 18–44 years of age, before and after pregnancy: United States, 1990. *Journal of the American Academy of Nurse Practitioners, 9,* 323–326.

Lee, I.-M and Paffenbarger, R.S. (1992). Change in body weight and longevity. *The Journal of the American Medical Association, 268,* 2045–2049.

Lee, I.-M, Paffenbarger, R.S., Jr., and Hsieh, C.C. (1991). Physical activity and risk of developing colorectal cancer among college alumni. *Journal of the National Cancer Institute, 83,* 1324–1329.

Lee, I.-M. (1994). Physical activity, fitness, and cancer. In C. Bouchard, R. Shephard, and T. Stephens (Eds.) *Physical Activity, Fitness, and Health: International Proceedings and Consensus Statement* (pp. 814–831). Champaign, IL: Human Kinetics.

Leon, A., Connett, J., Jacobs, D., and Rauramaa, R. (1987). Leisure-time physical activity levels and risk of coronary heart disease and death: The Multiple Risk Factor Intervention Trial. *Journal of the Amercian Medical Association, 258,* 2388–2395.

Leong, K.S. and Wilding, J.P. (1999). Obesity and diabetes. *Baillieres Best Practices Reseach Clinical Endocrinology Metabolism, 13,* 221–237.

Li, C.Q., Windsor, R.A., Perkins, L., Goldenberg, R.L., and Lowe, J.B. (1993). The impact on infant birth weight and gestational age of cotinine-validated smoking reduction during pregnancy. *Journal of the American Medical Association, 269,* 1519–1524.

Lin, B.H. and Frazao, E. (1997). Nutritional quality of foods at and away from home. *Food Review, 20,* 33–40.

Lindsted, K., Tonstad, S., and Kuzma, J. (1991). Self-report of physical activity and patterns of mortality in Seventh-Day Adventist men. *Journal of Clinical Epidemiology, 44,* 355–364.

Lissner, L., Johansson, S.E. Qvist, J., Rossner, S., and Wolk, A. (2000). Social mapping of the obesity epidemic in Sweden. *International Journal of Obesity and Related Metabolic Disorders, 24,* 801-805.

Lytle, L. and Achterberg, C. (1995). Changing the diet of America's children: What works and why? *Journal of Nutrition Education, 27,* 250–260.

Manson, J.E., Hu, F.B., Rich-Edwards, J.W., Colditz, G.A., Stampfer, M.J., Willett, W.C., Speizer, F.E., and Hennekens, C.H. (1999). A prospective study of walking compared with vigorous exercise in the prevention of coronary heart disease in women. *The New England Journal of Medicine, 341,* 650–658.

Marceau, M., Kouame, N., Lacourciere, Y., and Cleroux, J. (1993). Effects of different training intensities on 24 hour blood pressure in hypertensive subjects. *Circulation, 88,* 2803–2811.

Martinez, M.E., Giovannucci, E., Spiegelman, D., Hunter, D.J., Willett, W.C., Colditz, G.A. (1997). Leisure-time physical activity, body size, and colon cancer in women. Nurses' Health Study Research Group. *Journal of the National Cancer Institute, 89,* 948–955.

Marx, R., Aral, S., Rolfs, R., Sterk, C., and Kahn, J. (1991). Crack, sex, and STDs. *Sexually Transmitted Diseases,18,* 92–101.

Mason, J.B. and Levesque, T. (1996). Folate: effects on carcinogenesis and the potential for cancer chemoprevention. *Oncology, 10,* 1727–1736; 1742–1743.

Matsusaki, M., Ikeda, M., Tashiro, E., Koga, M., Miura, S., and Ideishi, M. (1992). Influence of workload on the antihypertensive effect of exercise. *Clinical and Experimental Pharmacology and Physiology, 19,* 471–479.

McCrory, M.A., Fuss, P.J., Hays, N.P., Vinken, A.G., Greenberg, A.S. and Roberts, S.B. (1999) Overeating in America: Association between restaurant food consumption and body fatness in healthy adult men and women ages 19 to 80. *Obesity Research, 7*, 564–571.

McCrory, M.A., Fuss, P.J., Saltzman, E., Roberts, S.B. (2000). Dietary determinants of energy intake and weight regulation in healthy adults. *Journal of Nutrition, 130 (2S Suppl)*, 276S–279S.

McGinnis, J.M. and Foege, W.H. (1993). Actual causes of death in the United States. *Journal of the American Medical Association, 270*, 2207–2212.

McTiernan, A., Stanford, J.L., Weiss, N.S., Daling, J.R., and Voigt, L.F. (1996). Occurrence of breast cancer in relation to recreational exercise in women age 50–64 years. *Epidemiology, 7*, 598–604.

Meade, T.W., Imeson, J., and Stirling, Y. (1987). Effects of changes in smoking and other characteristics on clotting factors and the risk of ischaemic heart disease. *Lancet, 2* (8566), 986–988.

Meis, P.J., Goldenberg, R.L., Mercer, G., Moawad, A., Das, A., McNellis, D., Johnson, F., Iams, J.D., Thom, E., and Andrews, W.W. (1995). The preterm prediction study: Significance of vaginal infections. *American Journal of Obstetrics and Gynecology, 173*, 1231–1235.

Mertens, I.L. and Van Gaal, L.F. (2000). Overweight, obesity, and blood pressure: The effects of modest weight reduction. *Obesity Research, 8*, 270–278.

Miller, B., Monson, B., and Norton, M. (1995). The effects of forced sexual intercourse on white female adolescents. *Child Abuse and Neglect, 19*, 1289–1301.

Minor, M. (1991). Physical activity and management of arthritis. *Annals of Behavioral Medicine, 13*, 117–124.

Mittendorf, R., Longnecker, M.P., Newcomb, P.A., Dietz, A.T., Greenberg, E.R., Bogdan, G.F., Clapp, R.W., and Willett, W.C. (1995). Strenuous physical activity in young adulthood and risk of breast cancer (United States). *Cancer Causes and Control, 6*, 347–353.

Mokdad, A., Serdula M.K., Dietz, W.H., Bowman, B.A., Marks, J.S., and Koplan J.P. (1999). The spread of the obesity epidemic in the United States, 1991–1998. *Journal of the American Medical Association, 282*, 1519–1522.

Mokdad, A., Serdula, M.K., Dietz, W.H., Bowman, B.A., Marks, J.S., and Koplan, J.P. (2000). The continuing epidemic of obesity in the United States. *Journal of the American Medical Association, 284*, 1650–1651.

Morrison, C., Schwingl, P., and Cates, W.J. (1997). Sexual behavior and cancer prevention. *Cancer Causes and Control, 8*, S21–S25.

Murphy, G.P., Mettlin, C., Menck, H., Winchester, D.P., and Davidson, A.M. (1994). National patterns of prostate cancer treatment by radical prostatectomy: Results of a survey by the American College of Surgeons Commission on Cancer. *Journal of Urology, 152*, 1817–1819.

Murray, C. and Lopez, A. (1996). *The global burden of disease.* Geneva: World Health Organization.

Must, A., Spandano, J., Coakley, E.H., Field, A.E., Colditz, G., and Dietz, W.H. (1999) The disease burden associated with overweight and obesity. *Journal of the American Medical Association, 282*, 1523–1529.

National Cancer Institute. (1986). *Cancer Control Objectives for the Nation: 1985–2000. National Cancer Institute Monographs 2.* Bethesda, MD: U.S. Department of Health and Human Services.

National Heart Lung Blood Institute Obesity Task Force (1998) Clinical guidelines on the identification, evaluation, and treatment of overweight and obesity in adults—the evidence report. *Obesity Research, 6 (suppl. 2),* 51S–209S.

National Research Council (NRC). (1989). *Diet and Health: Implications for Reducing Chronic Disease Risk.* Washington, DC: National Academy Press.

National Task Force on the Prevention and Treatment of Obesity (2000). Overweight, obesity, and health risk. *Archives of Internal Medicine, 160,* 898–904.

NCHS (National Center for Health Statistics) (1998a). *Health, United States, 1998: With Socioeconomic Status and Health Chartbook.* Hyattsville, MD: U.S. Dept. of Health and Human Services.

NCHS (National Center for Health Statistics) (1998b). *SEER Cancer Statistics Review, 1973–1995.* Bethesda, MD: National Cancer Institute.

Nelson, M.E., Fiatarone, M.A., Morganti, C.M., Trice, I., Greenberg, R.A., and Evans, W.J. (1994). Effects of high-intensity strength training on multiple risk factors for osteoporotic fractures. *Journal of the American Medical Association, 272,* 1909–1914.

NIAAA (National Institute on Alcohol Abuse and Alcoholism) (1993). *Alcohol and cancer,* (Alcohol Alert no. 21-1993). Bethesda, MD: U.S. Department of Health and Human Services.

NIH (National Institutes of Health) (1993). Methods for voluntary weight loss and control. *Annals of Internal Medicine, 119,* 764–770.

NIH (National Institutes of Health) (1994). Optimal Calcium Intake. *NIH Consensus Statement, 12,* 1–31.

NIH (National Institutes of Health) (1997a). Management of Hepatitis C. *NIH Consensus Statement, 15,* 1–41.

NIH (National Institutes of Health) (1997b). Breast Cancer Screening for Women Ages 40–49. *NIH Consensus Statement, 15,* 1–35.

O'Malley, P.M., Johnston, L.D., and Bachman, J.F. (1998). Alcohol use among adolescents. *Alcohol Health and Research World, 22,* 85–93.

Omenn, G.S., Goodman, G.E., Thornquist, M.D., Balmes, J., Cullen, M.R., Glass, A., Keogh, J.P., Meyskens, F.L., Jr., Valanis, B., Williams, J.H., Jr., Barnhart, S., Cherniack, M.G., Brodkin, C.A., and Hammar, S. (1996) Risk factors for lung cancer and for intervention effects in CARET, the Beta-Carotene and Retinol Efficacy Trial. *Journal of the National Cancer Institute, 88,* 1550–1559.

Oster, G., Thompson, D., Edelsberg, J., Bird, A.P., and Colditz, G.A. (1999). Lifetime health and economic benefits of weight loss among obese persons. *American Journal of Public Health, 89,* 1536–1542.

Owusu, W., Willett, W.C., Ascherio, A., Spiegelman, D., Rimm, E.B., Feskanich, D., and Colditz, G. (1998). Body anthropometry and the risk of hip and wrist fractures in men: results from a prospective study. *Obesity Research, 6,* 12–19.

Owusu, W., Willett, W.C., Feskanich, D., Ascherio, A., Spiegelman, D., and Colditz, G.A. (1997). Calcium intake and the incidence of forearm and hip fractures among men. *Journal of Nutrition, 127,* 1782–1787.

Paffenbarger, R., Jr., Hyde, R., Wing, A., Lee, I.-M, Jung, D., and Kampert J. (1993). The association of changes in physical activity level and other lifestyle characteristics with mortality among men. *New England Journal of Medicine*, *328*, 538–545.

Panush, R.S. and Lane, N.E. (1994). Exercise and the musculoskeletal system. *Baillieres Clinical Rheumatology*, 8, 79–102.

Pate, R.R., Long, B.J., and Heath, G. (1994). Descriptive epidemiology of physical activity in adolescents. *Pediatric Exercise Science*, 6, 434–447.

Pearl, R. (1926). *Alcohol and Longevity*. New York: Alfred A. Knopf.

Pirkle, J.L., Flegal, K.M., Bernert, J.T., Brody, D.J., Etzel, R.A., and Maurer, K.R. (1996). Exposure of the US population to environmental tobacco smoke: The Third National Health and Nutrition Examination Survey, 1988 to 1991. *Journal of the American Medical Association*, *275*, 1233–1240.

Pi-Sunyer, F.X. (1993). Medical hazards of obesity. *Annals of Internal Medicine*, *119*, 655–660.

Popham, R., Schmidt, W., and Israelstam, S. (1984). Heavy alcohol consumption and physical health problems: A review of epidemiologic evidence. In R.G. Smart, H.D. Cappell, F.B. Glaser, and Y. Israel (Eds.) *Recent Advances in Alcohol and Drug Problems*, No. 8, 149–182. New York: Plenum Press.

Potter, J. (1997). Hazards and benefits of alcohol. *New England Journal of Medicine*, *337*, 1763–1764.

Ravussin, E., Lillioja, S., Knowler, W.C., Christin, L., Freymond, D., Abbott, W.G., Boyce, V., Howard, B.V., and Bogardus, C. (1988). Reduced rate of energy expenditure as a risk factor for body-weight gain. *New England Journal of Medicine*, *318*, 467–472.

Reichman, M.E. (1994). Alcohol and breast cancer. *Alcohol Health and Research World*, *18*, 182–184.

Renaud, S., Beswick, A., Fehily, A., Sharp, P., and Elwood, P. (1992). Alcohol and platelet aggregation: the Caerphilly prospective heart disease study. *American Journal of Clinical Nutrition*, *55*, 1012–1017.

Ries, L.A.G., Miller, B.A., and Hankey, B.F (Eds.) (1996). *SEER Cancer Statistics Review, 1973–1993. National Cancer Institute*, (NIH Pub. No. 94-2789).

Rimm, E.B., Stampfer, M.J., Ascherio, A., Giovannucci, E., Colditz, G.A., and Willett, W.C. (1993). Vitamin E consumption and the risk of coronary heart disease in men. *New England Journal of Medicine*, *328*, 1450–1456.

Rimm, E.B., Stampfer, M.J., Giovannucci, E., Ascherio, A., Spiegelman, D., Colditz, G.A., and Willett, W.C. (1995). Body size and fat distribution as predictors of coronary heart disease among middle-aged and older US men. *American Journal of Epidemiology*, *141*, 1117–1127.

Rimm, E.B., Ascherio, A., Giovannucci, E., Spiegelman, D., Stampfer, M.J., and Willett, W.C. (1996). Vegetable, fruit, and cereal fiber intake and risk of coronary heart disease among men. *Journal of the American Medical Association*, *275*, 447–451

Rimm, E., Williams, P., Fosher, K., Criqui, M., and Stampfer, M. (1999). A biological basis for moderate alcohol consumption and lower coronary heart disease risk: A meta-analysis of effects on lipids and hemostatic factors. *British Medical Journal*, *319*, 1523–1528.

Rissanen, A.M., Heliovaara, M., Knekt, P., Reunanen, A., and Aromaa, A. (1991). Determinants of weight gain and overweight in adult Finns. *European Journal of Clinical Nutrition*, *45*, 419–430.

Rockhill, B., Willett, W.C., Hunter, D.J., Manson, J.E., Hankinson, S.E., Spiegelman, D., Colditz, G.A. (1998). Physical activity and breast cancer risk in a cohort of young women. *Journal of the National Cancer Institute*, 90, 1155–1160.

Roizen, J. (1993). Issues in the epidemiology of alcohol and violence. In S. Martin (Ed.) *Alcohol and Interpersonal Violence: Fostering Multi-Disciplinary Perspectives*, (NIH publication no. 93-3496). U.S. Department of Health and Human Services, Public Health Service, National Institutes of Health, National Institute on Alcohol Abuse and Alcoholism.

Rose, G. (1992). *The Strategy of Preventive Medicine*. New York: Oxford University Press.

Saadatamand, F., Stinson, F.S., Grant, B.F., and Dufour, M.C. (1997). *Surveillance Report #45: Liver Cirrhosis Mortality in the United States: 1970–1994*. Rockville, MD: NIAAA Division of Biometry and Epidemiology, Alcohol Epidemiological Data System.

Schatzkin, A., Lanze, E., Freedman, L.S., Tangrea, J., Cooper, M.R., Marshall, J.R., Murphy, P.A., Selby, J.V., Shike, M., Schade, R.R., Burt, R.W., Kikendall, J.W., and Cahill, J. (1996). The polyp prevention trial. I Rationale, design, recruitment, and baseline participant characteristics. *Cancer Epidemiology Biomarkers Prevention*, 5, 375–383.

Scheen, A.J. (2000). From obesity to diabetes: Why, when and who? *Acta Clinica Belgica*, 55, 9–15.

Schmidt, W. (1980). Effects of alcohol consumption on health. *Journal of Public Health Policy*, 1, 25–40.

Schoenborn, C. and Marano, M.. (1988). *Current estimates from the National Health Interview Survey: United States, 1987*. Washington, DC: Government Printing Office.

Scholes, D., Stergachis, A., Heidrich, F., Andrilla, H., Holmes, K., and Stamm, W. (1996). Prevention of pelvic inflammatory disease by screening for cervical chlamydia infection. *New England Journal of Medicine*, 334, 1362–1366.

Seidell, J.C. (1995). Obesity in Europe: Scaling an epidemic. *International Journal of Obesity and Related Metabolic Disorders*, 19 (Suppl. 3), S1–S4.

Selhub, J., Jacques, P.F., Bostom, A.G., D'Agostino, R.B., Wilson, P.W., Belanger, A.J., O'Leary, D.H., Wolf, P.A., Schaefer, E.J., and Rosenberg, I.H. (1995). Association between plasma homocysteine concentrations and extracranial carotid-artery stenosis. *New England Journal of Medicine*, 332, 286–291.

Severson, R.K., Nomura, A.M.Y., Grove, J.S., and Stemmermann, G.N. (1989). A prospective analysis of physical activity and cancer. *American Journal of Epidemiology*, 130, 522–529.

Shephard, R. (1993). Exercise in the prevention and treatment of cancer: an update. *Sports Medicine*, 15, 258–280.

Shephard, R., Verde, T., Thomas, S., and Shek, P. (1991). Physical activity and the immune system. *Canadian Journal of Sport Science*, 16, 163–185.

Sherman, S.E., D'Agostino, R.B., Cobb, J.L., and Kannel, W.B. (1994). Physical activity and mortality in women in the Framingham Heart Study. *American Heart Journal*, 128, 879–884.

Shetty, P.S. (1997) Obesity and physical activity. Accessed on line February 23, 2001. http://www.nutritionfoundationin.org/ARCHIVES/APR97A.HTM

Shu, X.O., Hatch, M.C., Mills, J., Clemens, J., and Susser, M. (1995). Maternal smoking, alcohol drinking, caffeine consumption, and fetal growth: results from a prospective study. *Epidemiology*, 6, 115–120.

Simmons, G., Jackson, R., Swinburn, B., and Yee, R.L. (1996). The increasing prevalence of obesity in New Zealand: Is it related to recent trends in smoking and physical activity? *New Zealand Medical Journal, 109*, 90–92.

Slattery, M., Jacobs, D., and Nichaman, M. (1989). Leisure time physical activity and coronary heart disease death: the US Railroad Study. *Circulation, 79*, 304–311.

Slattery, M.L., Schumacher, M.C., Smith, K.R., West, D.W., and Abd-Elghany, N. (1988). Physical activity, diet, and risk of colon cancer in Utah. *American Journal of Epidemiology, 128*, 989–999.

Smith-Warner, S.A., Spiegelman, D., Yaun, S.S., van den Brandt, P.A., Folsom, A.R., Goldbohm, R.A., Graham, S., Holmberg, L., Howe, G.R., Marshall, J.R., Miller, A.B., Potter, J.D., Speizer, F.E., Willett, W.C., Wolk, A., and Hunter, D.J. (1998). Alcohol and breast cancer in women: A pooled analysis of cohort studies. *Journal of the American Medical Association, 279*, 535–540.

Snow-Harter, C., Shaw, J.M., and Matkin, C.C. (1996). Physical activity and risk of osteoporosis. In R. Marcus, D. Feldman, and J. Kelsey (Eds.) *Osteoporosis* (pp. 511–528). San Diego, CA: Academic Press.

Sonnenschein, E., Toniolo, P., Terry, M.B., Bruning, P.F., Kato, I., Koenig, K.L., and Shore, R.E. (1999). Body fat distribution and obesity in pre- and postmenopausal breast cancer. *International Journal of Epidemiology 28*, 1026-1031.

St. Louis, M.E., Wasserheit, J.N., and Gayle, H.D. (1997). Editorial: Janus considers the HIV pandemic—harnessing recent advances to enhance AIDS prevention. *American Journal of Public Health, 87*, 10–12.

Stamm, W. and Holmes, K. (1990). Chlamydia trachomatis infections in the adult. In K. Holmes, P.A. Mardh, P. Sparling, P. Weisner, W. Cates, S. Lemon et al. (Eds.) *Sexually Transmitted Diseases, 2nd edition* (pp. 181–193). New York: McGraw-Hill, Inc.

Stampfer, M.J., Hennekens, C.H., Manson, J.E., Colditz, G.A., Rosner, B., and Willett, W.C. (1993). Vitamin E consumption and the risk of coronary disease in women. *New England Journal of Medicine, 328*, 1444–1449.

Steinmetz, K.A. and Potter, J.D. (1991). Vegetables, fruit, and cancer. II. Mechanisms. *Cancer Causes and Control, 2*, 427–442.

Stock, J.L., Bell, M.A., Boyer, D.K., and Connell, F.A. (1997) Adolescent pregnancy and sexual risk-taking among sexually abused girls. *Family Planning Perspective, 29*, 200-203, 227.

Strunin, L. and Hingson, R. (1992). Alcohol, drugs, and adolescent sexual behavior. *International Journal of the Addictions, 27*, 129–146.

Strunin, L. and Hingson, R. (1993). Alcohol use and risk for HIV infection. *Alcohol Health and Research World, 17*, 35–38.

Substance Abuse and Mental Health Services Administration (1993). *Race/ethnicity, socioeconomic status, and drug abuse* (No. (SMA) 93-2062). Washington, DC: U.S. Department of Health and Human Services.

Tabar, L., Faberberg, G., Day, N., and Holmberg, L. (1987). What is the optimum interval between mammographic screening examinations? An analysis based on the latest results of the Swedish two-county breast cancer screening trial. *International Journal of Cancer, 55*, 547–551.

Tanne, J. (1998). US has epidemic of sexually transmitted disease. *British Medical Journal, 317*, 1616.

Taubes, G. (1997). The breast-screening brawl. *Science, 275*, 1056–1059.

Taubes, G. (1998). As obesity rates rise, experts struggle to explain why. *Science, 280*, 1367–1368.

Thor, P., Konturek, J., Konturek, S., and Anderson, J. (1985). Role of prostaglandins in control of intestinal motility. *American Journal of Physiology, 248*, G353–G359.

Thun, M., Peto, R., Lopez, A., Monaco, J.H., Henley, S.J., Heath, C.W., Jr., and Doll, R. (1997). Alcohol consumption and mortality among middle-aged and elderly US adults. *New England Journal of Medicine, 337*, 1705–1714.

Thune, I., Brenn, T., Lund, E., and Gaard, M. (1997). Physical activity and the risk of breast cancer. *New England Journal of Medicine, 336*, 1269–1275.

Towler, B., Irwig, L., Glasziou, P., Kewenter, J., Weller, D., and Silagy, C. (1998). A systematic review of the effects of screening for colorectal cancer using the faecal occult blood test, hemoccult. *British Medical Journal, 317*, 559–565.

Troiano, R.P. and Flegal, K.M. (1998). Overweight children and adolescents: Description, epidemiology, and demographics. *Pediatrics, 101*, 497–504.

Tseng, B.S., Marsh, D.R., Hamilton, M.T., and Booth, F.W. (1995). Strength and aerobic training attenuate muscle wasting and improve resistance to the development of disability with aging. *Journal of Gerontology, 50A*, 113–119.

U.S. Preventive Services Task Force (1989). *Guide to Clinical Preventive Services*. Philadelphia: Williams and Wilkins.

U.S. Preventive Services Task Force (1996). *Guide to Clinical Preventive Services, 2nd edition*. Washington, DC: U.S. Department of Health and Human Services.

USDA (U.S. Department of Agriculture), USDHHS (U. S. Department of Health and Human Services) (1995a). *Report of the Dietary Guidelines Advisory Committee on the Dietary Guidelines for Americans*. Beltsville, MD: U.S. Department of Agriculture, Agricultural Research Service.

USDA (U.S. Department of Agriculture), USDHHS (U. S. Department of Health and Human Services) (1995b). *Nutrition and Your Health: Dietary Guidelines for Americans*. Washington, DC: U.S. Government Printing Office.

USDA (U.S. Department of Agriculture) (1995a). *Dietary Guidelines for Americans. 4th edition*. (USDA Home and Garden Bulletin No. 232). Washington, DC: U.S. Department of Agriculture, Agricultural Research Service.

USDA (U.S. Department of Agriculture) (1995b). *The Healthy Eating Index* (USDA Publication CNPP-1). Washington, DC: U.S. Department of Agriculture, Center for Nutrition Policy and Promotion.

USDA (U.S. Department of Agriculture) (1996). *USDA finds more and more Americans eat out, offers tips for making healthier food choices*. (Press release). Available: http://www.ars.usda.gov/is/pr/eatout1196.htm [1999, November 11].

USDA (U.S. Department of Agriculture) (1997). *What we eat in America: Results from the 1994–96 Continuing Survey of Food Intakes by Individuals*. (Fact Sheet). Beltsville, MD: Agricultural Research Service, Human Nutrition Research Center, Food Surveys Research Group.

USDHHS (U.S. Department of Health and Human Services) (1980) *Behavioral and Psychosocial Issues in Diabetes: Proceedings of the National Conference*. B.A. Hamburg, L.F. Lipsett, G. E. Inoff, and A.L. Drash(Eds.). NIH publication no. 80-1993

USDHHS (U.S. Department of Health and Human Services) (1983). *The Health Consequences of Smoking: Cardiovascular Disease. A Report of the Surgeon General.* Rockville, MD: Centers for Disease Control, Center for Health Promotion and Education, Office on Smoking and Health.

USDHHS (U.S. Department of Health and Human Services) (1986). *The Health Consequences of Involuntary Smoking. A Report of the Surgeon General.* Rockville, MD: Centers for Disease Control, Center for Health Promotion and Education, Office on Smoking and Health.

USDHHS (U.S. Department of Health and Human Services) (1988a). *The Health Consequences of Smoking: Nicotine Addiction: A Report of the Surgeon General.* (DHHS publication no. (CDC) 88-8406). Rockville, MD: Centers for Disease Control, Center for Health Promotion and Education, Office on Smoking and Health.

USDHHS (U.S. Department of Health and Human Services) (1988b). *The Surgeon General's Report on Nutrition and Health.* (DHHS publication no. (PHS) 88-050210). Washington, DC: Public Health Service.

USDHHS (U.S. Department of Health and Human Services) (1989). *Reducing the Health Consequences of Smoking: 25 Years of Progress. A Report of the Surgeon General.* (DHHS publication no. (CDC) 89-8411). Atlanta, GA: Centers for Disease Control, National Center for Chronic Disease Prevention and Health Promotion, Office of Smoking and Health.

USDHHS (U.S. Department of Health and Human Services) (1990). *The Health Benefits of Smoking Cessation. A Report of the Surgeon General.* (DHHS publication no. (CDC) 90-8416). Rockville, MD: Centers for Disease Control, National Center for Chronic Disease Prevention and Health Promotion, Office on Smoking and Health.

USDHHS (U.S. Department of Health and Human Services) (1993). *Eighth Special Report to Congress on Alcohol And Health.* Bethesda, MD: National Institutes of Health, National Institute on Alcohol Abuse and Alcoholism.

USDHHS (U.S. Department of Health and Human Services) (1996). *Physical Activity and Health: A Report of the Surgeon General.* Atlanta, GA: Centers for Disease Control and Prevention, National Center for Chronic Disease Prevention and Health Promotion.

USDHHS (U.S. Department of Health and Human Services) (1997a). *Ninth Special Report to the U.S. Congress on Alcohol and Health from the Secretary of Human Services* (NIH publication no. 97-4017). Bethesda, MD: National Institutes of Health, National Institute on Alcohol Abuse and Alcoholism.

USDHHS (U.S. Department of Health and Human Services) (1997b). *Sexually Transmitted Disease Surveillance, 1996.* Atlanta, GA: Centers for Disease Control and Prevention, Division of STD Prevention.

USDHHS (U.S. Department of Health and Human Services) (2000). *Healthy People 2010: Understanding and improving health.* Washington, DC: U.S. Department of Health and Human Services.

USDHHS (U.S. Department of Health and Human Services). (1994). *Preventing Tobacco Use Among Young People. A Report of the Surgeon General.* Atlanta, GA: Centers for Disease Control, National Center for Chronic Disease Prevention and Health Promotion, Office on Smoking and Health.

USDHHS (U.S. Department of Health and Human Services). (1995). *The Physicians'* *Guide to Helping Patients with Alcohol Problems* (NIH publication no. 95-3769). Bethesda, MD: National Institutes of Health, National Institute on Alcohol Abuse and Alcoholism.

USEPA (U.S. Environmental Protection Agency) (1992). *Respiratory Health Effects of* *Passive Smoking: Lung Cancer and Other Disorders.* (EPA publication no. EPA/600/6-90/006F). Washington, DC: U.S. Government Printing Office.

Ventura, S.J., Peters, K.D., Martin, J.A., and Maurer, J.D. (1997). Births and deaths: United States, 1996. *Monthly Vital Statistics Report, 46.* Hyattsville, MD: National Center for Health Statistics.

Walsh, R.A. (1994). Effects of maternal smoking on adverse pregnancy outcomes: examination of the criteria of causation. *Human Biology, 66,* 1059–1092.

Wasson, J., Cushman, C., Bruskewitz, R., Littenberg, B., Mulley, A.G., Jr., and Wennberg, J.E. (1993). A structured literature review of treatment for localized prostate cancer. *Archives of Family Medicine, 2,* 487–493.

Whittemore, A.S., Wu-Williams, A.H., Lee, M., Zheng, S., Gallagher, R.P., Jiao, D.A., Zhou, L., Wang, X.H., Chen, K., Jung, D., Teh, C-Z., Chengde, L., Yao, X.J., Paffenbarger, R.S., Jr., and Henderson, B.E. (1990). Diet, physical activity and colorectal cancer among Chinese in North America and China. *Journal of the National Cancer Institute, 82,* 915–926.

Willett, W.C. (1998). Nutritional Epidemiology. In K.J. Rothman and S. Greenland (Eds.) *Modern Epidemiology* (pp. 623–642). Philadelphia: Lippincott-Raven Publishers.

Willett, W.C. and Ascherio, A. (1994). Trans fatty acids: Are the effects only marginal? *American Journal of Public Health, 84,* 722–724.

Willett, W.C., Manson, J.E., Stampfer, M.J., Colditz, G.A., Rosner, B., Speizer, F.E., and Hennekens, C.H. (1995). Weight, weight change, and coronary heart disease in women: Risk within the 'normal' weight range. *The Journal of the American Medical Association, 273,* 461–465.

Willett, W.C., Stampfer, M.J., Manson, J.E., Colditz, G.A., Speizer, F.E., Rosner, B.A., Sampson, L.A., and Hennekens, C.H. (1993). Intake of trans fatty acids and risk of coronary heart disease among women. *Lancet, 341,* 581–585.

Wu, A.H., Paganini-Hill, A., Ross, R.K., and Henderson, B.E. (1987). Alcohol, physical activity and other risk factors for colorectal cancer: a prospective study. *British Journal of Cancer, 55,* 687–694.

Zakhari, S. (1997). Alcohol and the cardiovascular system: Molecular mechanisms for beneficial and harmful action. *Alcohol Health and Research World, 21,* 21–29.

Ziegler, R.G., Mayne, S.T., and Swanson, C.A. (1996). Nutrition and lung cancer. *Cancer Causes and Control, 7,* 157–177.

4

Social Risk Factors

Among the greatest advances in elucidating the determinants of disease over the past two decades has been the identification of social and psychological conditions that seem to influence morbidity and mortality directly through physiological processes and indirectly via behavioral pathways. This chapter examines a set of sociopsychological factors for which substantial evidence exists for effects on health outcomes: socioeconomic status; social support and networks; occupational stress, unemployment, and retirement; social cohesion and social capital, and religious belief. Although it was previously believed that some diseases were caused by psychological states with little biological basis and that others were purely "physical," it is now understood that in almost all cases that distinction is false. Most psychosomatic diseases involve various genetic and environmental determinants, and all states of health and disease are influenced to some extent by psychosocial conditions. Disorders rarely have discrete causes.

This chapter reviews the evidence accumulated during the 1980s and 1990s, identifying strengths and weaknesses and identifying areas for future investigations as they relate to social conditions that are risk related or health promoting.

SOCIOECONOMIC STATUS

A strong and consistent finding of epidemiologic research is that there are health differences among socioeconomic groups. Lower mortality, morbidity, and disability rates among socioeconomically advantaged people have been observed for hundreds of years and have been replicated using various indicators of socioeconomic status (SES) and multiple disease outcomes (Kaplan and Keil, 1993; Syme and Berkman, 1976). Educational differentials in mortality have increased over the past three decades in this country (Feldman et al., 1989; Pappas et al., 1993; Tyroler et al., 1993). Moreover, formal comparisons of the mortality differences associated with education show that relationships between educational attainment and mortality are stronger in the United States than they are in most European countries (Kunst and Mackenbach, 1994).

Results from the National Longitudinal Mortality Study (NLMS) are representative of recent research that has documented the link between SES and health. The NLMS is a large national database on the U.S. noninstitutionalized population assembled from survey information collected between 1978 and 1985; deaths were ascertained using the National Death Index for 1979–1989 (Sorlie et al., 1995). Mortality was strongly associated with education, income, and occupation (Rogot et al., 1992; Sorlie et al., 1992, 1995). For example, among those aged 25–64, white men and women with 0–4 total years of education had age-adjusted death rates that were 66% and 44% higher, respectively, than those with 5 or more years of college. For African American men and women, the corresponding increases in mortality were 73% and 78%, respectively. Similar findings were observed when income was used as a proxy for SES. Age-adjusted death rates among white men and women with annual family incomes of less than $5,000 were 80% and 30% higher, respectively, than were those among their counterparts in households with incomes of $50,000 or more. As with education, even greater differentials were seen among African Americans: men in African American households earning less than $5,000 were twice as likely to die during follow-up than were those in families earning $50,000 or more. Poor African American women were 80% more likely to die than were wealthier women.

Socioeconomic differentials in mortality have been observed for many causes of death. The Multiple Risk Factor Intervention Trial (MRFIT) followed 320,909 white and African American men for 16 years (Davey Smith et al., 1996a,b). Median family income in ZIP code of residence was predictive of death from a variety of medical conditions in analyses adjusted for age, smoking status, blood pressure, serum cholesterol, previous myocardial infarction, and treatment for diabetes.

To assess the 11-year mortality risk associated with individual family income, Anderson et al. (1997) linked NLMS data to census tract information on income for 239,187 persons. Among persons aged 25-64, the mortality rate ratios (that is, the ratio of mortality rate at the low income to the mortality rate at high income) associated with individual family income were 2.03 for white men, 2.10 for African American men, 1.61 for white women, and 1.92 for African American women. The rate ratios associated with median census tract income, adjusting for individual-level income, were 1.26 for white men, 1.49 for African American men, 1.61 for white women, and 1.30 for African American women. Although family income had a stronger association with mortality than did median census tract income, the results indicate that community SES makes an independent contribution to mortality.

With regard to specific disease outcomes, the relationship between SES and cardiovascular disease has received the most attention. SES appears to be an important factor in the development and progression of cardiovascular disease (Kaplan and Keil, 1993), the leading cause of death in this country (National Center for Health Statistics, 1992). The British Whitehall study of civil servants found that those in the lowest grades of employment were at highest risk for heart disease (Marmot et al., 1991) and that low levels of personal control in the work environment could explain much of this association (Bosma et al., 1997; Marmot et al., 1997).

Perhaps the most striking finding that emerges from these analyses is the graded and continuous nature of the association between income and mortality, with differences persisting well into the middle-class range of incomes. This phenomenon also has been observed in several European investigations (Blane et al., 1997; Davey Smith et al., 1990; Macintyre, 1997; Macintyre et al., 1998). For example, in the Whitehall longitudinal studies (Davey Smith et al., 1990; Marmot et al., 1991), each employment grade had worse health and higher mortality than did the grade above it. Executive-grade civil servants (level 2) are not poor by any absolute standard, but they had higher mortality than did administrators (level 1). The fact that socioeconomic differences in health are not confined to segments of the population that are materially deprived in the conventional sense argues against an interpretation of socioeconomic differences simply as a function of absolute poverty. The pathways involved are likely to be complex; diverse explanations for the socioeconomic gradient in health have been proposed and examined.

Material Conditions

SES is clearly associated with the material condition of a person's life. However, there are many examples of people who live in relative deprivation who exhibit greater disease resistance and general health than would be expected from their circumstances. Access to medical care and exposure to specific environmental conditions must be considered.

Distribution of Medical Care

There is ample evidence that SES is strongly related to access to and quality of preventive care, ambulatory care, and high-technology procedures (Kaplan and Keil, 1993). It appears unlikely, however, that these factors account for more than a small percentage of the variation. Because causes of death that are purportedly "not amenable" to medical care show socioeconomic gradients similar to those of potentially treatable causes (Davey Smith et al., 1996a; Mackenbach et al., 1989), it has been argued that differential access to healthcare programs and services is not entirely responsible for socioeconomic differentials in health (Wilkinson, 1996).

Toxic Physical Environments

Despite enormous improvements in sanitary engineering, which have contributed to the sharp increase in life expectancy observed among all socioeconomic groups during the past century, the socioeconomic gradient in health status persists. It has been proposed that the SES gap is still attributable to effects of crowded and unsanitary housing, air and water pollution, inadequate food supply, poor working conditions, and other such deficits that disproportionately affect those in the lower socioeconomic strata. Studies that incorporate assessments of material deprivation and the physical environment will be important to sort out the degree to which this is an important pathway. However, inasmuch as the gradient in morbidity and mortality persists even between middle-class and well-to-do men and women and even in societies in which material conditions are very good, it seems unlikely that gradients are solely the result of these material circumstances.

Psychosocial Risk Factors

Considerable evidence links low SES to adverse psychosocial conditions. People who work in low-paid jobs are not only the most materially disadvantaged, but they also have higher job and financial insecurity; experience more unemployment, work injury, lack of control, and other social and environmental stressors; report fewer social supports; and more frequently have a cynically hostile or fatalistic outlook (Adler et al., 1994; Berkman and Syme, 1979; Bosma et al., 1997; House et al., 1988; Karasek and Theorell, 1990).

Psychosocial Context

The most successful interventions of the many clinical trials incorporated elements of social or organizational change to modify individual behavioral risk factors, such as alcohol and tobacco consumption, diet, and physical activity. Most behaviors are not randomly distributed in the population, but rather are socially patterned and often cluster with one another. Thus, many people who drink also smoke cigarettes, and those who follow health-promoting dietary practices also tend to be physically active. People who are poor, have low levels of education, or are socially isolated are more likely to engage in a wide array of risk-related behaviors and less likely to engage in health-promoting ones (Adler et al., 1994; Matthews et al., 1989). This patterned behavioral response led Link and Phelan (1995) to speak of situations that place individuals "at risk of risks."

Understanding why "poor people behave poorly" (Lynch et al., 1997a) requires recognition that specific behaviors once thought of as falling exclusively within the realm of individual choice occur in a social context. The social environment influences behavior by shaping norms; enforcing patterns of social control (which can be health promoting or health damaging); providing or not providing environmental opportunities to engage in particular behaviors; and reducing or producing stress, for which engaging in specific behaviors might be an effective short-term coping strategy (Berkman and Kawachi, 2000). Environments, especially social contexts, place constraints on individual choice. Incorporating the social context into behavioral interventions led to a new array of clinical trials that take advantage of communities, schools, and worksites to achieve behavioral change (see Sorensen et al., 1998; Chapter 6, this volume).

Relationship to Health-Related Behaviors and Biological Risk Factors

Given the fact that socioeconomic stressors are disproportionately concentrated in lower socioeconomic groups (McLeod and Kessler, 1990), it is not surprising that many investigations indicate an inverse relationship between SES and adverse health behaviors (such as smoking, physical inactivity, less nutritious diets, and excessive alcohol consumption), and between SES and biological risk factors (such as high blood pressure, high serum cholesterol and fibrinogen, and obesity; Davey Smith et al., 1996a,b; Kaplan and Keil, 1993; Lynch et al., 1997a; Marmot et al., 1991). Statistical adjustment for such biological and behavioral risk factors generally leads to attenuation of excess mortality among lower groups. However, socioeconomic gradients still persist (Davey Smith et al., 1996a,b; 1990; Haan et al., 1987; Marmot et al., 1991). For example, in the MRFIT study (Davey Smith et al., 1996a,b), stratification by smoking status revealed similar gradients in income and coronary heart disease for smokers and nonsmokers.

Conceptualization and Measurement of SES

Commonly used measures of SES in epidemiologic studies include education, income, and occupation (Liberatos et al., 1988; Lynch and Kaplan, 2000; Morgenstern, 1985), but some work suggests that additional measures of wealth might be important and that increased attention should be paid to gender and life course issues (Anderson and Armstead, 1995; Lynch and Kaplan, 2000). In the social sciences, theoretical perspectives focus on different aspects of stratification. Social class as described by Weber (1946) has three domains: (1) class, by which he meant ownership and economic resources; (2) status, by which he meant prestige, community ranking, or honor; and (3) political power. This tripartite definition has led many social scientists to identify multiple indicators of social class. In the United States, these three domains are often assessed by income or wealth to tap economic resources and occupational rankings based on prestige to tap status. Political power per se is rarely assessed. Because occupationally based scales are often unavailable in the United States, most measures are based on income and education. In contrast, in Europe occupationally based scales are the most common indicators of social class. Common measures in Europe include the Erikson-Goldthorpe-Portocarero scheme. This scheme was developed to facilitate international comparisons of social stratification. It is still rarely used in the United States because routine data on the key elements are not commonly collected. (Kunst et al., 1998). Several reviews have outlined common measures of SES in the United States (Berkman and MacIntrye, 1997).

It is possible that different aspects of SES may lead to poor health through different pathways. For instance, income may influence outcomes very directly through material resources whereas occupational-based rankings may impact job-related psychosocial stresses and education may influence health-related behaviors. However, because these aspects of SES are usually highly correlated with each other, these distinct pathways are extremely difficult to identify. Thus, disentangling distinct effects of education or income for example remains a major challenge.

Almost all studies of income and health have measured income at only one point in adulthood. That fails to capture the health effects of sustained exposure to low income, to account for transitions into and out of low-income groups, or to allow for exploration of dynamic interrelationships between health and income. There is considerable volatility in income during adulthood: 26–39% of U.S. residents aged 45–65 experience income reductions of at least 50% in some 11-year period (Duncan et al., 1996), suggesting a need to measure income at multiple points in time (for example, through socioeconomic trajectories or careers). Lynch et al. (1997b) found significantly worse health outcomes among persons with sustained, as opposed to transitory, economic hardship.

General Susceptibility versus Disease Specificity

It has been argued that unfavorable socioeconomic position increases susceptibility to disease in general, and potential biological mechanisms of stress-related immune suppression and neuroendocrine activation have been postulated to account for this phenomenon (McEwen, 1998). However, within the general pattern of increased mortality, there is marked heterogeneity of the strength of the associations observed (Davey Smith et al., 1996a, b). Results from an examination of site-specific cancer mortality (Davey Smith et al., 1991) suggest that, although general susceptibility might be operative, research on disease-specific pathways should not be neglected.

Reverse Causation and Social Selection

The idea that poor health might lead to a worsening of SES rather than the other way around suggests a "reverse-causation" or "social-selection" hypothesis. If the less healthy are more likely to experience downward social mobility or are less likely to be upwardly mobile, the result will be a concentration of ill people in the lower social classes. Although evidence of reverse causation is strong for some conditions (most notably schizophrenia and other severe mental illnesses), such selection appears to have a relatively small influence on the overall socioeconomic gradient of health (Black et al., 1988; Marmot et al., 1995, 1987). Commonly cited evidence against the social-selection hypothesis includes the tendency of educational attainment, a measure not affected by illness that occurs after early adulthood, to be as strongly predictive of adult health outcomes as are other SES measures. Moreover, in longitudinal surveys, SES-related mortality differentials generated by social selection would be greatest early in the follow-up period if social selection were operative, but this has not been observed (Fox et al., 1985).

It is nevertheless possible that conditions operating at an early age— say between birth and entry into the workforce—are important in shaping social positions observed in adulthood and in influencing adult health directly (Lynch et al., 1997a). Early influences might shape developmental biology (Chapter 2), the lives people lead, and the environments in which they live and work as adults.

SOCIAL NETWORKS AND SOCIAL SUPPORT

A social network is the web of social relationships that surround an individual and the structural characteristics of that web. Many researchers have measured social networks in a general way that taps the degree to which an individual is integrated into society. Examples include the degree to which an individual participates in voluntary associations or the number of friends a person has. Social support is a distinct function of social relationships; it is clear that not all relationships are supportive. Other functions of networks can influence health outcomes, including patterns of social influence, social engagement, and person-to-person contacts (which can promote the spread of infectious diseases; Berkman and Glass, 2000).

People form ties with others from the moment they are born. The survival of newborns depends on their attachment to and nurturance by others over an extended period (Baumeister and Leary, 1995). The need to belong does not stop in infancy, but rather affiliation and nurture and social relationships are essential for physical and psychological well-being throughout life (Cohen and Syme, 1985; Seeman, 1996). Affirmative social interactions—those that satisfy the need for autonomy, competence, and relatedness—are related to feeling understood and appreciated (Reis and Judd, 2000). Cognitive or interpersonal deficits in childhood and adolescence can further impair individual ability to acquire the social and instrumental skills people need to avoid life stressors and achieve age-appropriate social roles.

Positive Social Relations

Initial assessments of social isolation (or integration) emphasized objective features of social support, such as the size or density of one's social network and frequency of contact with relatives and friends. Subsequent studies elaborated more subjective or functional aspects, such as the perception of emotional and instrumental support or the amount of assistance provided by others (Cohen, 1988; Cohen and Wills, 1985; Vaux, 1988). Research on social support has increasingly differentiated into specific substantive areas, such as the role of social support in stress and coping (Thoits, 1995), social support in family relationships (Pierce et al., 1996), social support and personality (Pierce et al., 1997), and social support in differential survival from particular health challenges, such as myocardial infarction (e.g., Ruberman et al., 1984), or cancer (e.g., Spiegel et al., 1989).

Buffering

One concept used to explain how social support affects health is buffering. For example, stress-induced decrements in immune function have been shown by research on medical students undergoing exams, but the decline was particularly pronounced for those lacking social buffers—those who reported being lonely (Glaser et al., 1992; Kiecolt-Glaser et al., 1994). Research involving people going through major life transitions (such as loss of a spouse or birth of a child) illustrates that social networks and social support influence the coping process and buffer the effects of stressors on health (Hirsch and Dubois, 1992; Rhodes et al., 1994; Walker et al., 1977).

Promoting Health-Enhancing Behaviors

Other research examines possible mechanisms, such as the extent to which significant others promote and encourage positive health practices (Berkman, 1995; Taylor et al., 1997). For example, social integration could enhance the beneficial effects of restorative behaviors, such as sleep. Sleep is a quintessential active restoration performed without immediate social contact. Although lonely individuals in one study slept as many hours as did socially embedded people, responses to the Pittsburgh Sleep Quality Index (Buysse et al., 1989) revealed that lonely individuals reported poorer sleep quality, longer sleep latency, and greater daytime dysfunction due to sleepiness than did socially embedded individuals. Other data confirm that lonely people sleep less efficiently, take slightly longer to fall asleep, evidence longer rapid eye movement latency, and awaken more frequently during the night than do embedded individuals (Cacioppo et al., 2000). Another study (Lewis and Rook, 1999) found that control in social relationships (that is, influencing and regulating social networks) was associated with more health-enhancing behavior, but with greater distress.

Altering Physiological Processes

Extensive research explores the underlying physiological roots through which social ties influence health (e.g., Berkman, 1995; Cohen and Herbert, 1996; Kang et al., 1998; Kiecolt-Glaser et al., 1994; Seeman, 1996; Seeman and McEwen, 1996; Uchino et al., 1996). Meta-analyses of the experimental literature support the hypothesis that perceived social isolation is associated with physiological adjustments, with the most reliable effects found for blood pressure, catecholamines, and aspects of cellular and humoral immune function (Seeman and McEwen, 1996; Uchino et al., 1996). In a study of carotid arthrosclerosis in middle-aged men, higher intima media thickness of the carotid artery was found in those who lived alone than in those who cohabited—even after controlling for age, health status, education, saturated fat consumption, and smoking (Helminen et al., 1995). The biological effects of loneliness are evident even after controlling for common individual personality differences (e.g., extraversion, neuroticism) in intervention studies designed to reduce social isolation and improve physiological functioning (Cacioppo et al., 2000; Uchino et al., 1996). People's beliefs, attitudes, and values pertaining to others appear to be especially important, as subjective indices of social isolation have been found to be more powerful predictors of stress and health than are objective indices (e.g., Uchino et al., 1996).

The relationship between social ties and the onset and progression of infectious disease has received growing attention recently. Socially sup- portive relationships appear to have beneficial effects on primary immune system parameters that regulate host resistance (Esterling et al., 1996; Kiecolt-Glaser et al., 1994; Uchino et al., 1996). Cohen et al. (1997) tested their hypothesis that diversity of network ties is related to suscepti- bility to cold. Participants were given nasal drops containing rhinovirus or placebo and monitored for the development of colds. Those who re- ported more types of social ties (e.g., spouse, parent, friend, workmate, and so on) were less susceptible to colds, produced less mucus, fought infection more efficiently, and shed less virus; moreover, susceptibility to infection decreased in a linear manner with increasing diversity of the social network. Further evidence that social ties mediate primary immune system parameters comes from a study by Theorell et al. (1995), who tracked the decline in the count of CD4 cells of the immune system over a 5-year period among a cohort of HIV-infected men in Sweden. The count declined more rapidly in men who reported lower "availability of attach- ments" at baseline.

Although research on the physiological pathways that could link net- works to health is just developing, researchers have documented associa- tions among social integration and social support and several physiologi- cal mechanisms related to health outcomes, including cardiovascular reactivity and neuroendocrine and immune function (Seeman, 1996; Uchino et al., 1996). In one of the few observational studies to link social support and neuroendocrine measures in humans, Seeman et al. (1994) found that older men and women who reported more frequent emotional support excreted less epinephrine, norepinephrine, and cortisol in their urine.

Several experimental studies have investigated the link between the social relationship and cardiovascular reactivity. Kamarck et al. (1990) found that participants asked to complete a laboratory task alone exhib- ited significantly greater systolic blood pressure and heart rate reactivity than did those who were allowed to have a friend with them. Lepore et al. (1993) varied the degree of social support available to participants asked to give a speech. The three social conditions were to give the speech alone, to give it in the presence of a nonsupportive confederate, and to give it in the presence of a supportive confederate. Participants in the last group exhibited the smallest increase in systolic pressure, followed by par- ticipants who gave their speeches alone. Links between neuroendocrine

measures, cardiovascular reactivity, and blood pressure and social relationships might constitute potential pathways by which social networks, support, and engagement influence important health outcomes.

Establishing and Maintaining Long-Term Resources

Researchers looking at attachment in early and later life and at close
personal relationships have described some features of deep, meaningful,
loving human connections (Ryff and Singer, 2000). Numerous investigators have examined the nature of affect in intimate relationships, its development over time, and related expressions of emotion during marital
interaction (e.g., Carstensen et al., 1995, 1996; Gottman, 1994; Gottman
and Levenson, 1992). Collectively, research on interpersonal flourishing
gives greater attention to the emotional upside of significant social relationships and their consequences for improved health (see Ryff and Singer,
1998, 2000; Taylor et al., 2000). Individuals on positive relationship pathways (positive ties with parents during childhood, intimate ties with
spouse in adulthood) are less likely to show high allostatic load than are
people on negative relationship pathways, and such relational strengths
appear to offer protection against cumulative economic adversity (Singer
and Ryff, 1999).

Negative Social Relations

Isolation

Over the past 20 years, 13 large prospective cohort studies in the
United States, Scandinavia, and Japan have shown that people who are
isolated or disconnected from others are at increased risk of dying prematurely. For example, in a study in Alameda County, California (Berkman
and Syme, 1979), men and women who had few ties to others (assessed
using an index of contacts with friends and relatives, marital status, and
church and group membership) were 1.9–3.1 times more likely to die in a
9-year follow-up period (1965–1974) than were those who had many more
contacts. The relative risks[1] associated with social isolation were not cen-

---

[1]Relative risk is the proportion of diseased people among those exposed to the relevant
risk factor divided by the proportion of diseased people among those not exposed to the
risk factor.

tered in one cause of death. Those who had few social ties were at increased risk of dying from ischemic heart disease; cerebrovascular and circulatory disease; cancer; and a final category that included respiratory, gastrointestinal, and all other causes of death. Several other studies, both in the United States and across the world, have replicated the basic observation that social isolation increases the relative risk of mortality (Berkman, 1995; Berkman and Kawachi, 2000; Blazer, 1982; Cohen, 1988; House et al., 1982, 1988; Kaplan et al., 1988; Orth-Gomer and Johnson, 1987; Pennix et al., 1997; Schoenbach et al., 1986; Seeman et al., 1988, 1993, 1996; Sugisawa et al., 1994; Welin et al., 1985).

Powerful epidemiologic evidence consistently supports the notion that social ties, especially intimate ties and emotional support provided by them, promote increased survival and better prognosis among people with serious cardiovascular disease (Berkman et al., 1992; Case et al., 1992; Krumholz et al., 1998; Orth-Gomer et al., 1988; Oxman et al., 1995; Ruberman et al., 1984; Williams et al., 1992). Most studies find that social networks are related more strongly to mortality than to the incidence of myocardial infarction (MI) (Kawachi et al., 1996; Reed et al., 1983; Vogt et al., 1992; but see Orth-Gomer et al., 1993). A similar pattern of associations between social integration and incidence versus recovery from stroke has been observed (Colantonio et al., 1992, 1993; Friedland and McColl, 1987; Glass and Maddox, 1992; McLeroy et al., 1984; Morris et al., 1993). For example, although social integration was not associated with the incidence of stroke in an elderly cohort (Colantonio et al., 1992), poststroke recovery after 6 months was significantly related to prestroke social integration (Colantonio et al., 1993). Socially isolated people exhibited worse functional status 6 months after a stroke (Glass et al., 1993), as measured by impairments in activities of daily living and frequency of nursing home placement.

Adverse Interactions

Being part of a social network, however, can have harmful as well as positive consequences, because the value to the individual of such ties depends upon the character of that network as well as on the strength of those ties. Membership in networks, for example, provides access to domestic, economic, and informational resources (Uehara, 1990). If a person is tied to a tightly knit group, the resources available through that group, especially informational resources, could be limited. Sometimes people who have weak ties have access to more resources than those who are tightly connected to a group with limited means (Pescosolido, 1986, 1991; Uehara, 1990).

Furthermore, not all social connections are beneficial. While both positive and negative interactions can affect psychological well-being, the negative interactions are generally more strongly linked (Ingersoll-Dayton et al., 1997; Rook, 1984). Studies of adult relationships have examined not only their contributions to intimacy (Berscheid and Reis, 1998) and well-being (Meyers and Diener, 1995; Sternberg and Hojat, 1997), but also their adverse consequences: divorce and bereavement (Kiecolt-Glaser et al., 1998), poor interpersonal relationships (Baumeister and Leary, 1995), and dispositional and cognitive factors that contribute to loneliness and depression (Marangoni and Ickes, 1989). One study of older adults in long-term marriages, for example, showed that 30 minutes of conflict discussion was associated with changes in cortisol, adrenocorticotropic hormone, and norepinephrine in women, but not in men (Kiecolt-Glaser et al., 1997). Other studies linked marital conflict and high blood pressure (Ewart et al., 1991), elevated plasma catecholamine concentrations (Malarkey et al., 1994), and autonomic activation (Levenson et al., 1993). Caregivers of relatives with progressive dementia are characterized by impaired wound-healing compared with controls matched for age and family income (Kiecolt-Glaser et al., 1995, 1998). Social conflicts have been shown to increase susceptibility to infection (Cohen et al., 1998; Glaser et al., 1999).

Family characteristics that could undermine the health of children and adolescents include a family environment that is conflictual, angry, violent, or abusive; parent/child relationships that are unresponsive and lacking in cohesiveness, warmth, and emotional support; and parenting styles that are either overly controlling and dominating or that offer little imposition of rules and structure (Taylor et al., 1997). Long-term exposure to such conditions contributes to deficits in emotional understanding, difficulties with appropriate expression of emotion, increased emotional reactivity to conflict, and maladaptive coping strategies for managing stressful events in general.

OCCUPATIONAL FACTORS

The workplace is an important source of adverse and protective health effects alike. A consistent body of research has emerged over the past two decades to show that work conditions (job demands, control, latitude) and trends in work, such as downsizing and unemployment, are related to health (Karasek and Theorell, 1990). Workplace investigations also have identified protective factors—such as the ability to develop social ties at work—that help guard against the adverse mental and health effects of work stress (Buunk and Verhoeven, 1991).

Job Strain

Since Karasek introduced the "demand/control" model to characterize the psychosocial work environment (Karasek and Theorell, 1990), many empirical studies have tested the predictive validity of the model with respect to the physical health of workers. Job strain—the combination of a psychologically demanding workplace and low job control—is hypothesized as leading to adverse health outcomes. Studies using both dimensions generally have provided better predictions than studies using either dimension alone. However, job control—the opportunity to use and develop skills and to exert authority over workplace decisions— emerged as the more robust component of a health-promoting work environment.

In reviewing the literature on the relationship between job strain and cardiovascular disease, Schnall et al. (1994) reported that 17 of 25 studies found that lack of job control significantly predicted adverse outcomes, whereas only 8 of 23 studies found that high psychological demands did so. Studies published in the past 5 years bolster the importance of job control (for example, Bosma et al., 1997, 1998; Johnson et al., 1996; North et al., 1996; Theorell et al., 1998). A recent population-based case/control study found that low job control was associated with incidence of first MI among employed Swedish men 45–64 years old, although the association was somewhat weakened by adjustment for social class (blue- or white-collar status; Theorell et al., 1998). A decrease in job control during the 10 years preceding MI was also significantly predictive of increased cardiovascular risk, as was job strain, even after adjustment for multiple covariates, including history of chest pain and shift, night, or overtime work. High psychological demand did not consistently predict MI onset in this cohort. In agreement with findings from other studies, the relationships between low job control and MI were strongest among younger respondents (under 55 years old) and among blue-collar workers. Empirical evidence of the adverse effect of low job control among women is sparse because few studies have been done among women.

Siegrist (1996) recently developed an effort/reward imbalance model of job stress that postulates that high-effort conditions (characterized by high job demands and psychological immersion in work) are balanced against three sources of rewards: money, esteem, and "occupational-status control" (promotion prospects and job security). The emphasis is on the balance between work-related costs and gains rather than on specific job task characteristics, as in the demand/control model. Effort/reward imbalance and low job control were independent predictors of incident coronary heart disease among British civil servants in models adjusted for age, employment grade, negative affectivity, and coronary risk profile (Bosma et al., 1998). Relative risk ratios for high-effort and low-reward conditions ranged from 2.59 to 3.63, depending on sex and specific coronary end point.

Unemployment

Several longitudinal epidemiologic studies have examined the relationship between unemployment and mortality (Kasl and Jones, 2000). Three reports from a national survey by the British Office of Population Censuses and Surveys were based on a 10-year follow-up of British men (Moser et al., 1984, 1986, 1987). Men seeking work during the week before the 1971 census had a higher age-adjusted mortality than would be expected from the rates in the total sample; after adjustment for social class, the standardized mortality ratio[2] (SMR) was 121. Particularly high mortality was observed for suicide (SMR, 169). Statistical adjustment for possible prior differences in health status was not possible. A shorter follow-up of men after the 1981 census confirmed the earlier findings but obtained a somewhat lower adjusted SMR of 112.

Additional studies using similar methods have been conducted in Sweden (Stefansson, 1991), Finland (Martikainen, 1990), Denmark (Iversen et al., 1987), and Italy (Costa and Segnan, 1987). Unemployment appears to be associated with SMRs of 150–200, adjusted for age and social class. Cause-specific analyses suggest that suicides, accidents, vio-

---

[2]Standardized mortality ratio is the ratio of the observed to the expected number of deaths multiplied by 100.

lent deaths, and alcohol-related deaths tend to be especially high, but that they do not completely account for the excess mortality. Adjustments for various indicators of health status reduce estimates much less than do adjustments for sociodemographic characteristics, but available health status indicators in these studies are quite limited. Sex differences were examined in two of the studies: the Danish data showed no difference in magnitude of effect attributable to unemployment, whereas the Swedish data showed a much weaker effect on women (SMR, 114). Results from the U.S. National Longitudinal Mortality Study (Sorlie and Rogot, 1990) are not consistent with the European data. Among those aged 45–64, the age-, education-, and income-adjusted SMRs due to unemployment were 107 for men and 81 for women; neither statistic was significantly different from the null value of 100. The discrepancy is not easily explained, inasmuch as the "social safety net" that protects the unemployed is believed to be stronger in Europe than in the United States (Kasl and Jones, 2000).

The British Regional Heart Study (Morris et al., 1994) followed men 40–59 years old who had been continuously employed for at least 5 years before initial screening. The respondents were contacted again 5 years later and asked about changes in employment since the initial screening. They were then followed for an additional 5.5 years for mortality. Compared with the continuously employed men, those with some unemployment (but not due to illness, according to self-report) had an age-adjusted relative risk of 1.59. Further adjustment for social class, smoking, alcohol use, and preexisting disease at initial screening slightly reduced the relative risk to 1.47. Men who were "unemployed or retired due to illness" had an adjusted relative risk of 3.14; this high relative risk reveals the inadequacy of using standard adjustments for health status measurements made while the men were all continuously employed. Baseline health status probably should be updated in such studies or, at a minimum, supplemented with reports of illness-related reasons for not working.

As discussed for SES, the causation-versus-selection question is raised here as well; it is not clear whether unemployment causes excess mortality or whether background variables (such as social class and poor pre-existing health) cause both unemployment and mortality (Kasl and Jones, 2000). To add further complexity, some studies find weaker associations between unemployment and mortality when the regional unemployment rate is high (Iversen et al., 1987; Martikainen and Valkonen, 1996).

Physical Morbidity

Studies of unemployment and physical morbidity introduce a new concern not applicable to mortality studies: the measurement of health status outcomes (Kasl and Jones, 2000). Physical symptoms and complaints, for instance, might result from psychological distress rather than from some underlying physical condition. Conversely, distress could lower the threshold for reporting existing physical symptoms. Moreover, measures based on seeking or receiving medical care could indicate differences in illness behavior rather than in underlying illness.

Morris and Cook (1991) reviewed longitudinal studies of factory closures. Their findings show that the job loss experience exerts a negative effect on physical health. In a prospective study of closure of a sardine factory in Norway (Westin, 1990; Westin et al., 1988, 1989), the rates of disability pension over a 10-year follow-up period were higher than were rates at a similar factory nearby that remained open. The pensions were supposedly "granted for medical conditions only," but it is difficult to know exactly what was being assessed and what health status differences would have been observed with other types of measurements. In a Canadian study of factory closure (Grayson, 1989), former employees reported about 2.5 times more ailments during a 27-month follow-up than the expected average. The higher prevalence was for a wide range of conditions, such as headaches, acute respiratory ailments, ulcers, arthritis, vision and hearing disorders, and dental troubles. Only heart disease, asthma, and endocrine diseases showed no significant differences. The authors offered the interpretation that the data indicated higher levels of stress that produce "a series of symptoms that people mistake for illness itself."

Biological and Behavioral Risk Factors

Studies of biological indicators of stress reactivity and cardiovascular-disease risk (Kasl and Jones, 2000) provide consistent evidence of their acute sensitivity to some aspect of the unemployment experience, particularly anticipation of job loss. However, chronic adverse changes in neuroendocrine and cardiovascular measures in relation to enduring unemployment are infrequently documented (Kasl and Jones, 2000).

Evidence on the impact of unemployment on health behaviors is mixed. Longitudinal data from the British Regional Heart Study (Morris et al., 1992, 1994) showed only an increase in weight attributable to unemployment; there was no evidence of an effect on cigarette or alcohol use. Higher levels of smoking and heavy drinking were in fact predictive of later unemployment in this study. But analysis of panel data from the U.S. Epidemiologic Catchment Area study suggested that the 1-year incidence of clinically significant alcohol abuse was greater among those who had been laid off than among those who had not been laid off (Catalano et al., 1993). The available evidence does not distinguish between the causation theory (unemployment led to alcohol use) and the selection theory (those who used alcohol were more likely to be laid off) (Dooley et al., 1992; Kasl and Jones, 2000).

Threatened Job Loss

The impact of threatened job loss has received increased attention recently. Foremost among the recent investigations are those of the Whitehall II cohort of British civil servants (Ferrie et al., 1995, 1998). White-collar workers under threat of major organizational change (elimination or transfer to the private sector) showed adverse changes in self-rated health, long-standing illness, sleep patterns, number of physical symptoms, and minor psychiatric morbidity. Only health-related behaviors did not show an adverse change. Longitudinal data on male Swedish shipyard workers threatened with job loss and on stably employed controls (Mattiasson et al., 1990) showed that serum cholesterol concentrations increased significantly among the former group. The increase was greater among those with increases in cardiovascular risk factors, particularly weight and blood pressure. However, no significant differential trends over time were seen for weight, blood pressure, or blood glucose. In a study of Finnish government workers (Vahtera et al., 1997), downsizing was associated with increased medically certified sick leave. Among American automobile workers (Heaney et al., 1994), extended periods of job insecurity were associated with increased physical symptoms. However, workers who remain in an organization after a downsizing do not experience a decline in well-being despite an increase in work demands (Parker et al., 1997).

Retirement

Negative health consequences associated with retirement have not been demonstrated (Kasl and Cobb, 1980; McGoldrick, 1989; Minkler, 1981; Moen, 1996). To the contrary, the evidence shows an absence of an adverse effect (Kasl and Jones, 2000).

Older studies (Palmore et al., 1984) tended to show neither adverse effects nor benefits. Some specific variables, such as subjective global evaluations of one's health, might show improvement, but this was seen as a function of reinterpreting one's health in the absence of physical demands on the job. More recent studies (Gall et al., 1997; Midanik et al., 1995; Ostberg and Samuelsson, 1994; Salokangas and Jowkamaa, 1991) tend to show some benefits of retirement, primarily in the psychological domain and in health behaviors. A study of older steelworkers forced to retire early because of downsizing did not show any adverse effects on their health (Gall et al., 1997; Gillanders et al., 1991). Loss of a job close to normal retirement age might have only small negative effects, if any.

There is no question that poor health leads to early or involuntary retirement (McGoldrick, 1989; Moen, 1996). This makes it difficult to test the proposition that, although planned and "on-schedule" retirement does not have negative consequences, it is the unplanned, involuntary, "off-schedule" retirement that should have adverse effects, because the downward health status trajectory that precipitated the retirement manifests itself as poor health status after retirement.

Men who choose to continue working well beyond the conventional retirement age are an unusual group, in good health and with a strong work commitment (Parnes and Sommers, 1994). It would be of interest to study the effects of mandatory retirement in this group rather than in blue-collar workers, who usually prefer to retire early (and usually do so if retirement benefits are adequate). But members of such occupational groups as doctors, judges, and farmers who continue working beyond typical retirement age are not easily recruited into a study of mandatory retirement (Kasl and Jones, 2000).

SOCIAL INEQUALITIES

Health and economic status are closely related (Wilkinson, 1996); indicators of health worsen as affluence decreases. The existence of inequality—a property of the population in question—has important consequences for the health of individuals and groups.

People and Places

The United States is among the richest countries in the world, yet it is also one of the least equal in distribution of its wealth (Atkinson et al., 1995). In 1968, the wealthiest 20% of U.S. households earned on average

$73,754, compared with $7,202 earned by households in the bottom 20%. In 1994, the inflation-adjusted average income of the top 20% had jumped to $105,945, whereas the average income of the bottom 20% had grown to only $7,762 (Brown et al., 1997). The best-off 1% of the American population owns 40–50% of the nation's wealth (Hacker, 1997; Wolff, 1995). The poverty rate at the bottom of the economic hierarchy has remained stable during the past three decades; today, some 36.5 million Americans (13.7%) are officially poor.

At a national level, the hypothesis linking income inequalities and health would predict that two countries with the same average income but different income distributions would experience different patterns of mortality; the country with the more equitable distribution having a higher life expectancy overall. Cross-national studies support an association between income equality and population longevity. For example, in a cross-sectional examination of 11 countries belonging to the Organisation for Economic Co-operation and Development (OECD), Wilkinson (1986) found a strong negative correlation ($R = -0.81$, $P < .0001$) between income inequality, as measured by the Gini coefficient, and life expectancy. The Gini coefficient is the most widely used measure of income distribution and theoretically ranges from 0 (perfect equality) to 1 (perfect inequality). Similarly, a high positive correlation ($R = 0.86$, $P < .001$) was found between the life expectancy of nine OECD countries and the proportion of national income accruing to the least well-off 70% of the population (Wilkinson, 1992). By itself, the gross national product per capita[3] could explain less than 10% of the variance in life expectancy (Wilkinson, 1992).

Income inequality within the United States has been linked to adverse health outcomes. Kaplan et al. (1996) and Kennedy et al. (1996) independently examined the relationship between degree of household income inequality in the 50 states and state-level variation in mortality. Kaplan et al. (1996) used as their measure of income distribution the share of total income earned by the bottom 50% of households in each state. If all incomes were equivalent, the bottom half of households would account for half the aggregate income. In reality, the income earned by the bottom half ranged only from 17.5% to 23.6% of the total income. A strong correlation ($R = -0.62$, $P < 001$) was found between this measure

---

[3]Gross national product per capita is the dollar value of a country's yearly output of goods and services divided by its population. It reflects the average income of a country's citizens.

of inequality and age standardized mortality. The association was observed in men and women and in whites and African Americans. Kennedy et al. (1996) examined two measures of income distribution: the Gini coefficient[4] and the Robin Hood index. The Robin Hood index is the proportion of aggregate income that must be redistributed from rich to poor households to attain perfect equality of incomes. Both measures were strongly correlated with age-adjusted total and cause-specific mortality. Adjusting for poverty rates and median income, a 1% increase in the Robin Hood index was associated with an excess mortality of 21.7 per 100,000 (95% CI, 6.6-36.7), which suggests that even a modest reduction in inequality could have important public health consequences. Income inequality was associated not only with higher total mortality but also with infant mortality and rates of death from coronary heart disease, cancer, and homicide. The findings persisted after controlling for urban rural proportion and for such health behavior variables as cigarette-smoking rates. Lynch et al. (1998) observed a relationship between income inequality and mortality at the level of U.S. metropolitan areas.

Although income inequality is strongly correlated with poverty (R = 0.73), the adverse effect of income inequality on health outcomes does not appear to be entirely explained by a *compositional* effect (places that exhibit income inequality have greater concentrations of poor people, who in turn have higher mortality risk). There is also evidence of a *contextual* effect of income inequality directly on individual health (Kennedy et al., 1998; Soobader and LeClere, 1999; Wilkinson, 1992). Kennedy et al. (1998) conducted a multilevel (individual ecologic) analysis of the effects of income inequality on individual self-rated health, adjusting for individual household income and other characteristics, such as educational attainment, smoking, overweight, and access to health care. People residing in states with the greatest income inequality were 1.25 times more likely to report being in only fair or poor health than were those living in the most egalitarian states. The effect of income inequality was statistically significant and independent of absolute income.

At least three pathways have been proposed to account for the rela-

---

[4]The Gini Coefficient is a measure of inequality of a frequency distribution calculated from the ratio of the area between the Lorenz curve and the 45-degree line and the area above the 45-degree line. The Lorenz curve plots the cumulative percentage of a population against the cumulative percentage of a variable such as income. A straight line indicates perfect equality and would have a Gini coefficient of zero.

tionship between income inequality and health: underinvestment in human capital (Kaplan, 1996); disruption of social cohesion by income disparities, which leads to disinvestment in social capital (Kawachi and Kennedy, 1997; Kawachi et al., 1997a); and direct psychological pathways, for example, frustration and envy created by invidious social comparisons (the relative-deprivation hypothesis) (Kawachi et al., 1994; Wilkinson, 1996). These are briefly described below.

Underinvestment in Human Capital

Kaplan (1996) reported striking correlations between degree of income inequality and indicators of human capital investment. States with the highest income inequality (as measured by the proportion of total household income received by the less well-off 50%) spent a smaller proportion of their budgets on education and showed poorer educational outcomes, ranging from worse reading and mathematics proficiency to higher high school dropout rates.

Erosion of Social Cohesion

Kawachi et al. (1997b) tested the association between income inequality and social cohesion at the population level. People living in states with high income disparities tend to be more mistrustful of each other (R = 0.71) and to belong to fewer civic organizations (R = –0.41). Both indicators were strongly correlated with age-adjusted mortality (R = 0.79 for social mistrust, R = –0.49 for civic-association membership, P < .05 for both). The authors speculated that income inequality erodes social cohesion, with adverse consequences for public health.

Relative Deprivation

Few epidemiologic studies directly connect frustrated expectations to health outcomes. Dressler (1996) coined the term "cultural consonance in lifestyle" to refer to the degree to which individuals succeed in achieving the lifestyle considered customary for their community. To the extent that individuals strive for and fail to meet the cultural ideal, negative health consequences follow. The degree of departure from cultural consonance is a strong predictor of systolic blood pressure, even after adjustment for established clinical risk factors for hypertension, including age, sex, obesity, occupation, education, and income (Dressler, 1996). The adverse consequences of relative deprivation are not confined to the psychological realm. As societies become more prosperous, material needs increase not just because people think they need more when their neighbors have more, but also for practical reasons. Many consumer goods introduced as luxury items (such as automobiles and telephones) gradually become necessities. In the early 1900s, when cities were organized on the assumption that residents would get around on foot or by streetcar, the automobile was considered a luxury. As car ownership became more prevalent, public transportation atrophied, and many employers, businesses, and families relocated to areas that were accessible only by car. In many places today it is extremely difficult, if not impossible, to work, shop, or socialize without a car (Jencks, 1992).

Race and Discrimination

Although whites and African Americans experienced substantial improvements in life expectancy at all ages throughout the 20th century, substantial gaps remain in life expectancy, morbidity, and functional status. The data suggest a temporal lag in life expectancies between the 2 groups in the United States. Life expectancy at birth for African Americans in 1990 was the same as it was for whites in 1950. Even after controlling for income, African American men and women have lower life expectancy than do whites at every income level (see for example Anderson et al., 1997; Geronimus et al., 1996).

Those differences, which are often substantial across a diversity of health outcomes, are commonly reduced but remain significant when indicators of socioeconomic status are considered. This phenomenon has led researchers to investigate the health effects of discrimination itself. Aspects of discrimination might influence health through any number of mechanisms, including socioeconomic position. However, conceptualizing discrimination (whether it applies to racial or ethnic minorities, women, homosexuals, or groups of different ages) as a stressful experience that can influence disease processes is a major advance in scientific thinking over the past decade.

Discrimination is defined as "the process by which a member, or members, of a socially defined group is, or are, treated differently (especially unfairly) because of his/her/their membership of that group" (Jary and Jary, 1995). Conceptually, the pathways by which discrimination can affect health involve exposure, susceptibility, and response to economic and social deprivation, toxic substances and hazardous conditions (physical, chemical, and biological agents), socially inflicted trauma (mental, physical, or sexual, ranging from verbal to violent), targeted marketing of legal and illegal psychoactive substances and other commodities, and inadequate health care by facilities and by specific providers (including access to care, diagnosis, and treatment) (Krieger, 2000).

Public health researchers have only recently begun to quantify the health effects of discrimination. Krieger (2000) outlines three approaches to studying these effects: indirect comparison of health outcomes of subordinate versus dominant groups without having specific information on discrimination; self-reported discrimination and its relation to health outcomes; and assessment of population-level experience of discrimination and health. The second and third approaches, although not without problems, can shed light on the specific aspects of discrimination with health consequences.

Krieger and Sidney (1996) investigated the relationship between self-reported racial discrimination and blood pressure among 4086 African American and white 25–34-year-old participants in the Coronary Artery Risk Development in Young Adults study, a prospective, multisite, community-based investigation. Among African Americans, systolic blood pressure was significantly increased, by 2–4 mm Hg (millimeters of mercury), among working-class men and women; in professional women reporting substantial discrimination; and among working-class men and women reporting no discrimination, when compared with those reporting moderate discrimination. Conversely, among professional men, blood pressure was more than 4 mm Hg *lower* among those reporting no discrimination.

One interpretation of why a self-report of no racial discrimination was associated with increased blood pressure among working-class African American women and men and professional African American women but lower blood pressure among professional African American men is that the meaning of "no discrimination" could be related to social position, in this case, sex and class. For people with more power and resources, a no might truly mean no. Among more disenfranchised people, a no might reflect internalized oppression. In such cases, a disjuncture between words and somatic evidence could be an instance of a pathogenic manifestation of experiences that people cannot readily describe. Adding plausibility to that interpretation are the results of two smaller studies, both of which found higher blood pressure among members of groups sub-jected to discrimination (African American women in one, white gay men in the other) who said that they had experienced no versus moderate discrimination (Krieger, 1990; Krieger and Sidney, 1997).

The third approach, measuring population-level experiences of dis-crimination and health effects, is illustrated by a study on the relationship of African American residential segregation and political empowerment with infant postneonatal mortality (the death rate of infants 2-12 months old) (LaVeist, 1992). Degree of residential segregation was assessed with a widely used index, the percentage of African Americans who would need to relocate to make the ratio of African Americans to whites in every neighborhood the same as that for the city as a whole. *Relative political power* was defined as the ratio of the proportion of African American representatives on the city council to the proportion of the voting-age population that was African American. *Direct political power* was defined as the percentage of city council members who were African American. Increased neonatal mortality was independently associated with higher levels of segregation, with poverty, and with lower levels of relative (but not direct) political power, even when controlling for intra city allocation of municipal resources (for example, per capita spending by neighborhoods on health, public safety, firefighting, streets, and sewers). Population mea-sures of economic participation and political empowerment developed for other subordinate groups (for example, United Nations Development Programme, 1996) have not yet been used in epidemiologic studies. Other neighborhood effects also have been reported in relation to blood pressure (Diez-Roux et al., 1997).

Multilevel analyses have not examined discrimination and health. It is plausible that residential segregation could modify perceptions and ef-fects of individually reported experiences of discrimination. This would be an important new phase of research.

Social Cohesion and Social Capital

Social integration can be conceived of as both an individual and a societal characteristic (Kawachi and Kennedy, 1997). A socially integrated individual has many social connections, in the form of intimate social contacts (spouse, friends, relatives) and more extended connections (membership in religious groups and other voluntary associations). At the group level, a socially cohesive society is one that is endowed with stocks of "social capital," which consists partly of moral resources, such as trust between citizens and norms of reciprocity.

More socially integrated societies seem to have lower rates of crime, suicide, mortality from all causes, and better overall quality of life (Kawachi and Berkman, 2000; Kawachi and Kennedy, 1997; Wilkinson, 1996). Kawachi et al. (1997b) analyzed social capital indicators across the United States in relation to state-level death rates. Social capital indicators were created from data gathered in the General Social Surveys conducted of the National Opinion Research Center in 1986-1990. Respondents in 39 states were asked to count the number of memberships in a variety of voluntary organizations, including church groups, sports groups, hobby groups, fraternal organizations, and labor unions. The per capita density of membership in voluntary groups was inversely correlated with age-adjusted mortality from all causes (R = –0.49, P < .0001). Adjusting for household poverty, an increase in average per capita group membership by 1 unit was associated with a decrease in age-adjusted mortality of 66.8 deaths per 100,000. Density of civic association membership and levels of interpersonal trust (percentage of citizens endorsing the expectation that altruistic behaviors will be returned in kind at some future time) were also important indicators of social capital. Level of distrust was strikingly correlated with age-adjusted mortality (R = 0.79, P < .0001). Lower levels of trust were associated with higher rates of most major causes of death, including coronary heart disease, cancer, cerebrovascular disease, unintentional injury, and infant mortality.

Kawachi et al. (1999) also carried out a multilevel study of the relationship between the above indicators of state-level social capital and individual self-rated health. A strength of this study was the availability of information on individual medical and behavioral confounding variables, including health insurance coverage, cigarette-smoking and overweight, and on sociodemographic characteristics, such as household income, education and whether one lived alone. Even after adjustment for those variables, people residing in states with low social capital were more likely to report fair or poor health. The odds ratio[5] for fair or poor health associated

---

[5]The odds ratio is a comparison of the presence of risk factors for a disease in a sample of diseased subjects and non diseased controls; the number of people with disease who were exposed to a risk factor (Ie) over those with disease who were not exposed (Io) divided by those without diseases who were exposed (Ne) over those without who were not exposed (No): (Ie/Io) / (Ne/No).

with living in areas with the lowest as opposed to the highest levels of interpersonal trust was 1.41.

There are several plausible mechanisms by which social cohesion might influence health through contextual effects (Kawachi and Berkman, 2000). At the neighborhood level, social capital might influence health behaviors by promoting more rapid diffusion of health information, increasing the likelihood that healthy norms of behavior are adopted, and exerting control over deviant health-related behavior. Sampson et al. (1997) provide evidence that "collective efficacy," or the extent to which neighbors are willing to exert social control over deviant behavior, plays an important role in preventing crime and delinquency. A similar process might operate to prevent other forms of unhealthy behavior, such as adolescent smoking, drinking, and drug abuse. Neighborhood social capital also could affect health by increasing access to local services and amenities; evidence from criminology suggests that socially cohesive neighborhoods are more successful at uniting to ensure that budget cuts do not disrupt local services (Sampson et al., 1997). Finally, neighborhood social capital could influence health through direct psychosocial pathways by providing social support and acting as the source of self-esteem and mutual respect, for example. Variations in the availability of psychosocial resources at the community level might explain the anomalous finding that individuals with few social ties but who reside in socially cohesive communities—such as East Boston (Seeman et al., 1993), African Americans in rural Georgia (Schoenbach et al., 1986), or Japanese Americans in Hawaii (Reed et al., 1983)—do not appear to suffer the same adverse health consequences as do socially isolated people living in less cohesive communities (Kawachi and Berkman, 2000). At the state level, it appears that more cohesive states produce more egalitarian patterns of political participation, which result in policies that ensure the security of all residents (Kawachi and Kennedy, 1997).

RELIGIOUS BELIEF

Longitudinal studies published in the past decade demonstrate the health benefits of religious involvement. For example, among residents of Alameda County, California, attendance at places of worship was associated with a lower 28-year mortality (Strawbridge et al., 1997). Residents of religious kibbutzim in Israel had a 40% lower 16-year mortality from cardiovascular disease than did those living on secular kibbutzim (Kark et al., 1996). The 6-month mortality after elective open-heart surgery was significantly lower among patients with strong religious faith than it was among their nonreligious counterparts (Oxman et al., 1995). In a community-based sample of elderly residents of New Haven, Connecticut, religious group membership protected elderly Christians and Jews against death in the month before their religious holidays during a 6-year period (Idler and Kasl, 1992). In that cohort, those who never or rarely attended religious services had nearly twice the stroke rate of those who attended weekly during the same period (Colantonio et al., 1992). Frequent religious attendance also predicted better physical function 8–12 years later, even after controlling for baseline function (Idler and Kasl, 1997).

Those longitudinal studies show that lower mortality and morbidity rates among those frequently attending religious services are partly but not entirely explained by improved health practices and increased social contacts deriving from attendance or by confounding due to baseline health status (i.e., selection). Nevertheless, evidence from some of the more methodologically sound studies indicates that the health-promoting effects of private worship or spirituality (such as prayer or scripture-reading at home, or subjective feelings of religious commitment) appears to be weaker than that of attendance at services (e.g., Idler and Kasl, 1997). However, this field is relatively new and more research is needed to determine how religious attendance is associated with good health. This complex topic is only briefly touched on here; a comprehensive analysis of the impact of spirituality and religion on health is beyond the scope of this report.

REFERENCES

Adler, N., Boyce, T., Chesney, M., Cohen, S., Folkman, S., Kahn, R., and Syme, L. (1994). Socioeconomic status and health: the challenge of the gradient. *American Psychologist, 49*, 15–24.

Anderson, N.B., and Armstead, C.A. (1995). Toward understanding the association of socioeconomic status and health: A new challenge for the biopsychosocial approach. *Psychosomatic Medicine, 57*, 213–225.

Anderson, R.T., Sorlie, P., Backlund, E., Johnson, N., and Kaplan, G.A. (1997). Mortality effects of community socioeconomic status. *Epidemiology, 8*, 42–47.

Atkinson, A.B., Rainwater, L., and Smeeding, T.M. (1995). *Income Distribution in OECD Countries: Evidence from the Luxembourg Income Study*. Paris: Organization for Economic Cooperation and Development.

Baumeister, R.F. and Leary, M.R. (1995). The need to belong: Desire for interpersonal attachments as a fundamental human motivation. *Psychological Bulletin 117*, 497–529.

Berkman, L. (1995). The role of social relations in health promotion. *Psychosomatic Medicine, 57(3)*, 245–254.

Berkman, L. and Glass, T. (2000). Social integration, social networks, social support and health. In L. Berkman and I. Kawachi (Eds.) *Social Epidemiology*. New York: Oxford University Press.

Berkman, L. and Kawachi, I. (Eds.) (2000). *Social Epidemiology*. New York: Oxford University Press.

Berkman, L. and Syme, S. (1979). Social networks, host resistance, and mortality: A nine-year follow-up of Alameda County residents. *American Journal of Epidemiology, 109*, 186–204.

Berkman, L.F. (1995). The role of social relations in health promotion. *Psychosomatic Medicine, 57*, 245–254.

Berkman, L.F. and Macintyre, S. (1997) The measurement of social class in health studies: old measures and new formulations. In M. Kogevinas, N. Pearce, M. Susser, and P. Boffetta (Eds.). *Social Inequalities and Cancer, IARC Scientific Publications No. 138* (pp. 51–64). Lyon: International Agency for Research on Cancer.

Berkman, L. F., Leo-Summers, L., and Horwitz, R.I. (1992). Emotional support and survival after myocardial infarction: A prospective, population-based study of the elderly. *Annals of Internal Medicine, 117*, 1003–1009.

Berscheid, E. and Reis, H.T. (1998). Attraction and close relationships. In D.T. Gilbert, S.T. Fiske, and G. Lindzey (Eds.) *The Handbook of Social Psychology, Vol. 2, 4th edition* (pp. 193–281). Boston: McGraw-Hill..

Black, D., Morris, J.N., Smith, C., Townsend, P., and Whitehead, M. (1988). *Inequalities in Health: The Black Report; the Health Divide*. London: Penguin Group.

Blane, D., Bartley, M., and Davey Smith, G. (1997). Disease aetiology and materialistic explanations of socioeconomic mortality differentials. *European Journal of Public Health, 7*, 385–391.

Blazer, D. (1982). Social support and mortality in an elderly community population. *American Journal of Epidemiology, 115*, 684–694.

Bosma, H., Marmot, M.G., Hemingway, H., Nicholson, A.C., Brunner, E., and Stansfeld, S.A. (1997). Low job control and risk of coronary heart disease in Whitehall II (prospective cohort) study. *British Medical Journal, 314*, 558–565.

Bosma, H., Peter, R., Siegrist, J., and Marmot, M. (1998). Two alternative job stress models and the risk of coronary heart disease. *American Journal of Public Health, 88*, 68–74.

Brown, L.R., Renner, M., and Flavin, C. (1997). *Vital Signs 1997*. New York: W.W. Norton and Company.

Buunk, B.P. and Verhoeven, K. (1991). Companionship and support at work: A microanalysis of the stress-reducing features of social interactions. *Basic and Applied Social Psychology, 12*, 243–258.

Buysse, D.J., Reynolds, C.F., 3rd, Monk, T.H., Berman, S.R., Kupfer, D.J. (1989). The Pittsburgh Sleep Quality Index: a new instrument for psychiatric practice and research. *Psychiatry Research, 28*, 193–213.

Cacioppo, J.T., Ernst, J.M., Burleson, M.H., McClintock, M.K., Malarkey, W.B., Hawkley, L.C., Kowalewski, R.B., Paulsen, A., Hobson, J.A., Hugdahl, K., Spiegel, D., and Bernston, G.G. (2000). Lonely traits and concomitant physiological processes: The MacArthur social neuroscience studies. *International Journal of Psychophysiology, 35*, 143–154.

Carstensen, L.L., Gottman, J.M., and Levenson, R.W. (1995). Emotional behavior in long-term marriage. *Psychology and Aging, 10*, 140–149.

Carstensen, L.L., Graff, J, Levenson, R.W., and Gottman, J.M. (1996). Affect in intimate relationships: The developmental course of marriage. In C. Magai and S.H. McFadden, (Eds.) *Handbook of Emotion, Adult Development, and Aging* (pp. 227–247). San Diego, CA: Academic Press.

Case, R. B., Moss, A.J., Case, N., McDermott, M., and Eberly, S. (1992). Living alone after myocardial infarction. *Journal of the American Medical Association, 267*, 515–519.

Catalano, R., Dooley, D., Wilson, G., and Hough, R. (1993). Job loss and alcohol abuse: A test using data from the Epidemiologic Catchment Area Project. *Journal of Health and Social Behavior, 34*, 215–225.

Cohen, S. (1988). Psychosocial models of the role of social support in the etiology of physical disease. *Health Psychology, 7*, 269–297.

Cohen, S. and Herbert, T.B. (1996). Health psychology: Psychological factors and physical disease from the perspective of human psychoneuroimmunology. *Annual Review of Psychology 47*, 113–142.

Cohen, S. and Syme, L. (Eds.). (1985). *Social support and health.* Orlando, FL: Academic Press.

Cohen, S. and Wills, T.A. (1985). Stress, social support, and the buffering hypothesis. *Psychology Bulletin, 98*, 310–357.

Cohen, S., Doyle, W.J., Skoner, D.P., Rabin, B.S., and Gwaltney, J.M., Jr. (1997). Social ties and susceptibility to the common cold. *Journal of the American Medical Association, 277*, 1940–1944.

Cohen, S., Frank, E., Doyle, W.J., Skoner, D.P., Rabin, B.S., and Gwaltney, J.M., Jr. (1998). Types of stressors that increase susceptibility to the common cold in healthy adults. *Health Psychology, 17*, 214–223.

Colantonio, A., Kasl, S., and Ostfeld, A. (1992). Depressive symptoms and other psychosocial factors as predictors of stroke in the elderly. *American Journal of Epidemiology, 136*, 884–894.

Colantonio, A., Kasl, S.V., Ostfeld, A.M., and Berkman, L.F. (1993). Psychosocial predictors of stroke outcomes in an elderly population. *Journal of Gerontology, 48*, S261–S268.

Costa, G. and Segnan, N. (1987). Unemployment and mortality. *British Medical Journal (Clinical Research Edition) 294*, 1550–1551.

Davey Smith, G., Leon, D., Shipley, M.J., and Rose, G. (1991). Socioeconomic differentials in cancer among men. *International Journal of Epidemiology, 20*, 339–345.

Davey Smith, G., Neaton, J.D., Wentworth, D., Stamler, R., and Stamler, J. (1996a). Socioeconomic differentials in mortality risk among men screened for the Multiple Risk Factor Intervention Trial. II. Black men. *American Journal of Public Health, 86*, 497–504.

Davey Smith, G., Shipley, M.J., and Rose, G. (1990). Magnitude and causes of socioeconomic differentials in mortality: Further evidence from the Whitehall Study. *Journal of Epidemiology and Community Health, 44*, 265–270.

Davey Smith, G., Wentworth, D., Neaton, J.D., Stamler, R., and Stamler, J. (1996b). Socioeconomic differentials in mortality risk among men screened for the Multiple Risk Factor Intervention Trial. I. White men. *American Journal of Public Health, 86*, 486–496.

Diez-Roux, A.V., Nieto, F.J., Muntaner, C., Tyroler, H.A., Comstock, G.W., Shahar, E., Cooper, L.S., Watson, R.L., and Szklo, M. (1997). Neighborhood environments and coronary heart disease: A multilevel analysis. *American Journal of Epidemiology, 146,* 48–63.

Dooley, D., Catalano, R., and Hough, R. (1992). Unemployment and alcohol disorder in 1910 and 1990: Drift versus social causation. *Journal of Occupational and Organizational Psychology, 65,* 277–290.

Dressler, W.W. (1996). Culture and blood pressure: Using consensus analysis to create a measurement. *Cultural Anthropology Methods, 8,* 6–8.

Duncan, C., Jones, K., and Moon, G. (1996). Health related behavior in context—a multi level modelling approach. *Social Science and Medicine, 42,* 817–830.

Esterling, B.A., Kiecolt-Glaser, J.K., and Glaser, R. (1996). Psychosocial modulation of cytokine-induced natural killer cell activity in older adults. *Psychosomatic Medicine, 58,* 264–272.

Ewart, C.K., Taylor, C.B., Kraemer, H.C., and Agras, W.S. (1991). High blood pressure and marital discord: Not being nasty matters more than being nice. *Health Psychology, 10,* 155–163.

Feldman, J., Makuc, D., Kleinman, J., and Cornoni-Huntley, J. (1989). National trends in educational differentials in mortality. *American Journal of Epidemiology, 129,* 919–933.

Ferrie, J., Shipley, M., Marmot, M., Stansfeld, S., and Davey Smith, G. (1995). Health effects of anticipation of job change and non-employment: Longitudinal data from the Whitehall II study. *British Medical Journal, 311,* 1264–1269.

Ferrie, J., Shipley, M., Marmot, M., Stansfeld, S., and Davey Smith, G. (1998). The health effects of major organisational change and job insecurity. *Social Science and Medicine, 46,* 243–254.

Fox, A.J., Goldblatt, P.O., and Jones, D.R. (1985). Social class mortality differentials: Artefact, selection or life circumstances? *Journal of Epidemiology and Community Health, 39,* 1–8.

Friedland, J. and McColl, M. (1987). Social support and psychosocial dysfunction after stroke: Buffering effects in a community sample. *Archives of Physical Medicine and Rehabilitation, 68,* 475–480.

Gall, T., Evans, D., and Howard, J. (1997). The retirement adjustment process: Changes in the well-being of male retirees across time. *Journals of Gerontology. Series B, Psychological Sciences and Social Sciences, 52,* 110–117.

Geronimus, A.T., Bound, J., Waidmann, T.A., Hillemeier, M.M., Burns, P.B. (1996) Excess mortality among blacks and whites in the United States. *New England Journal of Medicine, 335,* 1552–1558.

Gillanders, W., Buss, T., Wingard, E., and Gemmel, D. (1991). Long-term health impacts of forced early retirement among steelworkers. *Journal of Family Practice, 32,* 401–405.

Glaser, R., Kiecolt-Glaser, J.K. Bonneau, R.H., Malarkey, W., Kennedy, S., and Hughes, J. (1992). Stress-induced modulation of the immune response to recombinant hepatitis B vaccine. *Psychosomatic Medicine, 54,* 22–29.

Glaser, R., Rabin, B., Chesney, M., Cohen, S., and Natelson, B. (1999). Stress-induced immunomodulation: Implications for infectious diseases? *Journal of the American Medical Association, 281,* 2268–2270.

Glass, T., and Maddox, G.L. (1992). The quality and quantity of social support: Stroke recovery as psycho-social transition. *Social Science and Medicine, 34*, 1249–1261.

Glass, T.A., Matchar, D.B., Belyea, M., and Feussner, J.R. (1993). Impact of social support on outcome in first stroke. *Stroke, 24*, 64–70.

Gottman, J.M. (1994). *What Predicts Divorce? The Relationship Between Marital Processes and Marital Outcomes.* Hillsdale, NJ: Lawrence Erlbaum Associates.

Gottman, J.M. and Levenson, R.W. (1992). Marital processes predictive of later dissolution: behavior, physiology, and health. *Journal of Personality and Social Psychology, 63*, 221–233.

Grayson, J. (1989). Reported illness after CGE closure. *Canadian Journal of Public Health, 80*, 16–19.

Haan, M., Kaplan, G., and Camacho, T. (1987). Poverty and health: Prospective evidence from the Alameda County Study. *American Journal of Epidemiology, 125*, 989–998.

Hacker, A. (1997). *Money: Who Has How Much and Why.* New York: Scribner.

Heaney, C., Israel, B., and House, J. (1994). Chronic job insecurity among automobile workers: effects on job satisfaction and health. *Social Science and Medicine, 38*, 1431–1437.

Helminen, A., Rankinen, T., Mercuri, M., and Rauramaa, R. (1995). Carotid atherosclerosis in middle-aged men. Relation to conjugal circumstances and social support. *Scandinavian Journal of Social Medicine, 23*, 167–172.

Hirsch B.J. and DuBois, D.I. (1992). The Relation of Peers Social Support and Psychological Symptomatology during the Transition to Junior High School: A Two-year Longitudinal Analysis. *American Journal of Community Psychology, 20*, 333-347.

House, J., Robbins, C., and Metzner, H. (1982). The association of social relationships and activities with mortality: Prospective evidence from the Tecumseh Community Health Study. *American Journal of Epidemiology, 116*, 123–140.

House, J.S., Landis, K.R., and Umberson, D. (1988). Social relationships and health. *Science, 241*, 540–545.

Idler, E. and Kasl, S. (1992). Religion, disability, depression and the timing of death. *American Journal of Sociology, 97*, 1052–1079.

Idler, E. and Kasl, S. (1997). Religion among disabled and nondisabled persons. II. Attendance at religious services as a predictor of the course of disability. *Journal of Gerontology. Series B, Psychological Sciences and Social Sciences, 52*, S306–S316.

Ingersoll-Dayton, B., Morgan, D., and Antonucci, T. (1997). The effects of positive and negative social exchanges on aging adults. *Journals of Gerontology. Series B, Psychological Sciences and Social Sciences, 52*, S190–S199.

Iversen, L., Andersen, O., Andersen, P., Christoffersen, K., and Keiding, N. (1987). Unemployment and mortality in Denmark, 1970–80. *British Medical Journal, 295*, 879–884.

Jary, D. and Jary, J. (1995). *Collins Dictionary of Sociology, 2nd edition.* Glasgow, UK: Harper Collins.

Jencks, C. (1992). *Rethinking Social Policy: Race, Poverty, and the Underclass.* Cambridge: Harvard University Press.

Johnson, J.V., Stewart, W., Hall, E.M., Fredlund, P., and Theorell, T. (1996). Long-term psychosocial work environmental and cardiovascular mortality among Swedish men. *American Journal of Public Health, 86*, 324–331.

Kamarck, T.W., Manuck, S.B., and Jennings, J.R. (1990). Social support reduces cardiovascular reactivity to psychological challenge: A laboratory model. *Psychosomatic Medicine*, 52, 42–58.

Kang, D.H., Coe, C.L., Karaszewski, J., and McCarthy, D.O. (1998). Relationship of social support to stess responses and immune function in healthy and asthmatic adolescents. *Research in Nursing and Health*, 21, 11–28.

Kaplan, G. (1996). People and places: Contrasting perspectives on the association between social class and health. *International Journal of Health Services*, 26, 507–519.

Kaplan, G., Salonen, J., Cohen, R., Brand, R., Syme, S., and Puska, P. (1988). Social connections and mortality from all causes and cardiovascular disease: Prospective evidence from eastern Finland. *American Journal of Epidemiology*, 128, 370–380.

Kaplan, G.A. and Keil, J.E. (1993). Socioeconomic factors and cardiovascular disease: A review of the literature. *Circulation*, 88, 1973–1998.

Kaplan, G.A., Pamuk, E., Lynch, J.W., Cohen, R.D., and Balfour, J.L. (1996). Inequality in income and mortality in the United States: Analysis of mortality and potential pathways. *British Medical Journal*, 312, 999–1003.

Karasek, R. and Theorell, T. (1990). *Healthy Work*. New York: Basic Books.

Kark, J., Shemi, G., Friedlander, Y., Martin, O., Manor, O., and Blondheim, S. (1996). Does religious observance promote health? Mortality in secular vs. religious kibutzim in Israel. *American Journal of Public Health*, 86, 341–346.

Kasl, S. and Cobb, S. (1980). The experience of losing a job: Some effects on cardiovascular functioning. *Psychotherapy and Psychosomatics*, 34, 88–109.

Kasl, S. and Jones, B. (2000). The impact of job loss and retirement on health. In L. Berkman and I. Kawachi (Eds.) *Social Epidemiology*. New York: Oxford University Press.

Kawachi, I. and Berkman, L.(2000). Social cohesion, social capital and health. In L. Berkman and I. Kawachi (Eds.) *Social Epidemiology*. New York: Oxford University Press.

Kawachi, I. and Kennedy, B.P. (1997). Socioeconomic determinants of health: Health and social cohesion: Why care about income inequality? *British Medical Journal*, 314, 1037–1040.

Kawachi, I., Colditz, G.A., Ascherio, A., Rimm, E.B., Giovannucci, E., Stampfer, M.J., and Willett, W.C. (1996). A prospective study of social networks in relation to total mortality and cardiovascular disease in men in the U.S.A. *Journal of Epidemiology and Community Health*, 50, 245–251.

Kawachi, I., Kennedy, B., Lochner, K., and Prothrow-Stith, D. (1997b). Social capital, income inequality, and mortality. *American Journal of Public Health*, 87, 1491–1498.

Kawachi, I., Kennedy, B.P., and Lochner, K. (1997a). Long live community: Social capital as public health. *The American Prospect*, 35, 56–59.

Kawachi, I., Kennedy, B.P., Glass, R. (1999). Social capital and self-rated health: A contextual analysis. *American Journal of Public Health*, 89, 1187–1193

Kawachi, I., Levine, S., Miller, S.M., Lasch, K., and Amick, B.C.I. (1994). *Income Inequality and Life Expectancy: Theory, Research, and Policy*. Boston: The Health Institute, New England Medical Center.

Kennedy, B.P., Kawachi, I., and Prothrow-Stith, D. (1996). Income distribution and mortality: Cross-sectional ecologic study of the Robin Hood Index in the United States. *British Medical Journal*, 312, 1004–1007.

Kennedy, B.P., Kawachi, I., Glass, R., and Prothrow-Stith, D. (1998). Income distribution, socioeconomic status, and self rated health in the United States: Multilevel analysis. *British Medical Journal, 317*, 917–921.

Kiecolt-Glaser, J.K., Glaser, R., and Cacioppo, J.T. (1997). Marital conflict in older adults: Endocrinological and immunological correlates. *Psychosomatic Medicine, 59*, 339–349.

Kiecolt-Glaser, J.K., Malarkey, W.B., Cacioppo, J.T., and Glaser, R. (1994). Stressful personal relationships: Immune and endocrine function. In R. Glaser and J. Kiecolt-Glaser (Eds.) *Handbook of Human Stress and Immunity* (pp. 321–339). San Diego: Academic Press.

Kiecolt-Glaser, J.K., Marucha, P.T., Malarkey, W.B., Mercado, A.M., Glaser, R. (1995). Slowing of wound healing by psychological stress. *Lancet, 346*, 1194–1196.

Kiecolt-Glaser, J.K., Page, G.G., Marucha, P.T., MacCallum, R.C., and Glaser, R. (1998). Psychological influences on surgical recovery. Perspectives from psychoneuroimmunology. *American Psychologist, 53*, 1209–1218.

Krieger, N. (1990). Racial and gender discrimination: Risk factors for high blood pressure? *Social Science and Medicine, 30*, 1273–1281.

Krieger, N. (2000). Discrimination and health: A U.S. perspective on concepts, methods, and measures for epidemiologic research on health consequences of embodying racism, sexism, and other forms of social inequality. In L. Berkman and I. Kawachi (Eds.) *Social Epidemiology*. New York: Oxford University Press.

Krieger, N. and Sidney, S. (1996). Racial discrimination and blood pressure: The CARDIA study of young black and white adults. *American Journal of Public Health, 86*, 1370–1378.

Krieger, N., and Sidney, S. (1997). Prevalence and health implications of anti-gay discrimination: A study of black and white women and men in the CARDIA cohort. Coronary Artery Risk Development in Young Adults. *International Journal of Health Services, 27*, 157–176.

Krumholz, H.M., Butler, J., Miller, J., Vaccarino, V., Williams, C., Mendes, C.F., de Leon, C.F., Seeman, T.E., Kasl, S.V., and Berkman, L.F. (1998). The prognostic importance of emotional support for elderly patients hospitalized with heart failure. *Circulation, 97*, 958–964.

Kunst, A.E., Groenhof, F., Mackenbach, J.P., EU Working Group on socioeconomic inequalities in Health. (1998). Occupational class and cause specific mortality in middle aged men in 11 European countries: Comparison of population based studies. *British Medical Journal, 316*, 1636–1642.

Kunst, A.E. and Mackenbach, J.P. (1994). The size of mortality differences associated with educational level in nine industrialized countries. *American Journal of Public Health, 84*, 932–937.

LaVeist, T. (1992). The political empowerment and health status of African-Americans: Mapping a new territory. *American Journal of Sociology, 97*, 1080–1095.

Lepore, S.J., Mata Allen, K.A., and Evans, G.W. (1993). Social support lowers cardiovascular reactivity in an acute stressor. *Psychosomatic Medicine, 55*, 518–524.

Levenson, R.W., Carstensensen, L.L., and Gottman, J.M. (1993). Long-term marriage: Age, gender and satisfaction. *Psychology and Aging, 8*, 301–313.

Lewis, M.A. and Rook, K.S. (1999). Social control in personal relationships: Impact on health behaviors and psychological distress. *Health Psychology, 18*, 63–71.

Liberatos, P., Link, B.G., and Kelsey, J.L. (1988). The measurement of social class in epidemiology. *Epidemiologic Reviews, 10*, 87–121.

Link, B. and Phelan, J. (1995). Social conditions as fundamental causes of disease. *Journal of Health and Social Behavior (Spec No.)*, 80–94.

Lynch, J. and Kaplan, G.A. (2000). Socioeconomic position. In L.F. Berkman, and I. Kawachi (Eds.) *Social Epidemiology*. New York: Oxford University Press.

Lynch, J., Kaplan, G.A., Pamuk, E.R., Cohen, R.D., Heck, K.E., Balfour, J.L., and Yen, I.H. (1998). Income inequality and mortality in metropolitan areas of the United States. *American Journal of Public Health, 88*, 1074–1080.

Lynch, J.W., Kaplan, G.A., and Salonen, J.T. (1997a). Why do poor people behave poorly? Variation in adult health behaviors and psychological characteristics by stages of the socioeconomic life course. *Social Science and Medicine, 44*, 809–819.

Lynch, J.W., Kaplan, G.A., and Shema, S.J. (1997b). Cumulative impact of sustained economic hardship on physical, cognitive, psychological, and social functioning. *New England Journal of Medicine, 337*, 1889–1895.

Macintyre, S. (1997). The Black Report and beyond: What are the issues? *Social Science and Medicine, 44*, 723–746.

Macintyre, S., Ellaway, A., Der, G., Ford, G., and Hunt, K. (1998). Do housing tenure and car access predict health because they are simply markers of income or self-esteem? A Scottish study. *Journal of Epidemiology and Community Health, 52*, 657–664.

Mackenbach, J.P., Stronks, K., and Kunst, A.E. (1989). The contribution of medical care to inequalities in health: differences between socio-economic groups in decline of mortality from conditions amenable to medical intervention. *Social Science and Medicine, 29*, 369–376.

Malarkey, W.B., Kiecolt-Glaser, J.K., Pearl, D., and Glaser, R. (1994). Hostile behavior during marital conflict alters pituitary and adrenal hormones. *Psychosomatic Medicine, 56*, 41–51.

Marangoni, C. and Ickes, W. (1989). Loneliness: A theoretical review with implications for measurement. *Journal of Personal and Social Relationships, 6*, 93–128.

Marmot, M.G., Bobak, M., and Davey Smith, G. (1995). Explanations for social inequalities in health. In B. Amick, S. Levine, A.R. Tarlov, and D. Chapman Walsh (Eds.) *Society and Health* (pp. 172–210). New York: Oxford University Press.

Marmot, M.G., Bosma, H., Hemingway, H., Brunner, E., Stansfeld, S. (1997). Contribution of job control and other risk factors to social variations in coronary heart disease incidence. *Lancet, 350*, 235–239.

Marmot, M.G., Davey Smith, G., Stansfield, S., Patel, C., North, F., Head, J., White, I., Brunner, E., and Feeney, A. (1991). Health inequalities among British civil servants: The Whitehall II Study. *Lancet, 337*, 1387–1393.

Marmot, M.G., Kogevinas, M., and Elston, M.A. (1987). Social/economic status and disease. *Annual Review of Public Health, 8*, 111–135.

Martikainen, P. (1990). Unemployment and mortality among Finnish men, 1981–5. *British Medical Journal, 301*, 407–411.

Martikainen, P. and Valkonen, T. (1996). Excess mortality of unemployed men and women during a period of rapidly increasing unemployment. *Lancet, 348*, 909–912.

Matthews, K., Kelsey, S., Meilahn, E., Kuller, L.H., and Wing, R.R. (1989). Educational attainment and behavioral and biologic risk factors for coronary heart disease in middle-aged women. *American Journal of Epidemiology, 129*, 1132–1144.

Mattiasson, I., Lindegarde, F., Nilsson, J., and Theorell, T. (1990). Threat of unemployment and cardiovascular risk factors: Longitudinal study of quality of sleep and serum cholesterol concentrations in men threatened with redundancy. *British Medical Journal, 301,* 461–465.

McEwen, B.S. (1998). Protective and damaging effects of stress mediators. *New England Journal of Medicine, 338,* 171–179.

McGoldrick, A. (1989). Stress, early retirement, and health. In K. Markides and C. Cooper (Eds.) *Aging, Stress and Health* (pp. 91–118). Chichester, UK: John Wiley.

McLeod, J. and Kessler, R. (1990). Socioeconomic status differences in vulnerability to undesirable life events. *Journal of Health and Social Behavior, 31,* 162–172.

McLeroy, K.B., DeVellis, R., DeVellis, B., Kaplan, B., and Toole, J. (1984). Social support and physical recovery in a stroke population. *Journal of Social and Personal Relationships, 1,* 395–413.

Meyers, D.J. and Diener, E. (1995). Who is happy? *Psychological Science, 6,* 10–19.

Midanik, L., Soghikian, K., Ransom, L., and Tekawa, I. (1995). The effect of retirement on mental health and health behaviors: The Kaiser Permanente Retirement Study. *Journals of Gerontology. Series B, Psychological Sciences and Social Sciences, 50,* S59–S61.

Minkler M. (1981). Research on the health effects of retirement: An uncertain legacy. *Journal of Health and Social Behavior 22,* 117–130.

Moen, P. (1996). A life course perspective on retirement, gender and well-being. *Journal of Occupational Health Psychology, 1,* 131–144.

Morgenstern, H. (1985). Socioeconomic factors: Concepts, measurement and health effects. In A. Ostfeld, and E. Eaker (Eds.) *Measuring Psychosocial Variables in Epidemiological Studies of Cardiovascular Disease* (pp. 3– 36). Bethesda, MD: National Institutes of Health.

Morris, J. and Cook, D. (1991). A critical review of the effect of factory closures on health. *British Journal of Industrial Medicine, 48,* 1–8.

Morris, J., Cook, D., and Shaper, A. (1992). Non-employment and changes in smoking, drinking, and body weight. *British Medical Journal, 304,* 536–541.

Morris, J., Cook, D., and Shaper, A. (1994). Loss of employment and mortality. *British Medical Journal, 308,* 1135–1139.

Morris, P., Robinson, R., Andrzejewski, P., Samuels, J., and Price, T. (1993). Association of depression with 10-year poststroke mortality. *American Journal of Psychiatry, 150,* 124–129.

Moser, K., Fox, A., and Jones, D. (1984). Unemployment and mortality in the OCPS Longitudinal Study. *Lancet, 2* (8415), 1324–1329.

Moser, K., Fox, A., Jones, D., and Goldblatt, P. (1986). Unemployment and mortality: Further evidence from the OCPS Longitudinal Study 1971–1981. *Lancet, 1* (8477), 365–367.

Moser, K., Goldblatt, P., Fox, A., and Jones, D. (1987). Unemployment and mortality: comparison of the 1971 and 1981 longitudinal study census samples. *British Medical Journal, 294,* 86–90.

National Center for Health Statistics. (1992). *Vital Statistics of the United States, 1992.* Washington, DC: U.S. Government Printing Office.

North, F.M., Syme, S.L., Feeney, A., Shipley, M., and Marmot, M. (1996). Psychosocial work environment and sickness absence among British civil servants: The Whitehall II study. *American Journal of Public Health, 86,* 332–340.

Orth-Gomer, K. and Johnson, J. (1987). Social network interaction and mortality: A six year follow-up study of a random sample of the Swedish population. *Journal of Chronic Diseases, 40,* 949–957.

Orth-Gomer, K., Rosengren, A., and Wilhelmsen, L. (1993). Lack of social support and incidence of coronary heart disease in middle-aged Swedish men. *Psychosomatic Medicine, 55,* 37–43.

Orth-Gomer, K., Unden, A.L., and Edwards, M.E. (1988). Social isolation and mortality in ischemic heart disease. *Acta Medica Scandinavica, 224,* 205–215.

Ostberg, H., and Samuelsson, S. (1994). Occupational retirement in women due to age: Health aspects. *Scandinavian Journal of Social Medicine, 22,* 90–96.

Oxman, T.E., Freeman, D.H., Jr., and Manheimer, E.D. (1995). Lack of social participation or religious strength and comfort as risk factors for death after cardiac surgery in the elderly. *Psychosomatic Medicine, 57,* 5–15.

Palmore, E., Fillenbaum, G., and George, L. (1984). Consequences of retirement. *Journal of Gerontology, 39,* 109–116.

Pappas, G., Queen, S., Hadden, W., and Fisher, G. (1993). The increasing disparity in mortality between socioeconomic groups in the U.S. 1960–1986. *New England Journal of Medicine, 329,* 103–109.

Parker, S., Chmiel, N., and Wall, T. (1997). Work characteristics and employee well-being within a context of strategic downsizing. *Journal of Occupational Health Psychology, 2,* 289–303.

Parnes, H. and Sommers, D. (1994). Shunning retirement: Work experience of men in their seventies and early eighties. *Journal of Gerontology, 49,* S117–S124.

Pennix, B.W., van Tilburg, T., Kriegsman, D.M., Deeg, D.J., Boeke, A.J., and van Eijk, J.T. (1997). Effects of social support and personal coping resources on mortality in older age: The Longitudinal Aging Study, Amsterdam. *American Journal of Epidemiology, 146,* 510–519.

Pescosolido, B. (1986). Migration, medical care and the lay referral system: A network theory of adult socialization. *American Journal of Sociology, 51,* 523–590.

Pescosolido, B. (1991). Illness careers and network ties: A conceptual model of utilization and compliance. *Advances in Medical Sociology, 2,* 161–184.

Pierce, G.R., Lakey, B., Sarason, I.G., and Sarason, B.R. (Eds.) (1997). *Sourcebook of Social Support and Personality.* New York: Plenum Press.

Pierce, G.R., Sarason, B.R., and Sarason, I.G., (Eds.) (1996). *Handbook of Social Support and the Family.* New York: Plenum Press.

Reed, D., McGee, D., Yano, K., and Feinleib, M. (1983). Social networks and coronary heart disease among Japanese men in Hawaii. *American Journal of Epidemiology, 117,* 384–396.

Reis, H.T. and Judd, C.M. (Eds.) (2000). *Handbook of Research Methods in Social and Personality Psychology.* New York: Cambridge University Press.

Rhodes, J.E., Contreras, J.M., and Mangelsdorf, S.C. (1994). Natural mentor relationships among Latina adolescent mothers: Psychological adjustment, moderating processes, and the role of early parental acceptance. *American Journal of Community Psychology, 22,* 211–227.

Rogot, E., Sorlie, P., and Johnson, N. (1992). Life expectancy by employment status, income and education in the National Longitudinal Mortality Study. *Public Health Reports, 107,* 457–461.

Rook, K.S. (1984). The negative side of social interaction: impact on psychological well-being. *Journal of Personality and Social Psychology, 46,* 1097–1108.

Ruberman, W., Weinblatt, E., Goldberg, J., and Chaudhary, B. (1984). Psychosocial influences on mortality after myocardial infarction. *New England Journal of Medicine, 311,* 552–559.

Ryff, C.D. and Singer, B. (1998). The contours of positive human health. *Psychological Inquiry 9,* 1–28.

Ryff, C.D. and Singer, B. (Eds.) (2000). *Emotion, Social Relationships, and Health.* New York: Oxford University Press.

Salokangas, R. and Jowkamaa, M. (1991). Physical and mental health changes in retirement age. *Psychotherapy and Psychosomatics, 55,* 100–107.

Sampson, R.J., Raudenbush, S.W., and Earls, F. (1997). Neighborhoods and violent crime: A multilevel study of collective efficacy. *Science, 277,* 918–924.

Schnall, P., Landsbergis, P., and Baker, D. (1994). Job strain and cardiovascular disease. *Annual Review of Public Health, 15,* 381–411.

Schoenbach, V., Kaplan, B., Freedman, L., and Kleinbaum, D. (1986). Social ties and mortality in Evans County, Georgia. *American Journal of Epidemiology, 123,* 577–591.

Seeman, T. (1996). Social ties and health: the benefits of social integration. *Annals of Epidemiology, 6,* 442–451.

Seeman, T., Berkman, L., Blazer, D., and Rowe, J. (1994). Social ties and support as modifiers of neuroendocrine function. *Annals of Behavioral Medicine, 16,* 95–106.

Seeman, T., Berkman, L., Kohout, F., LaCroix, A., Glynn, R., and Blazer, D. (1993). Intercommunity variation in the association between social ties and mortality in the elderly: a comparative analysis of three communities. *Annals of Epidemiology, 3,* 325–335.

Seeman, T., Kaplan, G., Knudsen, L., Cohen, R., and Guralnik, J. (1988). Social network ties and mortality among the elderly in the Alameda County Study. *American Journal of Epidemiology, 126,* 714–723.

Seeman, T.E. and McEwen, B.S. (1996). Impact of social environment characteristics on neuroendocrine regulation. *Psychosomatic Medicine, 58,* 459–471.

Siegrist, J. (1996). Adverse health effects of high-effort/low-reward conditions. *Journal of Occupational Health Psychology, 1,* 27–41.

Singer, B. and Ryff, C.D. (1999). Hierarchies of life histories and associated health risks. *Annals of the New York Academy of Science, 896,* 96–115.

Soobader, M.J. and LeClere, F.B. (1999). Aggregation and the measurement of income inequality: Effects on morbidity. *Social Science and Medicine, 48,* 733–744.

Sorensen, G., Emmons, K., Hunt, M.K., and Johnston, D. (1998). Implications of the results of community intervention trials. *Annual Review of Public Health, 19,* 379–416.

Sorlie, P. and Rogot, E. (1990). Mortality by employment status in the National Longitudinal Mortality Study. *American Journal of Epidemiology, 132,* 983–992.

Sorlie, P., Backlund, E., and Keller, J.B. (1995). U.S. mortality by economic, demographic and social characteristics: the National Longitudinal Mortality Study. *American Journal of Public Health, 585,* 949–956.

Sorlie, P., Rogot, E., Anderson, R., Johnson, N., and Backlund, E. (1992). Black-white mortality differences by family income. *Lancet, 340*, 346–350.

Spiegel, D., Bloom, J.R., Kraemer, H.C., and Gottheil, E. (1989). Effect of psychosocial treatment on survival of patients with metastatic breast cancer. *Lancet 2 (8668)*, 888–891.

Stefansson, C. (1991). Long-term unemployment and mortality in Sweden, 1980–1986. *Social Science and Medicine, 32*, 419–423.

Sternberg, R.J. and Hojat, M. (Eds.) (1997). *Satisfaction in Close Relationships.* New York: Guilford.

Strawbridge, W., Cohen, R., Shema, S., and Kaplan, G. (1997). Frequent attendance at religious services and mortality over 28 years. *American Journal of Public Health, 87*, 957–961.

Sugisawa, H., Liang, J., and Liu, X. (1994). Social networks, social support and mortality among older people in Japan. *Journal of Gerontology, 49*, S3–13.

Syme, S. and Berkman, L. (1976). Social class, susceptibility and sickness. *American Journal of Epidemiology, 104*, 1–8.

Taylor, S.E., Kemeny, M.E., Reed, G.M., Bower, J.E., and Gruenewald, T.L. (2000). Psychological resources, positive illusions and health. *American Psychologist, 55*, 99–109.

Taylor, S.E., Repetti, R.L., and Seeman, T. (1997). Health psychology: What is an unhealthy environment and how does it get under the skin? *Annual Review of Psychology, 48*, 411–447.

Theorell, T., Blomkvist, V., Jonsson, H., Schulman, S., Berntrop E., and Stigendal, L. (1995). Social support and the development of immune function in human immunodeficiency virus infection. *Psychosomatic Medicine, 57*, 32–36.

Theorell, T., Tsutsumi, A., Hallquist, J., Reuterwall, C., Hogstedt, C., Fredlund, P., Emlund, N., and Johnson, J.V. (1998). Decision latitude, job strain, and myocardial infarction: A study of working men in Stockholm. The SHEEP Study Group. Stockholm Heart epidemiology Program. *American Journal of Public Health, 88*, 382–388.

Thoits, P.A. (1995). Stress, coping, and social support processes: Where are we? What next? *Journal of Health and Social Behavior, Extra Issue*, 53–79.

Tyroler, H.A., Wing, S., and Knowles, M.G. (1993). Increasing inequality in coronary heart disease mortality in relation to educational achievement profiles of places of residence, United States, 1962 to 1987. *Annals of Epidemiology, 3*, S51–S54.

Uchino, B.N., Cacioppo, J.T., and Kiecolt-Glaser, J.K. (1996). The relationship between social support and physiological processes: A review with emphasis on underlying mechanisms and implications for health. *Psychological Bulletin, 119*, 488–531.

Uehara, E. (1990). Dual exchange theory, social networks, and informal social support. *American Journal of Sociology, 96*, 521–557.

United Nations Development Programme (UNDP) (1996). *Human Development Report, 1996.* New York: Oxford University Press.

Vahtera, J., Kivimaki, M., and Pentti, J. (1997). Effect of organizational downsizing on health of employees. *Lancet, 350*, 1124–1128.

Vaux, A. (1988). Social and emotional loneliness: The role of social and personal characteristics. *Personality and Social Psychology Bulletin, 14*, 722–734.

Vogt, T.M., Mullooly, J.P., Ernst, D., Pope, C.R., and Hollis, J.F. (1992). Social networks as predictors of ischemic heart disease, cancer, stroke, and hypertension: incidence, survival and mortality. *Journal of Clinical Epidemiology*, *45*, 659–666.

Walker, K.N., MacBride, A., and Vachon, M.L.S. (1977). Social support networks and the crisis of bereavement. *Social Science and Medicine*, *11*, 35–41.

Weber, M. (1946). Class, status, party. In C.W. Mills (Ed.)and H. Gerth (Translator) *From Max Weber: Essays in Sociology*. New York: Oxford University Press, 180–195.

Welin, L., Tibblin, G., Svardsudd, K., Tibblin, B., Ander-Peciva, S., Larsson, B., and Wilhelmsen, L. (1985). Prospective study of social influences on mortality: The study of men born in 1913 and 1923. *Lancet*, *1 (8434)*, 915–918.

Westin, S. (1990). The structure of a factory closure: Individual responses to job loss and unemployment in a 10-year controlled follow-up study. *Social Science and Medicine*, *31*, 1301–1311.

Westin, S., Norum, D., and Schlesselman, J. (1988). Medical consequences of a factory closure: Illness and disability in a four-year follow-up study. *International Journal of Epidemiology*, *17*, 153–161.

Westin, S., Schlesselman, J., and Korper, M. (1989). Long-term effects of a factory closure: unemployment and disability during ten years' follow-up. *Journal of Clinical Epidemiology*, *42*, 435–441.

Wilkinson, R.G. (1992). Income distribution and life expectancy. *British Medical Journal*, *304*, 165–168.

Wilkinson, R.G. (1996). *Unhealthy Societies: The Afflictions of Inequality*. London: Routledge.

Wilkinson, R.G. (Ed.) (1986). *Class And Health: Research and Longitudinal Data*. London: Tavistock.

Williams, R., Barefoot, J., Califf, R., Haney, T., Saunders, W., Pryor, D., Hlatky, M.A., Siegler, I.C., and Mark, D.B. (1992). Prognostic importance of social and economic resources among medically treated patients with angiographically documented coronary artery disease. *Journal of the American Medical Association*, *267*, 520–524.

Wolff, E. (1995). *Top Heavy: A Study of the Increasing Inequality of Wealth in America*. New York: 20th Century Fund.

PART TWO

Health-Related Interventions

Recognition of the inequities in health status described in Chapter 4 has led to calls for a focus on an ecologic approach to health-related interventions. An ecologic approach recognizes that people live in social, political, and economic systems that shape behaviors and access to the resources they need to maintain good health (Brown, 1991; Gottlieb and McLeroy, 1994; Krieger, 1994; Krieger et al., 1993; Lantz et al., 1998; McKinlay, 1993; Sorensen et al., 1998; Stokols, 1992, 1996; Susser and Susser, 1996a,b; Williams and Collins, 1995; World Health Organization, 1986). There also is an effort to expand methods for evaluating interventions that incorporate an ecologic approach (Fisher, 1995; Green et al., 1995; Hatch et al., 1993; Israel et al., 1995; James, 1993; Pearce, 1996; Sorensen et al., 1998; Steckler et al., 1992; Susser, 1995).

The ecologic or social-systems perspective places the person in their primary social context and observes how he or she interacts with other important factors to affect and be affected by disease outcomes. The social context with the most immediate effects on disease management and with the greatest implications for intervention is the family, broadly defined (Campbell, 1986; Campbell and Patterson, 1995; Fisher et al., 1998). However, the ecologic perspective also emphasizes the importance of organizations, communities, and society as a whole.

Part Two presents relevant theoretical concepts and models and describes examples of interventions at the principal levels of the ecologic perspective, as described in Table 1-1 (individual, family, social network, organization, community, society). Note that those "levels" can describe either mechanisms that affect health status and disease etiology functioning at that level or the level at which a particular intervention is delivered. Thus, the distinction is made between community-wide interventions (which for the most part define community as a geographic place within which to carry out interventions that address individual-level behavior change relevant to health outcomes) and community-level interventions (which target social and structural changes associated with health status in the community as a whole).

Chapter 5 begins by presenting models and interventions relevant to the individual and family levels of the ecologic perspective. Chapter 6 then turns to the organization, community, and society levels. Chapter 7 reviews evaluation of the interventions and dissemination of health messages.

REFERENCES

Brown, E.R. (1991). Community action for health promotion: A strategy to empower individuals and communities. *International Journal of Health Services, 21*, 441–456.

Campbell, T.L. (1986). Family's impact on health: A critical review. *Family Systems Medicine, 4*, 135–328.

Campbell, T.L. and Patterson, J.M. (1995). The effectiveness of family interventions in the treatment of physical illness. *Journal of Marital and Family Therapy, 21*, 545–583.

Fisher, E.B. J. (1995). Editorial: The results of the COMMIT trial. *American Journal of Public Health, 85*, 159–160.

Fisher, L., Chesla, C.A., Bartz, R.J., Gilliss, C., Skaff, M.A., Sabogal, F., Kanter, R.A., and Lutz, C.P. (1998). The family and type 2 diabetes: A framework for intervention. *Diabetes Educator, 24*, 599–607.

Gottlieb, N.H. and McLeroy, K.R. (1994). Social health. In M.P. O'Donnell and J.S. Harris (Eds.) *Health Promotion in the Workplace, 2nd edition* (pp. 459–493). Albany, NY: Delmar.

Green, L.W., George, M.A., Daniel, M., Frankish, C.J., Herbert, C.J., Bowie, W.R., and O'Neill, M. (1995). *Study of Participatory Research in Health Promotion.* University of British Columbia, Vancouver: The Royal Society of Canada.

Hatch, J., Moss, N., Saran, A., Presley-Cantrell, L., and Mallory, C. (1993). Community research: partnership in Black communities. *American Journal of Preventive Medicine, 9*, 27–31.

Israel, B.A., Cummings, K.M., Dignan, M.B., Heaney, C.A., Perales, D.P., Simons-Morton, B.G., and Zimmerman, M.A. (1995). Evaluation of health education programs: current assessment and future directions. *Health Education Quarterly, 22*, 364–389.

James, S.A. (1993). Racial and ethnic differences in infant mortality and low birth weight: A psychosocial critique. *Annals of Epidemiology, 3*, 130–136.

Krieger, N. (1994). Epidemiology and the web of causation: Has anyone seen the spider. *Social Science and Medicine, 39*, 887–903.

Krieger, N., Rowley, D.L, Herman, A.A, Avery, B. and Phillips, M.T. (1993). Racism, sexism and social class: Implications for studies of health, disease and well-being. *American Journal of Preventive Medicine, 9*, 82–122.

Lantz, P.M., House, J.S., Lepkowski, J.M., Williams. D.R., Mero, R.P. and Chen, J. (1998). Socioeconomic factors, health behaviors, and mortality. *Journal of the American Medical Association, 279*, 1703–1708.

McKinlay, J.B. (1993). The promotion of health through planned sociopolitical change: Challenges for research and policy. *Social Science and Medicine, 36*, 109–117.

Pearce, N. (1996). Traditional epidemiology, modern epidemiology and public health. *American Journal of Public Health, 86*, 678–683.

Sorensen, G., Emmons, K., Hunt, M.K., and Johnston, D. (1998). Implications of the results of community intervention trials. *Annual Review of Public Health, 19*, 379–416.

Steckler, A.B., McLeroy, K.R., Goodman, R.M., Bird, S.T., and McCormick, L. (1992). Integrating qualitative and quantitative methods. *Health Education Quarterly, 19*, 1–8.

Stokols, D. (1992). Establishing and maintaining healthy environments: toward a social ecology of health promotion. *American Psychologist, 47*, 6–22.

Stokols, D. (1996). Translating social ecological theory into guidelines for community health promotion. *American Journal of Health Promotion, 10*, 282–298.

Susser, M. (1995). Editorial: The tribulations of trials—interventions in communities. *American Journal of Public Health, 85*, 156–58.

Susser, M. and Susser, E. (1996a). Choosing a future for epidemiology. I. Eras and paradigms. *American Journal of Public Health, 86*, 668–673.

Susser, M. and Susser, E. (1996b). From black box to Chinese boxes and eco-epidemiology. *American Journal of Public Health, 86*, 674–677.

Williams, D.R. and Collins, C. (1995). US socioeconomic and racial differences in health: patterns and explanations. *Annual Review of Sociology, 21*, 349–386.

World Health Organization (WHO). (1986). *Ottawa Charter for Health Promotion*. Copenhagen: WHO.

5

Individuals and Families: Models and Interventions

Human behavior plays a central role in the maintenance of health, and the prevention of disease. With an eye to lowering the substantial morbidity and mortality associated with health-related behavior, health professionals have turned to models of behavior change to guide the development of strategies that foster self-protective action, reduce behaviors that increase health risk, and facilitate effective adaptation to and coping with illness. Several decades of concerted effort to promote health and decrease risk through individual behavior change have produced successes, failures, and lessons learned.

This chapter addresses the models of behavior change and interventions designed to influence individual behaviors. It continues to explore the influence of family relationships on the management and outcomes of chronic disease.

MODELS OF BEHAVIOR CHANGE

Human behavior plays a central role in the maintenance of health and the prevention of disease. Growing evidence suggests that effective programs to change individual health behavior require a multifaceted approach to helping people adopt, change, and maintain behavior. For example, strategies for establishing healthy eating habits in children and adolescents might be quite ineffective for changing maladaptive eating behaviors—that is, when they are used to substitute one pattern for another—in the same population (e.g., Jeffery et al., 2000). Similarly, maintaining a particular behavior over time might require different strategies than will establishing that behavior in the first place (e.g., Ockene et al., 2000). Models of behavior change have been developed to guide strategies to promote healthy behaviors and facilitate effective adaptation to and coping with illness. Several models for individual behavior change are reviewed here.

Learning and Conditioning

Among the oldest, most widely researched, and yet most often misunderstood models of individual behavior applied to behavior change are those that deal with fundamental associative or classical conditioning and the related models of operant conditioning. Classical conditioning, pioneered by Pavlov, modifies behavior by repeatedly pairing a neutral stimulus with an unconditioned stimulus that elicits the desired response. Operant-conditioning builds on classical conditioning and focuses on the hypothesis that the frequency of a behavior is determined by its consequences (or reinforcements; Skinner, 1938). Although learning theory has been criticized for treating behavior in simplistic and mechanistic stimulus response terms, modern learning theory addresses complex components, including environmental cues and contexts, memory, expectancies, and underlying neurological processes related to learning (Rescorla, 1988). As Kehoe and Macrae (1998) note, today classical conditioning integrates cognition, brain science, associative learning, and adaptive behavior.

Classical conditioning introduced concepts that have been particularly important in the design of health-related interventions, such as reinforcement, stimulus–response relationships, modeling, cues to action, and expectancies. However, given the particular difficulty in maintaining behavior changes, the relapse of behaviors that have been eliminated (or "extinguished") by an intervention is of particular interest. Relapse of extinguished behaviors is a major problem in health-related behavior change interventions, especially those that target alcohol use, smoking, and diet (Dimeff and Marlatt, 1998; Marlatt and George, 1998; Perri et al., 1992; Wadden et al., 1998). Extinction initially was conceptualized as a process in which original learning, and therefore behavior, was unlearned or destroyed. That is, it was assumed that extinguished behavior would no longer be elicited by the environmental cues that originally evoked it. However, extensive research shows that extinction does not involve unlearning, but rather new learning that does not overwrite the original learning. Furthermore, the physical environment and social context in which extinction takes place, as well as such internal states as emotions, drug-related states, and time, will influence the process of extinction (Bouton, 1998, 2000).

Those findings have important implications for health-related behavior change. Specifically, the effectiveness of an intervention to reduce or eliminate a health risk, such as cigarette-smoking, will be limited to the extent that it is bound to the context in which it is delivered. As noted by Bouton (2000, p. 58), "the reformed smoker who once habitually smoked in a particular setting at work, or under the influence of a particular drug or alcohol, or in the presence of negative affect will be ready to lapse when cigarettes are made available in one of those contexts again. We now think of extinction as inherently context-specific, with the term 'context' being broadly defined."

One important implication of those findings is the importance of eliciting extinction in different contexts, including various physical environments, times, and emotional states. For example, extinction trials that are more widely spaced and in separate locations are more likely to be effective than core sessions that occur within short periods or in similar physical circumstances. Behavior change efforts should recognize the possible influence of contextual cues, identify the cues that might be involved, and help people avoid (or cope with) the contexts connected with the original health-compromising behavior, whether physical environments, interpersonal relationships, or negative emotional states. The learning of the new behavior (or extinction of the old) should take place in the contexts in which the person will need it the most.

There is another important difference between original learning and extinction, namely, that original learning of a behavior readily generalizes across contexts, whereas extinction does not (Bouton, 2000, p. 61):

> [F]irst-learned things seem much more likely to generalize over place and time. One implication of this is that if we really want to reduce cardiovascular risk, we should arrange a world in which healthy behaviors are the first things, not the second things, learned. One way of thinking about research on behavior change is that the organism seems to treat the second thing learned about a stimulus as a kind of exception to a rule. It is as if the learning and memory system is organized with a default assumption that the first-learned thing is correct, and everything else is conditional on the current context, place, or time.

That perspective provides support for the importance of preventive interventions that promote health-enhancing behaviors, as opposed to interventions designed to treat or change health-compromising behaviors.

The evidence that extinction depends on context is but one of several important results from basic research on learning and conditioning with important implications for explaining health-related behavior change. Closer ties between intervention research and basic learning theory and research could contribute to what O'Donohue (1998) called "third-generation behavior therapy," behavioral interventions that are informed by recent developments in learning theory and other fields of basic behavioral science.

Cognitive Social Learning

Cognitive social-learning theory (e.g., Bandura, 1977, 1986, 1997) proposes that reinforcements are not the sole determinants of behavior, but that behavior changes with observations of others. According to cognitive social-learning theory, the most important prerequisite for behavior change is a person's sense of self-efficacy or the conviction that one is able successfully to execute the behavior required to produce the desired outcome. People can feel susceptible to an illness, expect to benefit if they change their behavior, and perceive their social environment as encouraging the change, but if they lack a belief that they can indeed change, their efforts are not likely to succeed. Substantial empirical evidence suggests that self-efficacy beliefs (and the related concept of optimism) are reliable predictors of behavior, and that they mediate the effects of intervention on behavior change, including a number of health-related behaviors (e.g., Bandura et al., 1987; Ewart, 1995; Kaplan et al., 1994; Scheier et al., 1989; Wiedenfeld et al., 1990). A growing body of literature supports the importance of self-efficacy in initiation and maintenance of behavioral change (Bandura, 1977, 1986; Marlatt and Gordon, 1985; Strecher et al., 1986).

Self-regulation is a concept that derives from cognitive social learning theory (see Bandura, 1986; Baumeister et al., 1998; Carver and Scheier, 1998; Compas et al., 1999; Eisenberg et al., 1997), and it includes what many people call "will power." Self-regulation includes cognitive and behavioral processes that involve the initiation, termination, delay, modulation, modification, or redirection of a person's emotions, thoughts, behaviors, physiological responses, or environment (Compas et al., 1999). Self-regulation can be critical in such health-protective and health-maintaining behaviors as eating a healthy diet, engaging in regular exercise, and managing stress. Conversely, the failure or breakdown of self-regulatory efforts can be crucial in some risky behaviors, such as smoking, poor dietary management, and a sedentary lifestyle.

Although much research supports the utility of Social Learning Theory, limitations have been noted. It is difficult to evaluate the efficacy of theory-based interventions because the studies have involved only small numbers of subjects and the intervention designs have been very complex. In addition it is difficult to quantify and measure the conceptual elements of Social Learning Theory: self-efficacy, influence of observational learning, and emotional arousal.

Health Belief Model

One of the earliest theoretical models developed for understanding health behaviors was the health belief model (HBM; Hochbaum, 1958). The model was developed in the 1950s to explain why people did not engage in behaviors to prevent or detect disease early. It integrates elements of operant-conditioning and Cognitive Theory. Operant-conditioning theory focused on the hypothesis that the frequency of a behavior is determined by its consequences while Cognitive Theory gave more emphasis to expectations to explain behavior. For example, the desire to avoid becoming ill is a value, and belief that a specific health behavior can prevent an illness is an expectancy. Perceived susceptibility is the perception of personal risk of developing a particular condition, and it involves a subjective evaluation of risk rather than a rigorously derived level of risk. Perceived severity is the degree to which the person attributes negative medical, clinical, or social consequences to being diagnosed with an illness. Together, perceived susceptibility and perceived severity provide motivation for reducing or eliminating such threats. The type of action taken depends on perceived benefits (beliefs about the effectiveness of different actions) and perceived barriers (potential negative aspects of particular actions). People are thought to weigh an action's effectiveness in reducing a health threat against possible negative outcomes associated with that action.

The HBM has been applied, among other things, to influenza inoculation, screening for Tay-Sachs disease, exercise programs, nutrition programs, and smoking cessation (Strecher and Rosenstock, 1997). An important contribution of the model is the recognition that prevention requires people to take action in the absence of illness. This continues to be useful, for example, in explaining women's reluctance to perform breast self-examination or obtain mammograms (Rimer, 1990).

The limitations of the HBM are reviewed by Janz and Becker (1984). Perhaps the most critical of these is the lack of predictive value for some of its central tenets. For example, the perceived severity of a risk does not reliably predict protective health behaviors (Rimer, 1990). Moreover, the HBM is more descriptive than explanatory and does not presuppose or imply a strategy for change (Rosenstock and Kirscht, 1974). The predictive utility of the HBM and its applicability to behavior change can be improved by adding variables, such as self-efficacy, or by integrating it with other models.

Theory of Reasoned Action

The Theory of Reasoned Action was first proposed by Ajzen and Fishbein (1980) to predict an individual's intention to engage in a behavior at a specific time and place. The theory was intended to explain virtually all behaviors over which people have the ability to exert self-control. Factors that influence behavioral choices are mediated through the variable of behavioral intent. In order to maximize the predictive ability of an intention to perform a specific behavior, it is critical that measures of the intent closely reflect the measures of the behavior, corresponding in terms of action, target, context, and time.

Behavioral intentions are influenced by the attitude about the likelihood that the behavior will have the expected outcome and the subjective evaluation of the risks and benefits of that outcome. The predictive power of the model depends significantly on the identification of most or all of the salient outcomes associated with a given behavior for any particular target population.

Stages-of-Change Model/ Transtheoretical Model

Beginning with the first formulation of the HBM, Hochbaum (1958) assessed the "readiness" of adults to participate in screening. The inclusion of beliefs about susceptibility to illness and the personal benefits of screening was seen as an essential element in "readiness." The concept was expanded into more elaborate models, such as the Transtheoretical Model (also known as the Stages-of-Change Model) first proposed by Prochaska and DiClemente (1983). This model characterizes the continuum of steps that people take toward change and includes the activities or processes to move people from one stage to another. The earliest stage of behavior change starts with moving from being uninterested, unaware, or unwilling to change (precontemplation) to considering a change (contemplation). This is followed by the decision to take action (preparation) and the first steps toward the behavioral change (action). With determined action, the requirement for maintenance and relapses are recognized as part of the process. In addition to these temporal stages, the Transtheoretical Model encompassed the concepts of decision criteria, self-efficacy, and change processes (consciousness-raising, relief from negative emotions associated with unhealthy behavior, self-reevaluation, environmental reevaluation, committing to change, seeking support, substituting healthier alternative behaviors, contingency management, stimulus control, and recognizing supportive social norms; Prochaska et al., 1997). The Transtheoretical Model has been influential in research on smoking and was recently extended to other health risk behaviors (Prochaska et al., 1994).

The theoretical validity of the Stages-of-Change Model for behavior change is a matter of controversy (Budd and Rollnick, 1997; Sutton, 1996). Although early cross-sectional studies provided support for the theory (DiClemente et al., 1991; Fava et al., 1995), recent longitudinal studies did not support the Transtheoretical Model (Herzog et al., 1999; Sutton, 1996). Furthermore, multivariate analyses of several behavioral predictors demonstrate that the stages are weak predictors of cessation (Farkas et al., 1996; Pierce et al., 1998). Variables from cognitive social learning—such as outcome expectancy, self-efficacy, and behavioral self-control—appear to be better predictors of change than are the stages and associated processes (Bandura, 1997; Herzog et al., 1999).

Despite questions about its theoretical validity, the model has contributed to the recognition that most potential recipients of health-related behavior change efforts are not motivated to change. Population surveys show 80% of the target group in the "precontemplation" or "contemplation" stages. That result draws attention to the potential of approaches that increase motivation for health promotion and illness prevention. The development of innovative motivational programs to encourage less interested people to consider healthier lifestyles represents a new direction in health and behavior change (e.g., Miller and Rollnick, 1995).

Social Action Theory

One important example of a model that attempts to integrate individual psychological processes with social contextual factors is Social-Action Theory (Ewart, 1991), which builds on Social Cognitive-Learning Theory, models of self-regulation, processes of social interdependence and social interaction, and underlying biological processes to predict health-protective behaviors and outcomes (Ewart, 1991). It views the person as influenced by environmental contexts or settings to which he or she brings a particular temperament and biological context. Thus, a person's capacity to practice healthy eating habits and to exercise is influenced by access to health-enhancing foods and safe places to exercise and by internal goal structures, self-efficacy beliefs, and problem-solving skills.

In Social-Action Theory, biology and social and environmental contexts determine the success of interventions to promote individual behavior change (Ewart, 1991). Most behavioral research, however, has focused on individual strategies to facilitate desired changes, and less is known about how social and other contextual factors can be mobilized to promote behavior change. Social-Action Theory specifies mediating mechanisms that link organizational structures to personal health and incorporates key concepts from the earlier theoretical models, including self-efficacy and outcome expectancies. Some applications of social-action theory focus on the mechanisms and maintenance of behavior change (Ewart, 1990), again placing the focus on the influence of context on individual behavior.

Social-Action Theory provides a framework for multilevel approaches to health promotion and illness prevention. It offers a theoretical rationale for intervening in health policy and for creating environments that are conducive to self-protective choices. It provides an approach for defining public health goals and modifiable social and personal influences that can be used to encourage individual health-related behavior change. Social-Action Theory fosters interdisciplinary collaborations by incorporating and coordinating the perspectives of the biological, epidemiologic, social, and behavioral sciences.

Summary of Models for Behavioral Change

Strong conceptual models are available to guide the development, implementation, and evaluation of health-related behavior change interventions. While the models are useful constructs for thinking about behavioral change, they each have their limitations and each addresses different behavioral attributes. Furthermore, only rarely have these models been appropriately applied to interventions (IOM, 2001). The IOM report (2001) suggests that contextual and individual factors contributing to behavior should be fully surveyed and assessed from the perspective of the various models to gain insights from each as to pathways and barriers. It is prudent for researchers to look beyond specific models and to draw on general concepts of behavior change.

Recent advances in research on classical conditioning and self-regulation have important implications for establishing, reducing, and maintaining health-related behaviors. Establishing a stronger link with basic behavioral science promises to provide important directions for the continued development of health-related behavior interventions. Social Action Theory provides a promising way to integrate elements of several broad models in an attempt to account for health-related behavior change.

INTERVENTIONS TARGETED AT INDIVIDUALS

In response to mounting evidence that behaviors, such as cigarette-smoking and consumption of high-fat diets, are risk factors for chronic diseases, several studies target interventions for medically at-risk individuals. Some landmark clinical trials, such as the Multiple Risk Factor Intervention Trial (MRFIT Research Group, 1982), have contributed to our understanding of risk factors in disease. Trials also focus on psychosocial interventions after disease onset to improve treatment adherence and medical outcomes. Other interventions arise from the concept of population-attributable risk, which measures the amount of disease in the population that can be attributed to a given exposure (Marmot, 1994). A large number of people exposed to a small risk might generate more cases than will a small number exposed to a high risk (Rose, 1992), so that when risk is widely distributed in the population, small changes in behavior across an entire population can yield larger improvements in population-attributable risk than would larger changes among a smaller number of high-risk individuals (Marmot, 1994; McKinlay, 1995; Rose, 1992). Both approaches are described below.

Clinical Interventions

Clinical trials such as the Multiple Risk Factor Intervention Trial (MRFIT Research Group, 1982), the Lipid Research Clinics Coronary Primary Prevention Trials (Lipid Research Clinics Program, 1984a,b), and the Lifestyle Heart Trial (Ornish et al., 1990) have provided important contributions to the development of successful interventions and to the current understanding of risk factors for disease. Education and counseling can promote primary prevention measures reducing smoking and choosing a healthy diet. Interventions aimed at secondary prevention behaviors can influence early detection of illness. For instance, willingness to self-examine and participate in screening procedures is important for detection and treatment of cancer. Psychosocial interventions can improve people's coping skills and provide emotional support, thereby improving quality of life and medical outcomes among the chronically ill. The role of behavioral interventions for improving adherence to treatment is discussed below. Interventions addressing behavioral and psychosocial risk factors are also briefly reviewed.

Adherence

Adherence, the match between a patient's behavior and health care advice (Haynes et al., 1979), mediates the effectiveness of treatment recommendations, the scientific evaluation of treatment protocols, and even public health. For example, when treating bacterial infections, some patients stop taking antibiotics when symptoms stop, but before all the targeted bacteria are eradicated, resulting in relapse for the patient and the development of resistant bacteriological strains. Failure to follow medical recommendations for treatment is a common problem that is not without controversy. The term "adherence" has been increasingly used to replace the previous label of "compliance" to convey the patient's active participation in following a treatment regimen, rather than the patient's submission to a provider's directive (Roter et al., 1998). Between 30% and 70% of patients do not adhere effectively to treatment recommendations. Nonadherence to difficult behavioral recommendations, such as smoking cessation or following a restrictive diet, occurs in more than 80% of patients (National Heart, Lung, and Blood Institute [NHLBI], 1998). The reasons are varied: Providers sometimes fail to describe the treatment regimen clearly, resulting in confusion on the part of the patient. Patients may also not fully appreciate the consequences of nonadherence. Some regimens interfere with daily activities, particularly those requiring multiple doses each day, or those with special instructions regarding meals (e.g., take on empty stomach). Side effects, such as hair loss, can be embarrassing; others, such as dry mouth or gastrointestinal problems, can be uncomfortable. Insurance limits on reimbursement for treatments also can affect adherence. Nonadherence is more than failure to take medications as prescribed or to follow other recommendations for health behavior changes. One survey of oncologists (Hoagland et al., 1983) showed that failure to return for recommended outpatient treatments was the most frequent source of nonadherence. Adherence often depends on the nature of treatment. Therapies that are simple or that produce prompt relief of pain or symptoms typically result in high levels of adherence (Dunbar-Jacob et al., 2000). Adherence is usually poor if therapies last a long time, if they are preventive rather than curative, or if they are complicated. Patients who experience psychological problems or substance abuse are less likely to adhere (NHLBI, 1998).

Renewed attention has been given to non-adherence in recent years, led by concerns about the development of multi-drug-resistant tuberculosis (Cohen, 1997) and HIV (Chesney et al., 1999). Multidisciplinary research efforts are developing new self-report assessments of adherence that show significant relationships with biological outcomes. Electronic medication monitors, which are being used increasingly in research, provide more accurate estimates of adherence to medication regimens and suggest that patients overestimate their own adherence (Cramer et al., 1989) and that provider estimates of adherence are not better than chance (Haubrich et al., 1999).

Effective interventions have been developed to improve cooperation in the acute-care setting. For example, adjunctive nonpharmacologic analgesia involving self-hypnosis has been shown in two randomized trials to reduce pain, anxiety, patient-controlled medication use and episodes of hemodynamic instability and to reduce procedure time by 22% (Lang et al., 1996, 2000).

There have been surprisingly few studies of interventions that might enhance adherence (Shumaker et al., 1998). A recent systematic review of randomized trials of interventions to help patients adhere to medications revealed that successful interventions were those that were multifaceted, including such features as more convenient care, information, counseling, reminders, self-monitoring, reinforcements, and other forms of supervision and attention (Haynes et al., 1996). Relatively few studies have evaluated the benefits of interventions that require permanent lifestyle changes. The difficulties in sustaining the cessation of smoking, weight loss, or initiation of exercise are well recognized (Marlatt and George, 1998). The relapse rates, however, are not uniform for these behaviors. The rate of relapse from treatment of serious obesity is more than 90%, leading to revision of goals in its treatment to more modest but sustainable weight loss (Wadden et al., 1999), but half of those who stop smoking will remain completely abstinent for 2 years (Spiegel et al., 1993).

Addressing Psychosocial Risk Factors

As described in Chapter 2, depression is a risk factor for mortality from multiple causes. Furthermore, "distressed high utilizers" of medical care are substantially more likely to suffer from psychiatric disorders, including major depression, generalized anxiety disorder, and substance abuse (Von Korff et al., 1992). Poor adjustment to illness can increase the cost of medical care by as much as 75% (Browne et al., 1990). These problems make the development of programmatic interventions to provide psychosocial support both humane and expedient. Thus, providing appropriate psychotherapeutic and psychopharmacologic treatment for them not only can improve coping and reduce patient discomfort but also can make the delivery of medical care more efficient. The contributions of clinical behavioral and psychosocial interventions to diabetes, cancer, and heart disease are explored briefly. A recent chapter (Baum, 2000) from an Institute of Medicine (IOM) report provides further discussion of the influence of stress in cancer and cardiovascular disease.

Diabetes Mellitus. To reduce the incidence and severity of complications of diabetes, including vascular, coronary, renal, and neurologic disease, blood sugar must be carefully regulated. Adherence to medication regimens, glucose testing, exercise, and diet influences medical outcomes. Research indicates that coping skills and family stresses influence the management of diabetes (see Glasgow et al., 1999, for a review). Furthermore, depression is a serious co-occurring problem in diabetes (Glasgow et al., 1999; Jacobson, 1996; Lustman et al., 1992) that can affect glycemic control (Lustman et al., 2000). Several reviews and meta-analyses have demonstrated the effectiveness of educational approaches aimed at increasing knowledge, control, and self-efficacy among diabetics (Brown 1990, 1992, 1999; Hampson et al., 2000; Padgett et al., 1988). On the other hand, education did not consistently improve metabolic control (Grey, 2000). Psychosocial interventions (for example, enhancing coping skills and peer support) seem to provide greater success in improving both metabolic outcomes and quality of life (Grey, 2000; Grey et al., 1999). Educational interventions could be more effective when used in combination with behavioral psychosocial interventions (e.g., Brown, 1999, Clement, 1995). However, concerns exist that the beneficial changes might not be sustained long beyond the intervention (Brown, 1992).

Cancer. There is evidence that psychosocial interventions can improve quality of life, psychological adjustment, health status, and survival of cancer patients (see reviews by Andersen, 1992; Blake-Mortimer et al., 1999; Compas et al., 1998; Fawzy et al., 1995; Helgeson and Cohen, 1996; Meyer and Mark, 1995, Montazeri et al., 1998). A meta-analysis of 116 studies on the effects of psychoeducational care provided to adult cancer patients concludes that interventions affect anxiety, depression, and mood (Devine and Westlake, 1995). Another analysis of 45 psychosocial interventions showed statistically significant emotional benefits in adults (Meyer and Mark, 1995). Various interventions have been tested, including teaching specific methods of coping with the stress of cancer (Edgar et al., 1992; Fawzy et al., 1990; Telch and Telch, 1986), providing education and information (Manne et al., 1994), and providing social support and facilitating expression of emotions (Spiegel and Classen, 1995; Spiegel et al., 1981, 1989). Their relative effectiveness has been difficult to assess (Devine and Westlake, 1995; Fawzy, 1999; Meyer and Mark, 1995).

Some evidence supports the effectiveness of psychosocial interventions to improve medical outcomes and prolong survival (for reviews, see Creagan, 1999; Greer, 1999). Spiegel and colleagues (1998) found that psychosocial group treatment in metastatic cancer patients doubled survival time to an average of 18 months, from the point of randomization. A study by Richardson et al. (1990) showed that lymphoma and leukemia patients assigned to 1 of 3 educational and home-visiting supportive interventions had significantly longer survival than did patients allocated to routine care (control). The effect was sustained even when differences in medication adherence were controlled. In a study of 125 patients with metastatic melanoma, quality of life was found to be associated with duration of survival (Butow et al., 1999). A randomized controlled trial of 6 weeks of intensive group therapy aimed at developing active coping among 80 malignant melanoma patients significantly reduced mortality at 6-year follow-up (Fawzy et al., 1993). The mechanisms through which psychosocial interventions exert their effect is unknown, but it has been suggested that depression exacerbates symptoms (Evans et al., 1999) and that psychotherapy augments the immune response (for reviews, see Kiecolt-Glaser and Glaser, 1999; Spiegel et al., 1998). These results should be explored further and confirmed.

Although the potential of psychosocial intervention to slow the progression of cancer is promising, the literature is limited and several reports refute the hypothesis (for example, Cunningham et al., 1998; Gellert et al., 1993; Ilnyckyj et al., 1994; Linn et al., 1982; Morgenstern et al., 1984). One meta-analysis (Meyer and Mark, 1995) showed a small effect of psychosocial interventions on medical measures that was not statistically significant. Carefully designed studies are needed to clarify this issue.

Coronary Disease. Primary prevention can reduce the incidence of coronary disease (Chapter 3), but psychosocial interventions also can affect morbidity and mortality in at-risk patients. As described in Chapter 2, several studies have recently demonstrated that social isolation, depression, and type A personality traits—especially hostility—can mediate medical outcomes for patients with coronary disease (also see Rozanski et al., 1999; Williams and Littman, 1996). Evidence is increasing that psychosocial interventions after the onset of disease are effective supplements to routine cardiac care. One recent meta-analysis of 37 studies (Dusseldorp et al., 1999) found that psychoeducational programs reduced mortality by 34% and decreased recurrence of myocardial infarction by 29%. Another meta-analysis (Linden et al., 1996) of 23 clinical trials on coronary artery disease reported a similar significant reduction in morbidity and mortality with psychosocial interventions, especially during the first 2 years.

The interventions included in the analysis by Linden et al. (1996) were diverse but consistently positive. Powell and Thoresen (1988) found that counseling designed to reduce hostility and impatience typical in type A people reduced mortality among acute myocardial infarction patients who had less serious cardiac disease. Ornish et al. (1990) demonstrated that an intensive program of group support, stress management, moderate exercise, smoking cessation, and strict vegetarian diet resulted in a measurable reversal of coronary artery disease. Blumenthal et al. (1997a) found that stress management in coronary artery disease patients significantly reduced the subsequent risk of a cardiac event.

Many studies support psychosocial interventions, but other evaluations show no significant effects. Black et al. (1998) provided psychiatric evaluation and behavioral therapy to 380 cardiac patients and reported decreases in depression but not in rehospitalization rates. A clinical trial by Jones and West (1996) revealed no benefit from relaxation training and stress management. In contrast to the results of an earlier study that indicated that simply monitoring for psychological distress in cardiac patients reduced mortality (Frasure-Smith and Prince 1985), a follow-up study (Frasure-Smith et al., 1997) could not replicate the results and recommended against implementing such programs into routine care. The discrepancies among studies probably result from methodologic limitations, including small study sizes, varied interventions (some of which may not be behaviorally effective), indefinite clinical endpoints, and lack of intention-to-treat analyses. To address these limitations, a national multicentered clinical trial has been initiated (Enhancing Recovery in Coronary Heart Disease [ENRICHD], 1999), to determine the effects of psychosocial interventions on 3000 patients. Interventions will target depression and social isolation in patients with a recently diagnosed myocardial infarction. Endpoints will include mortality, nonfatal infarctions, cardiovascular hospitalizations, and changes in risk factor profiles (Blumenthal, 1997b; ENRICHD, 2000).

Addressing Behavioral Risk Factors

The primary care physician is in an optimal position to provide advice on healthy behaviors. Many studies have indicated that counseling by a primary care physician can be effective in changing the behaviors of patients but the approaches are varied. Several fundamental characteristics contribute to the effectiveness of these interventions. Recognition of differing patient needs is one fundamental characteristic of practices dedicated to enhancing beneficial behavior change. Some patients need only visual cues as a reminder to ask for help with smoking cessation, to obtain timely mammograms, to exercise more regularly, or to follow up for management of depression (Pronk and O'Connor, 1997; Rogers, 1995). Others respond more favorably to printed materials, coaching via telephone-based counseling, or classes. Some patients cannot change health-related behavior without one-on-one structured education and counseling supplemented by frequent reinforcement from their physicians. Multiple modalities of support are used in the practices that are most heavily committed to encouraging beneficial behavior change and that target individual patients (Oxman et al., 1995). Similarly, multiple methods are necessary to communicate with physicians and other clinical staff to encourage behavior change on their part that reinforces patient behavior change (Green et al., 1988; Greer, 1988). Chart reminders, computerized medical records with automated protocols, and physician and other staff education have all shown promise (Buntinx et al., 1993; Davis et al., 1995).

A second beneficial approach to behavioral intervention is the organizational leadership to decide to focus on a problem and devote energy and resources to it (Greer, 1988; Hammer and Champy, 1993; Oxman et al., 1995; Patti and Resneck, 1972; Rossi, 1992). A clinical practice that has an enhanced capacity to change patients' health-related behavior has leadership able to relate to the physician staff members and to engender enough emotional, internal, political, and economic support to drive behavior-change efforts toward success (Davis and Taylor-Vaisey, 1997). That presents a major challenge because most clinical practices are organized to deliver acute care rather than to change patients' behavior to prevent illness (Walsh and McPhee, 1992). Engaging busy practices to reach into new health promotion endeavors for which there is little economic reward is challenging, no matter how dedicated the leadership and clinical staff (Fishman et al., 1997). Rising to such a challenge tests the leadership and organizational adaptability of any practice that also must comply with innumerable legal, business, and clinical regulations and requirements. Many variables peculiar to a given practice—such as physician attitudes, local competitive pressures, staff morale, and socioeconomic needs of the patient population—can enhance or inhibit change in the practice toward a greater focus on prevention or other innovation (Crabtree et al., 1998). For example, changing practice patterns to document brief but consistent efforts to encourage smoking cessation initially proved beyond the reach of many good practices (Kottke et al., 1988).

Health care systems and practices in the United States are moving toward use of methods to increase the predictable quality and efficiency of medical care (Berwick, 1989; Carlin et al., 1996; Grimshaw and Russell, 1993, 1994; McDonald, 1976; Miller et al., 1998; Mittman et al., 1992). Current quality improvement models propose a more active and continuous method of identifying problems and testing interventions. This is a change from traditional methods of identifying faulty practices and practitioners by investigating clinical cases that have unsatisfactory outcomes (Balas et al., 1996). Rather than a list of poorly performing health providers, the result of a continuous improvement model can be a testable hypothesis that outlines a series of steps for caring for patients with specific problems that can result in measurable improvement in outcomes or processes (Crabtree et al., 1998; McBride et al., 1993; Solberg et al., 1997).

A simplified continuous-improvement model has four steps: (1) design a guideline with active participation of clinicians; (2) implement the guideline; (3) measure the outcomes; (4) study the outcomes, compared with what was expected, and redesign as needed (Mosser and Sakowski, 1996). Working with two large managed-care organizations, Solberg et al. (1998) conducted an RCT to assess the effectiveness of a process to help primary care clinics develop systems for the delivery of preventive services. Previous research showed that even when external technical assistance succeeded in increasing preventive services, the services declined to baseline when the assistance ended (Magnan et al., 1998). To build practices' internal capacity to initiate and manage change, the IMPROVE (Improving Prevention through Organization, Vision, and Empowerment) trial (Solberg et al., 1998) used organizational development approaches, such as continuous quality improvement and process consultation. The intervention facilitated the formation of continuous improvement teams that instituted prevention processes (Solberg et al., 1995). However, the extent to which patients in the intervention practices are actually receiving more preventive services has not been determined.

Clinical practice guidelines are formal statements that provide guidance to health care practitioners regarding specific clinical circumstances. Ideally, guidelines are based on the best available scientific evidence and clinical judgment. They should lead to the best patient outcomes and should steer clinicians away from unnecessary or extravagant interventions. The appeal of practice guidelines has led to remarkable growth in their development. An editorial in *Lancet* (Fletcher and Fletcher, 1998) describes beleaguered clinicians faced with more than 2000 sets of guidelines. However, guidelines lack standards of quality and have been developed by fragmented groups that might have different goals, motivations, and capabilities. Furthermore, guidelines are often outdated by the time they are released, often ignore patient preferences (Eddy, 1990), and often emphasize peer consensus rather than outcome evidence.

Many focused interventions to encourage health-related behavior change would benefit from population databases that keep track of patients' medical histories, behaviors, and attitudes. One fundamental factor for practice-based interventions is the availability of a database that defines the population served, accepts searches of health parameters or disease targets, and allows tracking of measurable changes in the defined health behavior or health outcome. An ideal database can link names, addresses, telephone numbers, diagnoses, pharmacy use, and other use of health care visits and educational resources (Redding et al., 1993). An example of a practice-based intervention that requires such a database is improving the diet and exercise patterns of poorly controlled diabetes mellitus patients and tracking their metabolic-outcome measurements for improvement (Thomson O'Brien et al., 1999). However, there has been little systematic research on the benefits of such databases in the United States. Practice databases are available primarily in large, well-organized practices and in staff model health-maintenance organizations whose physicians or other providers are paid salaries. They are not often used in smaller group practices because of the cost and personnel required to maintain them. Their use also raises major legal and ethical issues of privacy and confidentiality that have been the topic of several reviews (Gostin, 1997; Sweeney, 1997; Woodward, 1997) .

Need for Research on Practice

Much of the information in this section is based on evidence from uncontrolled trials and one-time interventions in large multispecialty group practices and well-organized staff model health maintenance organizations. Some of the information is based on the opinions of experts. Little of what is known about dissemination is based on well-controlled trials wherein a practice-level intervention is compared with reasonably controlled and parallel practice. Only occasional studies (e.g., Cohen et al., 1999; Cooper et al., 1997) have tried to assess interventions such as screening practices at the level of primary care physicians. Little research funding in the past has been applied to systematic evaluation of fundamental (systemic) changes in clinical practices that might support health-enhancing behavior change in defined populations. Future efforts should test various hypotheses that would encourage experimentation and practice-level interventions.

Population-Based Interventions

This section examines a sampling of studies that are representative of population-based intervention trials in a community, worksite, or school that are focused on changing individual behavior for primary prevention of disease. Given the importance of shifting the population distribution of disease risk, the effectiveness of interventions must be measured among the entire population for whom the intervention is intended, and not only among program participants. In addition, because of the importance of accounting for the influence of secular trends and for other factors not associated with the intervention that could affect behavior change, the studies discussed here included intervention and control conditions alike. Finally, to narrow the field of potential studies, a focus was given to those interventions conducted in the United States that targeted primary prevention of cancer or coronary heart disease, although the committee recognizes that considerable progress has been made using community interventions to address other public health problems.

Several early population-based community studies, including the Minnesota Heart Health Program (MHHP), the Stanford Five City Project (SFCP), and the Pawtucket Heart Health Program (PHHP), tracked changes in morbidity and mortality. For subsequent intervention studies, however, funding did not permit following participants long enough or in sufficient numbers to determine long-term costs and consequences of the interventions for survival, quality of life, or disease incidence. Instead, subsequent population-based intervention research rests on prior evidence linking behavioral outcomes to health benefits, such as reductions in morbidity and mortality (Chapter 3). Thus, for most population-based trials, behavior change is the primary outcome. The behaviors examined include dietary changes, tobacco use, and physical activity.

Community-wide Trials

Large-scale studies. Two early studies targeting cardiovascular disease prevention set the stage for population-based community intervention trials: the North Karelia Project (Puska et al., 1983) and the 1977 Stanford Three Community Study (Farquhar et al., 1977; Fortmann et al., 1981). Although the North Karelia Study was not done in the United States, it is included here because of its importance as a groundbreaking study of community intervention trials. The North Karelia Project grew out of that community's concern about having the highest heart attack risk worldwide (Blackburn, 1983; Keys, 1970; Verschuren et al., 1995). Results of a community-wide intervention implemented in North Karelia were compared with a reference area in eastern Finland. After 10 years, the net effects among middle-aged males included significant reductions in smoking, mean serum cholesterol concentrations, mean systolic blood pressure, and mean diastolic blood pressure; significant declines in mean systolic and diastolic blood pressure were observed among women (Puska et al., 1983). The study set the stage for community-wide intervention studies in the United States, the first of which was the Stanford Three Community Study (SHDPP). Initiated in 1972, that study demonstrated the feasibility and potential effectiveness of mass-media-based educational campaigns combined with intensive instruction of individuals in group or home classes directed at entire communities (Farquhar et al., 1977; Fortmann et al., 1981; Maccoby and Solomon, 1981). Significant reductions in cholesterol and saturated fat were reported at the conclusion of the intervention and were sustained during a 1-year maintenance period (Fortmann et al., 1981).

In the late 1970s, three large community-wide intervention trials were funded by the National Heart, Lung, and Blood Institute: SFCP (Farquhar et al., 1990), MHHP (Luepker et al., 1994), and PHHP (Carleton et al., 1995). All targeted change in risk factors for coronary heart disease (CHD), including high blood pressure, elevated blood cholesterol, cigarette-smoking, and obesity. None was randomized; rather, communities were matched to optimize comparability of study conditions (Murray, 1995). The multiple-risk-factor intervention trials varied in length from 5 to 7 years, and they tracked changes in morbidity and mortality beyond the intervention period. The interventions were aimed at raising public awareness of CHD risk factors through media education. Other objectives were to change risk-related behaviors through public education in schools, worksites, and other community organizations; educate health professionals; and initiate environmental change programs, such as labeling of foods sold in grocery stores and restaurants. For SFCP, significant effects were observed in blood cholesterol, smoking, and systolic and diastolic blood pressure; and decreases in risk—shown in composite risk factor indices— were significantly larger in the intervention than in the comparison communities (Farquhar et al., 1990). At the 3-year follow-up, the possibility was suggested of sustaining at least some observed outcomes, although the magnitude of the long-term effects was small (Winkleby et al., 1996). Fewer significant results were observed in MHHP and PHHP. MHHP reported significant effects for smoking prevalence among women and for physical activity (Luepker et al., 1994). PHHP resulted in smaller increases in body mass index in the intervention communities than in the controls; no other significant results were reported (Carleton et al., 1995).

In 1989, the National Cancer Institute (NCI), building on methods used in cardiovascular disease studies, launched the Community Intervention Trial (COMMIT) for Smoking Cessation (COMMIT, 1991). The trial used 11 matched pairs of communities across North America, and it was designed to test the effectiveness of a multifaceted, 4-year community intervention to encourage smokers, particularly heavy smokers, to achieve and maintain cessation (COMMIT, 1991, 1995a,b). A significant effect was observed among light-to-moderate smokers, and it appeared to be greater among a less-educated subgroup of participants (COMMIT, 1995a). There was no effect among heavy smokers (COMMIT, 1995a,b).

Although not a randomized, controlled intervention trial, the American Stop Smoking Intervention Study (ASSIST) was a large-scale, 7-year demonstration project building on randomized community-wide intervention trials. The intervention was implemented in 17 states through a partnership among NCI, the American Cancer Society, state health departments, and other organizations. The primary goal was to reduce smoking prevalence and cigarette consumption. To assess the results, investigators compared data from ASSIST and non-ASSIST states. Comprehensive tobacco control programs emphasized policy interventions, including indoor air, pollution, youth access, advertising, and tobacco taxes, as well as mass-media interventions and program services such as cessation classes (Manley et al., 1997a,b). Per capita consumption of cigarettes was comparable in ASSIST and non-ASSIST states before the beginning of the 1993 intervention. By 1996, smokers in ASSIST states were smoking 7% fewer cigarettes per capita. The intervention also included guidelines for raising cigarette excise taxes as a means of reducing consumption. Inflation-adjusted cigarette prices were nearly identical in both groups of states before 1993. Although the tobacco industry reduced prices during this period, in 1994 the average price was more than $0.12/pack higher in intervention than in control states (Manley et al., 1997a,b).

Small-scale studies. Several recent community-wide studies have borrowed principles from the early large cardiovascular disease prevention trials, but they have been implemented on a smaller scale and with smaller budgets. It might be difficult for such studies to achieve the necessary intensity and reach to show significant intervention effects. The Bootheel Heart Health Project, for example, was conducted in a six-county area in southeastern Missouri (Brownson et al., 1996). This rural area has the largest African American population in Missouri, and it is characterized by high rates of poverty and low education levels. The intervention was tailored to the community through the participation of local coalitions, each establishing its own priorities for intervention. The researchers conducted population-based cross-sectional surveys before and after the intervention to compare results in communities where there were coalitions against results from communities that did not have coalitions. Physical inactivity decreased and the prevalence of self-reported cholesterol screening increased in communities with active coalitions. Differences observed in self-reported weight gain were in the right direction, although not statistically significant. No differences were found for fruit and vegetable consumption or for smoking prevalence. Similar results were observed in the Heart to Heart Project, which reported decreases in dietary fat consumption and increases in cholesterol screening (Croft et al., 1994; Heath et al., 1995).

A more targeted definition of "community" was used in the Physical Activity for Risk Reduction (PARR) Project, conducted with residents of rental communities administered by the housing authority in Birmingham, Alabama (Lewis et al., 1993). PARR targeted physical inactivity among African Americans of low socioeconomic status who were residents of public housing, and it was evaluated in eight communities randomly assigned to intervention through a staged design ($n = 6$) and control ($n = 2$). Baseline assessments confirmed the low levels of physical activity in the target population. Despite using community residents as interviewers, however, there were substantial problems in obtaining participation from randomly selected households, particularly in the initial survey. Pre- and post-intervention physical activity scores were not significantly different in the intervention and control communities.

In a move toward ensuring greater community input, the Kaiser Family Foundation's Community Health Promotion Grant Program (CHPGP) offered communities substantial flexibility in developing program targets that were responsive to local needs and priorities. This program was designed to foster community health promotion efforts targeting cardiovascular disease, cancer, substance abuse, adolescent pregnancy, and injuries (Tarlov et al., 1987; Wagner et al., 1991). Comparisons among 11 intervention and 11 control communities, however, indicated little evidence of positive changes in the outcomes selected by the intervention communities (Wagner et al., 1991). That project illustrates the challenges of interpreting results when the intervention is not standardized across communities; the lack of consistency in the results was due at least in part to differences in the interventions (Cheadle et al., 1995).

Conclusions. The ability to draw conclusions on the basis of these trials is limited by their designs and methods. Only a few included an adequate number of communities to provide sufficient statistical power. Most studies used random samples for project evaluation, but the response rates varied widely, and few studies had adequate response rates. Most studies used nonvalidated self-report of behaviors as outcome measures. Few studies reported the results of process tracking. The assignment of multiple communities is expensive, and ultimately might require multicenter collaborations, such as that used in the COMMIT (1991) study.

Worksite Trials

In the past 15 years, an increasing number of health promotion studies have been conducted in workplaces and worksites are now considered important channels for delivery of interventions to reduce chronic disease among adult populations (Abrams, 1991; Abrams et al., 1994; Fielding, 1984; Heimendinger et al., 1990; Tilley et al., 1999). The U.S. Department of Health and Human Services conducted two National Surveys of Worksite Health Promotion Activities, one in 1985 and another in 1992 (USDHHS, 1985, 1992). In 1985, 66% of private worksites with 50 or more employees offered health promotion activities. This increased to 81% by 1992 (McGinnis, 1993). Many worksite trials have targeted cancer and cardiovascular disease risk factors either as discrete trials (Byers et al., 1995; Emmons et al., 1999; Glasgow et al., 1995, 1997; Heirich et al., 1993; Jeffery et al., 1993, 1994; Salina et al., 1994; Sorensen et al., 1992, 1996, 1999; Tilley et al., 1999) or within the context of larger community-wide trials (Glasgow et al., 1996; Sorensen et al., 1993). Most of those studies used individual behaviors as the primary outcome. Intervention methods included strategies to incorporate employee input and a variety of activities based on tested behavior change theories. The reported interventions ranged from more intensive group behavioral counseling sessions of varying duration and number and supervised exercise prescriptions to less intense interventions with a wider reach, such as mailed self-help materials and newsletters. Several of the programs achieved statistically significant effects on smoking cessation (Jeffery et al., 1993; Salina et al., 1994; Sorensen et al., 1993, 1996). Jeffery and colleagues (1994) reported that where worksites changed from unrestrictive to restrictive tobacco control policies during the course of the intervention, there were significant reductions in smoking among employees. In the Working Well trial (Sorensen et al., 1996), no trialwide differences in smoking cessation were observed, but one of the four participating study centers reported significant effects for 6-month abstinence rates. That study center was unique in that it integrated an occupational health focus into the health promotion intervention, thereby targeting a key concern of workers in the participating worksites (Sorensen et al., 1995).

The Working Healthy Project (WHP), a multi-risk-factor study that was part of the Working Well trial, showed significant increases in self-reported exercise behavior in the intervention group as compared with controls (Emmons et al., 2000). Dishman and colleagues (1998) reviewed 26 studies of worksite interventions targeting physical activity, including those that did and did not use the worksite as the unit of analysis. The poor scientific quality of the studies precludes judgment about whether such interventions can increase physical activity, and the researchers concluded that there is a need for studies that use valid designs and methods.

School Trials

Over the past two decades, extensive attention has been paid to health promotion and disease prevention among youth, particularly in schools. Schools provide an established setting in the community for reaching children and their families (Best, 1989; Perry et al., 1989; Stone and Perry, 1990; Stone et al., 1989). Several reviews summarize school-based smoking, physical activity, and nutrition education intervention trials from the 1980s and 1990s (Best, 1989; Contento et al., 1992; Flay et al., 1985; Stone et al., 1998). Some of those trials and analyses are reviewed here.

Reviews of youth smoking-control interventions generally conclude that social influence interventions can curb smoking onset (Best et al., 1988) although recent meta-analyses yielded a somewhat guarded picture of their efficacy. The first (Bruvold, 1993) found that effect sizes were largest for interventions that focus on social reinforcement, moderate for those with either a developmental orientation or a focus on increasing social norms, and small for interventions with a health information focus. A second meta-analysis (Rooney and Murray, 1996) reviewed 90 studies of school-based smoking prevention programs published in 1974–1991. They concluded that the influence of peer or social programs could be improved if they were delivered early in the transition from elementary to middle school (e.g., 6th grade), if same-age peer leaders were used, if they were part of a multicomponent health program, and if booster sessions were included in subsequent years. Although the average effects were small, with a reduction in smoking of as little as 5%, and only 20–30% under optimal conditions, school-based programs showed promise. The Life Skills Training (LST) program, a school-based intervention that teaches personal coping and social skills, has shown promising effects in both immediate and longer-term outcomes (Botvin et al., 1995). Dusenbury and Falco (1997) reported that the results of the 10 published studies of the LST program showed reductions up to 50% to 75% in tobacco, alcohol, and marijuana use at post-test, and a 6-year follow-up of over 4,000 participants indicated a 44% reduction in tobacco use.

Recognition of multilevel influences on smoking in youths has led to multifaceted interventions, including schoolwide media campaigns in combination with individual approaches. Such programs have been effective in reducing smoking prevalence throughout secondary school (Perry et al., 1992). A trial focusing on high-risk youths tested a combined program of mass media and standard school smoking prevention programs. This program was implemented in two schools; two other schools (the controls) had only the school program. At the 2-year followup, prevalence of smoking in the schools was compared; participants in the combined program showed a significantly lower prevalence of smoking than the controls (Flynn et al., 1997).

A recent school-based smoking prevention program (Peterson et al., 2000), The Hutchinson Smoking Prevention Project (HSPP), randomly assigned 40 school districts to experimental or control groups. Students were followed from grade 3 until 2 years after high school. An enhanced social-influence approach to the intervention was used, containing the 15 "essential elements" for school-based tobacco prevention developed by an NCI Advisory Panel (explained in Flay, 1985; Glynn, 1989). No significant differences between the control and experimental groups were evident at grade 12 or 2 years after high school suggesting that the intervention had little, if any, impact. The highly controlled, and well-designed nature of the study, including the high follow-up rates, high compliance with the intervention, the maintenance of the randomization by the school districts, well-matched control and treatment groups, and appropriate statistical analysis, strongly suggest that the failure to achieve change was a result of a failed intervention and not poor methodology. This conclusion implies that future interventions need to take a different approach, critically rethinking the interactions of biological, behavioral, and psychosocial risk factors at social and cultural contexts.

A review of the literature of school-based physical activity intervention research in 1980s and 1990s (Stone et al., 1998) found that the work was based on multiple theoretical approaches and incorporated simultaneous multicomponent interventions. In general, the studies found significant intervention effects for student knowledge and for psychosocial factors related to physical activity. Significant positive behavior changes were less common, but they were demonstrated in several studies (Dale et al., 1998; Homel et al., 1981; Killen et al., 1988; Leslie et al., 1998; Luepker et al., 1996; McKenzie et al., 1996; Sallis et al., 1999; Tell and Vellar, 1987). Two studies that conducted long-term follow-up found sustained significant differences up to 12 years after the intervention (Luepker et al., 1996; McKenzie et al., 1996; Tell and Vellar, 1987). The more extensive interventions typically had better results (Stone et al., 1998).

Most youth intervention programs to enhance physical activity have been conducted in school environments, typically through the physical education programs in elementary schools. The Child and Adolescent Trial of Cardiovascular Health (CATCH), a multicenter randomized trial for grades 3–5 involving 5,100 students in 96 schools, developed an intensive, teacher-based curriculum for enhancing health behaviors, including physical activity (Luepker et al., 1996). The program demonstrated significant differences in vigorous physical activity between experimental and control schools (Luepker et al., 1996); the differences were maintained three years after the intervention ended in the 5th grade (Stone et al., 1998).

Several school-based trials targeted dietary behaviors and found significant differences in knowledge, attitudes, and behavior change between intervention and control schools. Two exemplary programs are the Class of 1989 Study as part of the Minnesota Heart Health Program for 6th–12th graders (Kelder et al., 1994) and CATCH for 3rd–5th graders (Luepker et al., 1996; Perry et al., 1992). Both studies involved school-based interventions with large samples assessed for a long duration. Both interventions had beneficial effects on diet and eating habits (Nader et al., 1999); however, CATCH did not produce effects on physiological measures related to cardiovascular disease. In a review of interventions to promote healthy dietary behavior in children and adolescents, Perry et al. (1997) concluded that school-based nutrition education programs have been effective in improving aspects of children's eating behaviors, with positive effects also observed in physiological outcomes such as serum cholesterol.

Lessons from Behavioral Intervention Studies

There is clear evidence of efficacy of interventions to establish health-protective or health-enhancing behaviors, such as diet and physical activity; to reduce health-risk behaviors, such as smoking; and to facilitate adaptation to chronic illness, including cancer and heart disease. Yet the behavior changes frequently are difficult to maintain, which poses an important challenge to the field. The limited maintenance of behavioral change seen in initial intervention efforts may be due to the failure to take into account the contextual factors that allow relapse. Advances will require the practical application of new research on the role of contributing contextual factors that include intrapersonal, interpersonal, environmental, and temporal variables. A second challenge is the effective translation of trials to real-world settings. Generalization of effective interventions will require an expansion of the assessment of intervention outcomes delivered in diverse settings. Community-wide and organization-wide interventions have shown varied success. The findings are marred by poor designs and methods. In general, however, the interventions that were more broadly based and multifaceted were more likely to be effective. These challenges are not confined to advances in individual behavior change. As later chapters will reflect, similar challenges apply to all levels of interventions.

FAMILIES AND HEALTH

Another framework for examining health-related behavior change focuses on the family. The good influence of supportive family relationships is widely accepted in the scientific community (Broadhead et al., 1983; House et al., 1988; Uchino et al., 1996). Family relationships have greater emotional intensity than do most other social relationships, and research suggests that there is a substantive, positive association between the specific bonds within families and chronic-disease management and outcomes (Primomo et al., 1990).

The report defines a family as a group of intimates with strong emotional bonds (identification, attachment, loyalty, reciprocity, and solidarity) and a history and future as a group (Gilliss et al., 1989; Ransom and Vandervoort, 1973). In the United States, the incidence of a "traditional" family of a married couple with children has decreased from 40% of households in 1970 to only 25% in 1996 (US Bureau of the Census, 1998). Considering the family as the setting of disease management requires a definition of the family that is narrow enough to be useful in intervention but broad enough to include the multiple forms that families take in contemporary society. In this context, family members generally live together or close to one another. Our definition of family is not constrained by the number, configuration, sex, sexual orientation, age, or ethnicity of members (Doherty and Campbell, 1988; Holder et al., 1998). It assumes only three characteristics of family relationships: they persist over time, they are emotionally intense, and they involve high levels of intimacy in day-to-day life.

That definition sets family relationships apart from other social relationships that provide "social support." It identifies the family as a unique setting with powerful continuing relationships that assume levels of complexity and organization that go beyond the individual people involved. Family members create a shared social reality that is linked to health (Kleinman et al., 1978; Reiss, 1981), and it is in this environment that most disease management takes place—whether by the patient alone or with other family members (Ell, 1996).

Family and Disease Management

Chronic disease is a long-term stressor for patient and family members alike. The nature and intensity of this chronic stress has three important determinants. The first is the magnitude of the change required of the patient and family members—in their daily activities and in the way they relate to one another (Rolland, 1984). The second determinant is the capacity of the patient, within the circumstances of the family and its approach to life, to make these changes. Parents, spouses, and other family members are assumed to be the primary source of support, and their ability to meet the needs of the patient is often confounded by the distress that illness generates in other family members (Baider et al., 1996; Boss et al., 1990). Distressed household members are less able to provide support and also might need help themselves (Helgeson, 1994). Third, the availability of medical assistance and community resources for support of people with chronic disease can mitigate or exacerbate the stress of illness.

Secure and supportive close personal relationships help patients and other family members regulate the emotional distress that disease can engender (Saarni and Crowley, 1990; Schmoldt, 1989; Wyke and Ford, 1992). Conflicted family relationships, however, can interfere with regulation of emotion (Fiscella et al., 1997; Levenson and Gottman, 1983; Levenson et al., 1994). The body's homeostatic and allostatic regulatory systems connect emotional experience to the physiologic stress response (McEwen, 1998; Sapolsky et al., 1986), and the resulting changes in hormonal, immunologic, and neurochemical systems can influence the outcomes of chronic disease (Kiecolt-Glaser et al., 1997).

Family and Behavioral Risk Factors

Behavior also defines the influence of family relationships on chronic disease. Stable, secure, and mutual family relationships enhance consistent disease management behavior by permitting a sharing of the burdens associated with disease. Such relationships enhance joint "ownership" of disease, which often includes a partitioning of disease management responsibilities among the patients and others and reduces patients' emotional and behavioral burdens. A family-focused approach is likely to maximize intervention effectiveness, whether or not family members other than the patient are directly involved. For example, at the simplest level, patient-focused interventions to alter diet might be only minimally effective if the patient's spouse shops for food and prepares meals (Cousins et al., 1992).

INTERVENTIONS TARGETED AT FAMILY INTERACTIONS

Given the importance of family relationships, it is surprising that they have not been addressed more systematically and extensively in intervention research on the management of chronic disease. Table 5-1 indicates the relative amount of family-focused intervention research for several chronic diseases. Most family-based clinical-intervention research has concerned chronic diseases of childhood and adolescence (e.g., insulin-dependent diabetes, asthma). Family-focused intervention studies of dementia in the elderly (especially Alzheimer's disease) are increasing, but relatively less attention has been directed to family-focused interventions for diseases of adulthood. For example, of the diseases with the highest cost to the United States health-care system—cardiovascular disease, chronic obstructive pulmonary disease, asthma, and non-insulin-dependent diabetes—the latter two have been the subject of very little family-focused intervention research (Campbell and Patterson, 1995).

TABLE 5-1 Family Focused Intervention Research on Selected
Chronic Diseases[a]

Diseases of Childhood and Adolescence	Diseases of Adulthood and the Elderly
Cystic fibrosis[1]	Breast cancer[1]
Cancer[1]	Coronary arterial disease[1]
Insulin-dependent diabetes[2]	Hypertension[1]
Congenital heart disease[1]	Non-insulin-dependent diabetes[0]
Sickle-cell anemia[1]	Alzheimer's disease and other dementia[2]
Asthma[2]	Human immunodeficiency virus[0]
	Chronic obstructive pulmonary disease and asthma[0]

[a]Superscript numbers refer to amount of correlational and intervention research found in literature: 2 = considerable, 1 = some, 0 = little or none.

Interventions for Children and Adolescents with Chronic Disease

An organizational framework of family-focused interventions is help-ful for comparing outcomes across several diseases. Three categories are used here and defined in Table 5-2: psychoeducational interventions to provide information about the disease and methods for its management by multiple family members, modified psychoeducational interventions to strengthen and improve family relationship quality and functioning, and family therapy. These are described below with illustrative examples.

Psychoeducational Interventions

This is the most common type of family-focused intervention. It aims to increase family members' understanding of the disease and its manage-ment and to improve their capacity for management of the disease, in-cluding early recognition of the stress-induced changes occasioned by managing disease in the family setting and more effective adaptations that involve asking for help, reconfiguring expectations, reappropriating roles, and so on. Education and behavioral methods predominate. Parents and siblings of ill children are common targets for psychoeducational inter-

TABLE 5-2 Methods of Family-Focused Intervention

I.   Psychoeducational interventions with individual family members to facilitate disease management and to prevent maladjustment to the illness:
   •   *Psychoeducation* about the cause, course, and treatment of the disease; how the disease affects individuals and family relationships over time; and how to access the medical care system and other resources.
   •   *Cognitive and behavioral, problem-solving* methods, including specific programs to increase action-oriented coping, provide solutions to specific management problems, and provide techniques for managing psychological comorbidities of medical illness.
II. Interventions that affect family relationship quality and functioning:
   •   *Psychosocial interventions* with individual family members or with the family unit to strengthen relationships as a preventive intervention.
   •   *Multifamily groups* to provide psychoeducation and to strengthen family relationships as a preventive intervention.
   •   *Continuing screening* for patients and family members to detect depression, excessive anxiety, family conflict, and social isolation followed by secondary preventive interventions for individual family members, the family unit, or multifamily groups to prevent clinical dysfunction.
   •   *Family "support groups"* with well-defined goals and protocols, including self-help and leaderless groups for primary prevention and professionally led groups for secondary and tertiary preventive interventions.
III. *Family therapy* for seriously dysfunctional families only.
IV. *Reconfiguration of the health care team* to incorporate working with families to provide a continuing resource for the family as it manages over times—a setting where family members are known.

ventions, as are caregivers and their ailing adult relatives. A few interventions of this type targeted the families of adult patients. Secondary prevention—attempts to prevent recurrence, progression, or mortality among those with a disease—is the goal of most psychoeducational interventions.

For example, psychoeducational interventions for insulin-dependent diabetes have included groups for parents that run concurrently with groups for the children who are patients (McNabb et al., 1994; Mendez and Belendez, 1997; Thomas-Dobersen et al., 1993). Each of those randomized trials enrolled samples of 11–37 families with diabetic children. They included 6–14 weekly sessions aimed at adherence to treatment and coping with illness. No differences in metabolic control or self-care were found. However, improvement in disease knowledge and body image, decrease in barriers to adherence, and decrease in daily hassles were documented in the intervention groups.

There have been two well-controlled randomized trials of psychoeducational interventions for children with asthma. Tal et al. (1990) studied an intervention with 28 children and their families and found that patients in the intervention group took more responsibility for daily health care and demonstrated greater independence in the family than did patients in the control group. Medical outcomes were not assessed. Clark and colleagues (1984) randomly assigned 274 individuals to six 1-hour group sessions or to treatment as usual. One year later, the intervention group had fewer emergency room visits and better grades in school than did the control group.

One well-controlled study of a family-focused intervention for cystic fibrosis has been published (Bartholomew et al., 1997). It involved separate psychoeducational groups for parents, young children, school-age children, and adolescents, and it focused on increasing knowledge about cystic fibrosis, self-efficacy, self-management, and quality of life. Compared with controls, there were improvements in knowledge in all groups, improvements in self-efficacy in parents and children (but not adolescents), better management of the condition, and better health status of the children with cystic fibrosis in the first year after the intervention (Bartholomew et al., 1997).

There has been relatively little research on family interventions for childhood cancer. Two randomized trials of psychoeducational interventions focused on improving parental coping with the stress of the illness (Hoekstra-Weebers et al., 1998; Jay and Elliott, 1990). Each failed to show reduced patient distress, although the parents were less distressed in the study by Jay and Elliott (1990).

There have been two studies of family-focused interventions for children with congenital heart disease. Both were randomized trials of interventions that focused on decreasing distress related to cardiac procedures and their aftermath. Campbell and colleagues (1986) studied adjustment in children after they received cardiac catheterization. The study group, who received supportive counseling and stress management training, made a better adjustment than did a control group. The interventions were delivered separately for children and parents. Parental reports of stress were lower in the intervention group, but there were no differences in parents' or children's fear, affect, or cooperation during hospitalization.

A subsequent randomized intervention study of patients preparing for cardiac surgery compared individualized information and coping-skills training with routine presurgical information for primary caregivers and their children before and during hospitalization (Campbell et al., 1995). Children in the treatment group had a higher level of well-being with a gradual increase over time. There were no significant treatment effects on medical outcome measures or on children's or caregivers' anxiety. However, treatment group caregivers perceived themselves as substantially more competent to care for the children, and the intervention favorably affected the children's behavior in the hospital, at home, and at school.

Kaslow and colleagues (Collins et al., 1997; Kaslow and Brown, 1995; Kaslow et al., 1997) studied a family-focused intervention for sickle-cell disease. They developed a psychoeducational family intervention aimed at improving relationships in families of children and adolescents (aged 7–16 years) with sickle-cell disease. The intervention consisted of a culturally and developmentally sensitive manualized treatment in six sessions tailored to the needs and competencies of each child and family. It included education about the disease, provision of skills for enhancing stress management and coping, and methods to improve family and peer relationships. African American health-care counselors conducted all the interventions. Preliminary post-intervention results revealed that, compared with families randomly assigned to the usual control condition ($n = 20$), youth and their caretakers assigned to the experimental condition ($n = 20$) showed greater increases in knowledge about sickle cell disease. That change is important because treatment compliance has been found to be greater among patients who have a better understanding of the disease (Dunbar-Jacob et al., 2000). No reductions in psychological symptoms were noted for the children or caretakers at the end of the intervention. Six-month follow-up data were collected but have not been reported.

Interventions Affecting Family Relationship Quality and Functioning

This type of intervention focuses on family relationships and includes various methods to foster emotional expressiveness, reduce social isolation, prevent disease from dominating family life, help deal with loss, promote collaboration among family members, improve empathy, deal with stigma, reinforce developmental family roles, and resolve intrafamily conflict. Psychoeducation is often combined with family relationship interventions, which might be more effective than psychoeducation alone for secondary prevention. These interventions also appear to be helpful for tertiary prevention (reducing the duration and effects of established complications of disease and comorbid psychological disorders) when used selectively for reversing noncompliance with recommended treatments and for relieving subclinical psychological distress engendered by disease management burdens in patients and family members.

Children with newly diagnosed diabetes have been studied in individual families in intensive full-time programs (Sundelin et al., 1996), intensive home follow-up and crisis intervention (Galatzer et al., 1982), and weekly outpatient sessions with boosters at 6 and 12 months (Delamater et al., 1990). Sample sizes were 38, 223, and 36 families, respectively. Concentrations of hemoglobin A1C were used to monitor efficacy of the first and third of those interventions, with one confirmatory and one nonconfirmatory result, respectively. Improvement in family relationship quality was documented in the first two studies, and better treatment compliance was shown in the second. The interventions took place shortly after diagnosis, in contrast with the psychoeducational interventions described earlier, which were done at 1–5 years after diagnosis. The stronger effects of family relationship interventions on disease outcomes therefore might be attributable to timing rather than to type of intervention.

Interventions that affect family relationship quality and functioning in childhood asthma include those shown in a study by Hughes and colleagues (1991), in which 89 families had monthly sessions focused on supportive parent/child relationships and asthma management. As a group, children of the families randomly assigned to the intervention had better airway-function scores, fewer school absences, and fewer hospitalizations during the year after the intervention. The differences disappeared after that, so continuing reinforcement of family intervention might be needed to maintain the benefits.

In contrast with the need for chronic management of the medical problem in the diseases of childhood and adolescence described above, childhood cancer treatment is usually accompanied by a period of distress and disorganization followed by a general improvement in psychological health and family functioning as treatment demands lessen. Treatments can be traumatic, and symptoms of posttraumatic stress in patients and family members have been recognized as long-term sequelae. A study by Kazak and colleagues (1998) demonstrated effectiveness with a cognitive/behavioral, family-oriented intervention for parents that focused on decreasing the *child's* distress related to painful medical procedures. For this disease-management situation, that study supports an intervention that goes beyond psychoeducation alone to a relationship-focused intervention targeting the parents' interaction with the child.

The use of multifamily groups is an efficient way to provide psychoeducation and family-relationship-functioning interventions, although some families might not work optimally in a multifamily setting (Gonzalez et al., 1989). A randomized study of 32 families compared six weekly multifamily group sessions with usual care for children with insulin-dependent diabetes (Satin et al., 1989). The intervention focused on metabolic control and psychosocial function of the child and on family function. The children in the intervention group had better hemoglobin A1C, attitudes, and self-care behavior than did those in the control group.

Wamboldt and Levin (1995) reported the results of a multifamily group intervention delivered to 72 children with asthma and their families. The intervention lasted 5 hours, and was delivered on 2 consecutive days for 17 groups of families. It included education, support, and group discussion. Preintervention and postintervention assessments revealed an increase in family members' reports of feeling understood by others, feeling open to help with the illness, and having a stronger belief that it is helpful for family members to share their feeling about the illness with each other. No medical outcomes or long-term follow-up were reported. However, increased sense of support and increased belief that communication is useful are associated with improved disease outcomes in descriptive studies, so this intervention potentially could improve asthma management and outcome.

Another multifamily group intervention pilot project included 19 families of survivors of childhood cancer (Kazak et al., 1999). A combination of cognitive/behavioral approaches and manualized family therapy was used during four sessions delivered on 1 day. Success in decreasing symptoms of posttraumatic stress and anxiety in parents, siblings, and survivors was documented with preintervention and postintervention assessment.

Family Therapy

Family therapy has been used for secondary prevention, but it might be most appropriate for tertiary prevention. Screening programs can detect families in which serious psychological dysfunction predates the disease or complications of the chronic disease already constitute disorders to target for more intensive intervention.

A randomized trial of family therapy ($n = 25$) in the setting of poorly controlled childhood diabetes (Ryden et al., 1993) documented better metabolic control, improved behavioral symptoms, and better patient/ family relations associated with intervention. A pilot study of family problem-solving therapy in 14 families documented efficacy in increasing adherence to treatment for diabetes and in decreasing family conflict (Auslander, 1993).

Family therapy was associated with greater clinical improvement than was medical management alone in a small ($n = 17$) randomized study of children with severe asthma (Gustafsson et al., 1986). A larger study of children with severe asthma ($n = 32$) by Lask and Matthew (1979) documented lower daily wheezing scores and lower thoracic gas volumes in the intervention group than in the control group.

None of those studies had well-validated measures of family functioning, so it is unclear whether the interventions exerted their effects by improving family functioning. Indeed, inasmuch as both interventions also taught asthma management strategies, it is possible that the interventions did not directly change family functioning. In contrast, improvement in family communication and parental discipline was documented with preintervention and postintervention assessments of an intensive rehabilitation program that used family therapy and education for children with severe asthma (Weinstein et al., 1992).

Interventions for Adults and the Elderly with Chronic Disease

Chronic diseases of adulthood have received the least systematic attention with respect to family-focused interventions. There have been, however, many clinical reports and descriptive studies of informal interventions to assist families struggling with chronic disease. Most have been unsystematic and uncontrolled, but they indicate a growing recognition by the clinical community of the need to address family issues and of the utility of basing intervention in a family context. Although reported studies tend to use family-based intervention methods similar to those outlined for children and adolescents (psychoeducation and multifamily groups), there are so few studies on adults that categorizing them by method of intervention is not useful. The studies also appear somewhat scattered among several chronic diseases. Therefore, a few illustrative studies are reviewed below.

Pilot work on a family intervention during hospitalization of 56 stroke patients, which was followed up with telephone tracking for 3 months, showed decreased perceived criticism among family members and decreased use of health care, compared with standard medical follow-up. The study also showed a trend for improved performance of daily activities by stroke patients in the intervention group (Bishop et al., 1997; see also Glass et al., 2000).

Several descriptive studies indicate that spouse support is crucial for optimal risk reduction and management of existing heart disease. Family studies show that counseling about diet and exercise delivered to both marital partners reduced risk for both spouses over time (Family Heart Study Group, 1994; Knutsen and Knutsen, 1991). When interventions focused on changing the amount of support provided by the spouse, mixed results were found (Campbell and Patterson, 1995).

There have been five randomized, controlled trials of partner-supported smoking cessation. Although the data from descriptive studies show that such support is highly correlated with reduced smoking, most of the interventions were ineffective in increasing support or in reducing smoking (Campbell and Patterson, 1995). A similar pattern emerged in reducing the weight of obese patients (Black et al., 1990; Pearce et al., 1981). Involvement of spouses in cardiac-rehabilitation programs also has produced mixed results (Campbell and Patterson, 1995). It has been suggested that interventions to decrease patient smoking or promote weight loss might have failed for a couple of reasons: lack of integration of the social support intervention with other aspects of the treatment program (nicotine replacement, extrafamilial stressors, and so on) and failure to use a customized approach to address the complexities of married relationships.

A major study of a family intervention for hypertension (Morisky et al., 1983, 1985) is an exception to the trend of mixed findings. It demonstrated that a single home visit to develop a personalized plan for family medication and lifestyle changes resulted in improved patient compliance, reduced blood pressure, and reduced mortality. The responsiveness of hypertension to relationship-altering interventions was demonstrated by Ewart and colleagues (1984). Communication training of couples in which one member had hypertension decreased both blood pressure and hostility during discussion of a conflict compared to couples receiving treatment as usual.

Interventions for Caregivers

Caregivers face tremendous stress. It has been observed that family members caring for someone with progressive dementia are characterized by impaired wound-healing compared with controls matched for age and family income (Kiecolt-Glaser et al., 1995, 1998). Interventions to address this stress are challenging issues in health and behavior and deserves greater attention.

A series of reports by Mittleman et al. (1993, 1995, 1996) explored family-based interventions for the elderly with dementia. They demonstrated that an intervention with multiple members of the patient's family substantially improved caregiver well-being. The intervention also resulted in a significant delay in institutionalization of the demented elderly, compared with controls who received usual care. The intervention consisted of six psychoeducational sessions with individual families followed by long-term availability of the healthcare counselors to the family members. More studies on the effectiveness of interventions for caregivers are warranted.

Lessons from Family Intervention Studies

Family-focused interventions have multiple aims. They are intended to help family members agree on and collaborate in a program of disease management in ways that are consistent with their beliefs and operational style. Helping family members manage stress by preventing the disease from dominating family life and sacrificing normal developmental and personal goals is also important. Interventions help the family deal with the losses that chronic disease can create, mobilize the family's natural support system, provide education and support for family members, and reduce the social isolation and the resulting anxiety and depression accompanying disease management. Finally, interventions can provide new structure for the family, with adjustments of roles and expectations if needed, to ensure optimal patient self-care.

Studies of interventions that involve family members are more common in diseases of children than in diseases of adults. Most family-focused intervention studies of children's diseases have been conducted with groups of patients or groups of family members, not with whole families. Interventions have focused more on adherence to treatment and metabolic control than on family-behavior variables or family processes themselves. However, a few studies demonstrate improved family relationships associated with better health outcomes (for example, Delamater et al., 1990; Ryden et al., 1993; Satin et al., 1989). Results suggest that interventions focused on family relationships, rather than education of individual family members, might be a fruitful approach to improving the management of various chronic diseases in children and adolescents. Research on family interventions for management of chronic diseases in adults and the elderly is in its infancy and careful attention is needed to develop realistic and systematic trials. The available data suggest that recognizing and attending to the family relationship context adds considerably to improving the health and well-being of patients and family members struggling with the management of a chronic disease.

An increase in complexity occurs when a shift is made from addressing only the individual patient to addressing the broader social context in which the patient lives and in which the disease is managed. Accompanying the increased complexity, however, is the need to increase the flexibility of intervention approaches, the number of methods of intervention, and the number of risk and protective factors that are targeted for change so that the potential for effecting substantive improvement can be realized.

REFERENCES

Abrams, D. (1991). Conceptual models to integrate individual and public health interventions: The example of the workplace. In M. Henderson (Ed.) *Proceedings of the International Conference on Promoting Dietary Change in Communities* (pp. 173–194). Seattle: The Fred Hutchinson Cancer Center.

Abrams, D.B., Emmons, K.M., Linnan, L., and Biener, L. (1994). Smoking cessation at the workplace: Conceptual and practical considerations. In R. Richmond (Ed.) *International Perspective on Smoking* (pp. 137–169). Baltimore, MD: Williams and Wilkins.

Ajzen, I. and Fishbein, M. (1980). *Understanding attitudes and predicting social behavior.* Englewood Cliffs, NJ: Prentice-Hall.

Andersen, B.L. (1992). Psychosocial interventions for cancer patients to enhance quality of life. *Journal of Consulting and Clinical Psychology, 60,* 552–568.

Auslander, W.D. (1993). Brief family interventions to improve family communication and cooperation regarding diabetes management. *Diabetes Spectrum, 6,* 330–333.

Baider, L., Kaufman, B., Peretz, T., Manor, O., Ever-Hadani, P., and Kaplan-DeNour, A.K. (1996). Mutuality of fate: Adaptation and psychological distress in cancer patients and their partners. In L. Baider, C. Cooper, and A. Kaplan-DeNour (Eds.) *Cancer and the Family* (pp. 173–186). Chichester, England: John Wiley and Sons.

Balas, E.A., Boren, S.A., Brown, G.D., Ewigman, B.G., Mitchell, J.A., and Perkoff, G.T. (1996). Effect of physician profiling on utilization. Meta-analysis of randomized clinical trials. *Journal of General Internal Medicine, 11,* 584–590.

Bandura, A. (1977). Self-efficacy: Toward a unifying theory of behavior change. *Psychological Review, 84,* 191–215.

Bandura, A. (1986). *Social Foundations of Thought and Action: A Social Cognitive Theory.* Englewood Cliffs, New Jersey: Prentice-Hall.

Bandura, A. (1997). *Self-Efficacy: The Exercise of Control.* New York: W.H. Freeman and Co.

Bandura, A., O'Leary, A., Taylor, C.B., Gauthier, J., and Gossard, D. (1987). Perceived self-efficacy and pain control: Opioid and nonopioid mechanisms. *Journal of Personality and Social Psychology, 53,* 563–571.

Bartholomew, L.K., Czyzewski, D.I., Percel, G.S., Swank, P.R., and Sochrider, M.M. (1997). Self-management of cystic fibrosis: Short-term outcomes of the cystic fibrosis family education program. *Health Education and Behavior, 24,* 652–666.

Baum, A (2000) Behavioral and psychosocial intervention to modify pathophysiology and disease course. In B.D. Smedley and S.L. Syme (Eds.) *Promoting Health: Intervention Strategies from Social and Behavioral Research.* Institute of Medicine. (pp. 450-488).Washington, DC: National Academy Press.

Baumeister, R.F., Leith, K.P., Muraven, M., and Bratslavsky, E. (1998). Self-regulation as a key to success in life. In D. Pushkar and W.M. Bukowski, A.E. Schwartzman, D.M. Stack, and D.R. White, (Eds.) *Improving competence across the lifespan: Building interventions based on theory and research* (pp. 117–132). New York: Plenum Press.

Berwick, D.M. (1989). Continuous improvement as an ideal in health care. *New England Journal of Medicine, 320,* 53–56.

Best, J. (1989). Intervention perspectives on school health promotion research. *Health Education Quarterly, 16,* 301–306.

Best, J.A., Thomson, J., and Santi, S. (1988). Preventing cigarette smoking among school children. *Annual Review of Public Health, 9,* 161.

Bishop, D., Miller, I., Guilmette, T., Feldman, E., Ryan, C., Epstein, N., Muhand, J., Adams, J., Evans, R., Maynard, R., Stason, W., Seifer, R., Keitner, R., Weiner, D., Albro J. (1997). A pilot study evaluating the effectiveness of family intervention telephone tracking (FITT) in reducing sequelae of stroke. Abstract prepared for the *Symposium on Mental Health Sciences,* Rhode Island Hospital, Department of Psychiatry, Providence, RI.

Black, D.R., Gleser, L.J., and Kooyers, K.J. (1990). A meta-analytic evaluation of couples' weight loss programs. *Health Psychology, 9,* 330–347.

Black, J.L., Allison, T.G., Williams, D.E., Rummans, T.A., and Gau, G.T. (1998) Effect of intervention for psychological distress on rehospitalization rates in cardiac rehabilitation patients. *Psychosomatics, 39,* 134–143.

Blackburn, H. (1983). Research and demonstration projects in community cardiovascular disease prevention. *Journal of Public Health Policy, 4,* 398–422.

Blake-Mortimer, J., Gore-Felton, C., Kimerling, R., Turner-Cobb, J.M., and Spiegel, D. (1999). Improving the quality and quantity of life among patients with cancer: A review of the effectiveness of group psychotherapy. *European Journal of Cancer 35,* 1581–1586.

Blumenthal, J.A., Jiang, W., Babyak, M.A., Krantz, D.S., Frid, D.J., Coleman, R.E.; Waugh, R., Hanson, M., Appelbaum, M., O'Connor, C., and Morris, J.J. (1997a) Stress management and exercise training in cardiac patients with myocardial ischemia. Effects on prognosis and evaluation of mechanisms. *Archives of Internal Medicine, 157,* 2213–2223.

Blumenthal, J.A., O'Connor, C., Hinderliter, A., Fath, K., Hegde, S.B., Miller, G., Puma, J., Sessions, W., Sheps, D., Zakhary, B., and Williams, R.B. (1997b) Psychosocial factors and coronary disease. A national multicenter clinical trial (ENRICHD) with a North Carolina focus. *North Carolina Medical Journal, 58,* 440–444.

Boss, P., Caron, W., Horbal, J., and Mortimer, J. (1990). Predictors of depression in caregivers of dementia patients: Boundary ambiguity and mastery. *Family Process, 29,* 245–254.

Botvin, G.J., Baker, E., Dusenbury, L., Botvin, E.M., and Diaz, T. (1995). Long-term follow-up results of a randomized drug abuse prevention trial in a white middle-class population. *Journal of the American Medical Association, 273,* 1106–1112.

Bouton, M.E. (1998). The role of context in classical conditioning: Some implications for cognitive behavior therapy. In W. O'Donohue *Learning and Behavior Therapy* (pp. 59–84). Boston: Allyn and Bacon.

Bouton, M.E. (2000). A learning-theory perspective on lapse, relapse, and the maintenance of behavior change. *Health Psychology, 19,* 57–63.

Broadhead, W.E., Kaplan, B.H., James, S.A., Wagner, E.H., Schoenbach, V.J., Grimson, R., Heyden, S., Tibblin, G., and Gehlbach, S.H. (1983). The epidemiologic evidence for a relationship between social support and health. *American Journal of Epidemiology, 117,* 521–537.

Brown, S.A. (1990). Studies of educational interventions and outcomes in diabetic adults: a meta-analysis revisited. *Patient Education and Counseling, 16,* 189-215.

Brown, S.A. (1992). Meta-analysis of diabetes patient education research: variations in intervention effects across studies. *Research in Nursing and Health, 15,* 409–419.

Brown, S.A. (1999). Interventions to promote diabetes self-management: State of the science. *Diabetes Educator, 25* (6 suppl.), 52–61.

Browne, G.B., Arpin, K., Corey, P., Fitch, M., and Gafni, A. (1990). Individual correlates of health service utilization and the cost of poor adjustment to chronic illness. *Medical Care, 28,* 43–58.

Brownson, R.C., Smith, C.A., Pratt, M., Mack, N.E., Jackson-Thompson, J., Dean, C.G., Dabney, S., and Wilkerson J.C. (1996). Preventing cardiovascular disease through community-based risk reduction: The Bootheel Heart Health Project. *American Journal of Public Health, 86,* 206–213.

Bruvold, W.H. (1993). A meta-analysis of adolescent smoking prevention programs. *American Journal of Public Health, 83,* 872–880.

Budd, R.J. and Rollnick, S. (1997). The structure of the Readiness to Change Questionnaire: A test of Prochaska and DiClemente's transtheoretical model. *British Journal of Health Psychology, 2,* 365–376.

Buntinx, F., Winkens, R., Grol, R., and Knottnerus, J.A. (1993). Influencing diagnostic and preventive performance in ambulatory care by feedback and reminders. A review. *Family Practice, 10,* 219–228.

Butow, P.N., Coates, A.S., and Dunn, S.M. (1999) Psychosocial predictors of survival in metastatic melanoma. *Journal of Clinical Oncology 17,* 2256–2263.

Byers, T., Mullis, R., Anderson, J., Dusenbury, L., Gorsky, R., Kimber, C., Krueger, K., Kuester, S., Mokkad, A., and Perry, G. (1995). The costs and effects of a nutritional education program following work-site cholesterol screening. *American Journal of Public Health, 85,* 650–655.

Campbell, L.A., Clark, M., and Kirkpatrick, S. (1986). Stress management training for parents/children undergoing cardiac catheterization. *American Journal of Orthopsychiatry, 56,* 234–243.

Campbell, L.A., Kirkpatrick, S.E., Berry, C.C., and Lambertie, J.J. (1995). Preparing children with congenital heart disease for cardiac surgery. *Journal of Pediatric Psychology, 20,* 313–328.

Campbell, T.L. and Patterson, J.M. (1995). The effectiveness of family interventions in the treatment of physical illness. *Journal of Marital and Family Therapy, 21,* 545–583.

Carleton, R.A., Lasater, T.M., Assaf, A.R., Feldman, H.A., and McKinlay, S. (1995). The Pawtucket Heart Health Program: Community changes in cardiovascular risk factors and projected disease risk. *American Journal of Public Health, 85,* 777–785.

Carlin, E., Carlson, R., and Nordin, J. (1996). Using continuous quality improvement tools to improve pediatric immunization rates. *Journal on Quality Improvement, 22,* 277–288.

Carver, C.S. and Scheier, M.F. (1998). *On the Self-Regulation of Behavior.* New York: Cambridge University Press.

Cheadle, A., Psaty, B.M., Diehr, P., Koepsell, T., Wagner, E., Curry, S., and Kristal, A. (1995). Evaluating community-based nutrition programs: Comparing grocery store and individual-level survey measures of program impact. *Preventive Medicine, 24,* 71–79.

Chesney, M.A., Ickovics, J., Hecht, F.M., Sikipa, G., and Rabkin, J. (1999). Adherence: A necessity for successful HIV combination therapy. *AIDS, 13,* S271–S278.

Clark, N.M., Feldman, D., Wasilewski, Y., and Levison, M. (1984). Changes in children's school performance as a result of education for family management of asthma. *Journal of School Health, 54,* 143–145.

Clement, S. (1995). Diabetes self-management education. *Diabetes Care, 18,* 1204–1214.

Cohen, P. (1997). Tuberculosis. Rise of an old killer. *Health Services Journal, 107,* supplement 13.

Cohen, S.J., Robinson, D., Dugan, E., Howard, G., Suggs, P.K., Pearce, K.F., Carroll, D.D., McGann, P., and Preisser, J. (1999). Communication between older adults and their physicians about urinary incontinence. *Journal of Gerontology A Biological Science Medical Science, 54,* M34–M37.

Collins, M., Loundy, M.R., Brown, F.L., Hollins, L.D., Aldridge, Y., Eckman, J.E., and Kaslow, N.J. (1997). Applicability of criteria for empirically validated treatments to family interventions for pediatric sickle cell disease (SCD). *Journal of Developmental and Physical Disabilities, 9,* 293–309.

COMMIT (1991). Community intervention trial for smoking cessation (COMMIT): Summary of design and intervention. *Journal of the National Cancer Institute, 83,* 1620–1628.

COMMIT (1995a). Community intervention trial for smoking cessation (COMMIT). I. Cohort results from a four year community intervention. *American Journal of Public Health, 85,* 183–192.

COMMIT (1995b). Community intervention trial for smoking cessation (COMMIT). II. Changes in adult cigarette smoking prevalence. *American Journal of Public Health, 85,* 193–200.

Compas, B. E., Haaga, D. F. Keefe, F. J., Leitenberg, H., Williams, D.A. (1998). Sampling of empirically supported psychological treatments from health psychology: smoking, chronic pain, cancer, and bulimia nervosa. *Journal of Consulting and Clinical Psychology, 66,* 89–112.

Compas, B.E., Connor, J.K., Saltzman, H., Thomsen, A.H., and Wadsworth, M. (1999). Getting specific about coping: Effortful and involuntary responses to stress in development. In M. Lewis and D. Ramsay (Eds.) *Soothing and Stress* (pp. 229–256). Mahwah, NJ: Lawrence Erlbaum Associates.

Contento, I.R., Manning, A.D., and Shannon, B. (1992). Research perspective on school-based nutrition education. *Journal of Nutrition Education, 24,* 247–260.

Cooper, G.S., Fortinsky, R.H., Hapke, R., and Landefeld, C.S. (1997) Primary care physician recommendations for colorectal cancer screening. Patient and practitioner factors. *Archives of Internal Medicine 157,* 1946–1950.

Cousins, J.H., Rubovits, D.S., Dunn, J.K., Reeves, R.S., Ramirez, A.G., and Foreyt, J.P. (1992). Family versus individually oriented intervention for weight loss in Mexican American women. *Public Health Reports, 107,* 549–555.

Crabtree, B., Miller, W., Aita, V., Flocke, S.A., and Stange, K.C. (1998). Primary care practice organization and preventive services delivery: A qualitative analysis. *Journal of Family Practice, 46,* 404–409.

Cramer, J.A., Mattson, R.H., Prevey, M.L., Scheyer, R.D., and Ouellette, V.L. (1989). How often is medication taken as prescribed? A novel assessment technique. *Journal of the American Medical Association, 261,* 3273–3277.

Creagan, E.T. (1999). Attitude and disposition: Do they make a difference in cancer survival? *Journal of Prosthetic Dentistry, 82,* 352–355.

Croft, J.B., Temple, S.P., Lankenau, B., Heath, G.W., Macera, C.A., Eaker, E.D., and Wheeler, F.C. (1994). Community intervention and trends in dietary fat consumption among black and white adults. *Journal of the American Dietetic Association, 94,* 1284–1290.

Cunningham, A.J., Edmonds, C.V., Jenkins, G.P., Pollack, H., Lockwood, G.A., and Warr, D. (1998) A randomized controlled trial of the effects of group psychological therapy on survival in women with metastatic breast cancer. *Psychooncology, 7,* 508–517.

Dale, D., Corbin, C.B., and Cuddihy, T.F. (1998). Can conceptual physical education promote physically active lifestyles? *Pediatric Exercise Science, 10,* 97–109.

Davis, D.A. and Taylor-Vaisey, A. (1997). Translating guidelines into practice. A systematic review of theoretic concepts, practical experience and research evidence in the adoption of clinical practice guidelines. *Canadian Medical Association Journal, 157,* 408–416.

Davis, D.A., Thomson, M.A., and Haynes, R.B. (1995). Changing physician performance. A systematic review of the effect of continuing medical education strategies. *Journal of the American Medical Association, 274,* 700–705.

Delamater, A.M., Bubb, J., Davis, S.G., Smith, J.A., Schmidt, L., White, N.H., and Santiago, J.V. (1990). Randomized prospective study of self-management training with newly diagnosed diabetic children. *Diabetes Care, 13,* 492–498.

Devine, E.C. and Westlake, S.K. (1995) The effects of psychoeducational care provided to adults with cancer: meta-analysis of 116 studies. *Oncology Nursing Forum, 22 ,* 1369–1381.

DiClemente, C.C., Prochascka, J.O., Fairhurst, S.K., Velicer, W.F., Valesquez, M.M., and Rossi, J.S. (1991). The processes of smoking cessation: An analysis of precontemplation, contemplation, and preparation stages of change. *Journal of Consulting and Clinical Psychology, 59*, 295–304.

Dimeff, L.A. and Marlatt, G.A. (1998). Preventing relapse and maintaining change in addictive behaviors. *Clinical Psychology-Science and Practice, 5*, 513–525.

Dishman, R.K., Oldenburg, B., O'Neal, H., and Shephard, R.J. (1998). Worksite physical activity interventions. *American Journal of Preventive Medicine, 15*, 344–361.

Doherty, W.J., and Campbell, T.L. (1988). *Families and health.* Newbury Park, CA: Sage Publications.

Dunbar-Jacob, J., Erlen, J.A., Schlenk, E.A., Ryan, C.M., Sereika, S.M. and Doswell, W.M. (2000) Adherence in chronic disease. *Annual Review of Nursing Research, 18*, 48–90.

Dusenbury, L., and Falco, M. (1997). School-based drug abuse prevention strategies: From research to policy to practice. In R.P. Weissberg, T.P. Gullotta, R.L. Hampton, B.A. Ryan, and G.R. Adams (Eds.) *Enhancing Children's Wellness* (pp. 47–75). Thousand Oaks, CA: Sage.

Dusseldorp, E., van Elderen, T., Maes, S., Meulman, J., and Kraaij, V. (1999) A meta-analysis of psychoeduational programs for coronary heart disease patients. *Health Psychology, 18*, 506–519.

Eddy, D.M. (1990). Clinical decision making: From theory to practice. Anatomy of a decision. *Journal of the American Medical Association, 263*, 441–443.

Edgar, L., Rosberger, Z., and Nowlis, D. (1992). Coping with cancer during the first year after diagnosis. *Cancer, 69*, 817–828.

Eisenberg, N., Fabes, R.A., and Guthrie, I.K. (1997). Coping with stress: The roles of regulation and development. In Sharlene A. Wolchik and Irwin N. Sandler (Eds.) *Handbook of Children's Coping: Linking Theory and Intervention. Issues in Clinical Child Psychology.* (pp. 41–70). New York, NY: Plenum Press.

Ell, K. (1996). Social networks, social support and coping with serious illness: The family connection. *Social Science and Medicine, 42*, 173–183.

Emmons, K.M., Linnan, L.A., Shadel, W.G., Marcus, B., and Abrams, D.B. (1999). The Working Healthy Project: A worksite health-promotion trial targeting physical activity, diet, and smoking. *Journal of Occupational and Environmental Medicine, 41*, 545–555.

Emmons, K.M., Thompson, B., Sorensen, G., Linnan, L., Basen-Engquist, K., Biener, L., and Watson, M. (2000). The relationship between organizational characteristics and the adoption of workplace smoking policies. *Health, Education and Behavior, 27*, 483–501.

ENRICHD (1999) *Ask Me About Enriched,* vol. 1, issue 1. Accessed online October 9, 2000. http://www.bios.unc.edu/cscc/ENRI/enridesc.html

ENRICHD (2000) Enhancing recovery in coronary heart disease patients (ENRICHD): Study design and methods. *Am Heart Journal, 139*, 1–9.

Evans, D.L., Staab, J.P., Petitto, J.M., Morrison, M.F., Szuba, M.P., Ward, H.E., Wingate, B., Luber, M.P., and O'Reardon, J.P. (1999) Depression in the medical setting: Biopsychological interactions and treatment considerations. *Journal of Clinical Psychiatry, 60 (Suppl. 4)*, 40–55.

Ewart, C.K. (1990). A social problem-solving approach to behavior change in coronary heart disease. In S. Shumaker, E.B. Schron, J.K. Ockene, C.T. Parker, J.L. Probstfield, and J.M. Wolle (Eds.) *The Handbook of Health Behavior Change.* New York: Springer.

Ewart, C.K. (1991). Social action theory for a public health policy. *American Psychologist, 46,* 931–946.

Ewart, C.K. (1995). Self-efficacy and recovery from heart attack: Implications for a social cognitive analysis of exercise and emotion. In J.E. Maddux et al. (Eds.) *Self-efficacy, Adaptation, and Adjustment: Theory, Research, and Application* (pp. 203–226). New York: Plenum.

Ewart, C.K., Taylor, C.B., Kraemer, H.C., and Agras, W.S. (1984). Reducing blood pressure reactivity during interpersonal conflict: Effects of marital communication training. *Behavior Therapy, 15,* 473–484.

Family Heart Study Group. (1994). Randomized controlled trial evaluating cardiovascular screening and intervention in general practice: Principal results of British family heart study. *British Medical Journal, 308,* 313–320.

Farkas, A.J., Pierce, J.P., Zhu, S.H., Rosbrook, B., Gilpin, E.A., Berry, C., and Kaplan, R.M. (1996). Addiction versus stages of change models in predicting smoking cessation. *Addiction, 91,* 1271–1280.

Farquhar, J.W., Fortrmann, S.P., Flora, J.A., Taylor, B., Haskell, W.L., Williams, P.T., Maccoby, N., and Wood, P.D. (1990). Effects of community-wide education on cardiovascular disease risk factors. *Journal of the American Medical Association, 264,* 359–365.

Farquhar, J.W., Maccoby, N., Wood, P.D., Alexander, J.K., Breitrose, H., Brown, B.W., Jr., Haskell, W.L., McAlister, A.L., Meyer, A.J., Nash, J.D., and Stern, M.P. (1977). Community education for cardiovascular health. *Lancet, 1 (8023),* 1192–1195.

Fava, J.L., Velicer, W.F, and Prochaska, J.O. (1995). Applying the transtheoretical model to a representative sample of smokers. *Addictive Behaviors, 20,* 189–203.

Fawzy, F.I. (1999). Psychosocial interventions for patients with cancer: What works and what doesn't. *European Journal of Cancer, 35,* 1559–1564

Fawzy, F.I., Cousins, N., Fawzy, N.W., Kemeny, M.E., Elashoff, R., and Morton, D.A (1990). Structured psychiatric intervention for cancer patients. I. Changes over time in methods of coping and affective disturbance. *Archives of General Psychiatry, 47,* 720–725.

Fawzy, F.I., Fawzy, N.W., Arndt, L.A., and Pasnau, R.O. (1995). Critical review of psychosocial interventions in cancer care. *Archives of General Psychiatry, 52,* 100–113.

Fawzy, F.I., Fawzy, N.W., Hyun, C.S., Elashoff, R., Guthrie, D., Fahey, J.L., and Morton, D.L. (1993). Malignant melanoma. Effects of an early structured psychiatric intervention, coping, and affective state on recurrence and survival 6 years later. *Archives of General Psychiatry, 50,* 681–689.

Fielding, J. (1984). Health promotion and disease prevention at the worksite. *Annual Review of Public Health, 5,* 237–265.

Fiscella, K., Franks, P., and Shields, C.G. (1997). Perceived family criticism and primary care utilization: Psychosocial and biomedical pathways. *Family Process, 36,* 25–41.

Fishman, P., Von Korff, M., Lozano, P., and Hecht, J. (1997). Chronic care costs in managed care. *Health Affairs, 16,* 239–247.

Flay, B.R. (1985). Psychosocial approaches to smoking prevention: A review of findings, *Health Psychology, 4*, 449–488.

Flay, B.R., Ryan, K.B., Best, A., Brown, K.S., Kersell, M.W., d'Avernas, J.R., and Zanna, M.P. (1985). Are social-psychological smoking prevention programs effective? The Waterloo study. *Journal of Behavioral Medicine, 8*, 37–59.

Fletcher, S.W. and Fletcher, R.H. (1998). Development of clinical guidelines. *Lancet, 352*, 1876.

Flynn, B.S., Worden, J.K., Secker-Walker, R.H., Pirie, P.L., Badger, G.J., and Carpenter, J.H. (1997). Long-term responses of higher and lower risk youths to smoking prevention interventions. *Preventive Medicine, 26*, 389–394.

Fortmann, S.P., Williams, P.T., Hulley, S.B., Haskell, W.L., and Farquhar, J.W. (1981). Effect of health education on dietary behavior: The Stanford three community study. *American Journal of Clinical Nutrition, 34*, 2030–2038.

Frasure-Smith, N. and Prince, R. (1985) The ischemic heart disease life stress monitoring program: Impact on mortality. *Psychosom. Med. 47*, 431–445.

Frasure-Smith, N., Lesperance, F., Prince, R.H., Verrier, P., Garber, R.A., Juneau, M., Wolfson, C., and Bourassa, M.G. (1997) Randomised trial of home-based psychosocial nursing intervention for patients recovering from myocardial infarction. *Lancet, 350*, 473–479.

Galatzer, A., Amir, S., Gil, R., Karp, M., and Laron, Z. (1982). Crisis intervention in newly diagnosed diabetic children. *Diabetes Care, 5*, 414–419.

Gellert, G.A., Maxwell, R.M., and Siegel, B.S. (1993) Survival of breast cancer patients receiving adjunctive psychosocial support therapy: A 10-year follow-up study. *Journal of Clinical Oncology, 11*, 66–69.

Gilliss, C.L., Highly, B.L., Roberts, B.M., and Martinson, I.M. (1989). *Toward a Science of Family Nursing.* Menlo Park, CA: Addison-Wesley.

Glasgow, R.E., Fisher, E.B., Anderson, B.J., LaGreca, A., Marrero, D., Johnson, S.B., Rubin, R.R., and Cox, D.J. (1999). Behavioral science in diabetes. Contributions and opportunities. *Diabetes Care, 22*, 832–843.

Glasgow, R.E., Sorensen, G., Giffen, C., Shipley, R.H., Corbett, K., and Lynn, W. (1996). Promoting worksite smoking control policies and actions: The community intervention trial for smoking cessation (COMMIT) experience. *Preventive. Medicine, 25*, 186–194.

Glasgow, R.E., Terborg, J.R., Hollis, J.F., Severson, H.H., and Boles, S.M. (1995). Take Heart: Results from the initial phase of a work-site wellness program. *American Journal of Public Health, 85*, 209–216.

Glasgow, R.E., Terborg, J.R., Stycker, L.A., Boles, S.M., and Hollis, J.F. (1997). Take Heart II: Replication of a worksite health promotion trial. *Journal of Behavioral Medicine, 20*, 143–161.

Glass, T.A., Dym, B., Greenberg, S., Rintell, D., Roesch, C., and Berkman, L.F. (2000). Psychosocial intervention in stroke: Families in Recovery from Stroke Trial (FIRST). *American Journal of Orthopsychiatry, 70*, 169–181.

Glynn, T.J. (1989). Essential elements of school-based smoking prevention programs, *Journal of School Health, 59*, 181–188.

Gonzalez, S., Steinglass, P., and Reiss, R. (1989). Putting the illness in its place: Discussion groups for families with chronic medical illnesses. *Family Process, 28*, 69–87.

Gostin, L. (1997). Health care information and the protection of personal privacy: Ethical and legal considerations. *Annals of Internal Medicine, 127*, 683–690.

Green, L.W., Eriksen, M.P., and Schor, E.L. (1988). Preventive practices by physicians: Behavioral determinants and potential interventions. *American Journal of Preventive Medicine, 4*, S101–S107.

Greer, A.L. (1988). The state of the art versus the state of the science: The diffusion of new medical technologies into practice. *Internal Journal of Technology Assessment in Health Care, 4*, 5–26.

Greer, S. (1999). Mind–body research in psychooncology. *Advances Mind Body Medicine, 15*, 236–244.

Grey, M. (2000). Interventions for children with diabetes and their families. *Annual Review of Nursing Research, 18*, 149–170.

Grey, M., Kanner, S., and Lacey, K.O. (1999) Characteristics of the learner: Children and adolescents. *Diabetes Educator, 25 (6 Suppl)*, 25–33.

Grimshaw, J.M. and Russell, I.T. (1994). Achieving health gain through clinical guidelines II: Ensuring guidelines change medical practice. *Quality Health Care, 3*, 45–52.

Grimshaw, J.M. and Russell, I.T. (1993). Effect of clinical guidelines on medical practice: A systematic review of rigorous evaluations. *Lancet, 342*, 1317–1322.

Gustafsson, P.A., Kjellman, N.I., and Cederblad, M. (1986). Family therapy in the treatment of severe childhood asthma. *Journal of Psychosomatic Research, 30*, 369–374.

Hammer, M. and Champy, J. (1993). *Reengineering the Corporation*. New York: Harper Business.

Hampson, S.E., Skinner, T.C., Hart, J., Storey, L., Gage, H., Foxcroft, D., Kimber, A., Cradock, S., and McEvilly, E.A. (2000). Behavioral interventions for adolescents with type 1 diabetes: How effective are they? *Diabetes Care, 23*, 1416–1422.

Haubrich, R.H., Little, S.J., Currier, J.S., et al. (1999). The value of patient-reported adherence to antiretroviral therapy in predicting virologic and immunologic response. California Collaborative Treatment Group. *AIDS, 13*, 1099–1107.

Haynes, B., Taylor, D., and Sackett, D., (Eds.) (1979). *Compliance in Health Care*. Baltimore: Johns Hopkins University Press.

Haynes, R.B., McKibbon, K.A., and Kanani, R. (1996). Systematic review of randomised trials of interventions to assist patients to follow prescriptions for medications. *Lancet, 348*, 383–386.

Heath, G.W., Temple, S.P., Fuchs, R., Wheeler, F.C., and Croft, J.B. (1995). Changes in blood cholesterol awareness: Final results from the South Carolina Cardiovascular Disease Prevention Project. *American Journal of Preventive Medicine, 11*, 190–196.

Heimendinger, J., Thompson, B., Ockene, L., Sorensen, G., Abrams, D.B., Emmons, K., Varnes, J., Eriksen, M.P., Probart, C., and Himmelstein, J. (1990). Reducing the risk of cancer through worksite intervention. *Occupational Medicine: State of the Art Reviews (Vol. 7)*. Philadelphia: Henley and Belfus.

Heirich, M.A., Foote, A., Erfurt, J.C., and Konopka, B. (1993). Work-Site Physical Fitness Programs: Comparing the impact of different program designs on cardiovascular risks. *Journal of Occupational Medicine, 35*, 510–517.

Helgeson, V.S. (1994). The onset of chronic illness: Its effect on the patient-spouse relationship. *Journal of Social and Clinical Psychology, 12*, 406–428.

Helgeson, V.S. and Cohen, S. (1996). Social support and adjustment to cancer: Reconciling descriptive, correlational, and intervention research. *Health Psychology, 15*, 75–83.

Herzog, T.A., Abrams, D.B., Emmons, K.M., Linnan, L., and Shadel, W.G. (1999). Do processes of change predict smoking stage movements? A prospective analysis of the Transtheoretical Model. *Health Psychology, 4*, 369–375.

Hoagland, A.C., Morrow, G.R., Bennett, J.M., and Carnrike, C., Jr. (1983) Oncologists' views of cancer patient noncompliance. *American Journal of Clinical Oncology, 6*, 239–244.

Hochbaum, G.M. (1958). Public participation in medical screening programs: A socio-psychological study. Washington: U.S. Dept. of Health, Education, and Welfare.

Hoekstra-Weebers, J., Heuval, F., Jaspers, J., Kamps, W., and Klip, E. (1998). Brief Report: An intervention program for parents of pediatric cancer patients: A randomized controlled trial. *Journal of Pediatric Psychology, 23*, 207–214.

Holder, B., Turner-Musa, J., Kimmel, P.L., Alleyne, S., Kobrin, S., Simmens, S., Cruz, I., and Reiss, D. (1998). Engagement of African American Families in research on chronic illness: A multisystem recruitment approach. *Family Process, 37*, 127–151.

Homel, P.J., Daniels, P., Reid, T.R., and Lawson, J.S. (1981). Results of an experimental school-based health development program in Australia. *International Journal of Health Education, 4*, 263–270.

House, J.S., Landis, K.R., and Umberson, D. (1988). Social relationships and health. *Science, 241*, 540–545.

Hughes, D.M., McLeod, M., Garner, B., and Goldbloom, R.B. (1991). Controlled trial of a home and ambulatory program for asthmatic children. *Pediatrics, 87*, 54–61.

Ilnyckyj, A., Farber, J., Cheang, M., and Weinerman, B. (1994) A randomized controlled trial of psychotherapeutic intervention in cancer patients. *Annals of the Royal College of Physicians and Surgeons of Canada, 27*, 93–96.

IOM (Institute of Medicine) (2001). *Speaking of Health: Assessing Health Communication. Strategies for Diverse Populations.* C. Chrvala and S. Scrimshaw (Eds.). Washington, DC: National Academy Press.

Jacobson, AM. (1996). The psychological care of patients with insulin-dependent diabetes mellitus. *New England Journal of Medicine, 334*, 1249–1253.

Janz, N.K. and Becker, M.H. (1984). The Health Belief Model: A decade later. *Health Education Quarterly, 11*, 1–47.

Jay, S. and Elliott, C. (1990). A stress inoculation program for parents whose children are undergoing painful medical procedures. *Journal of Consulting and Clinical Psychology, 58*, 799–804.

Jeffery, R., French, S., Raether, C., and Baxter, J. (1994). An environmental intervention to increase fruit and salad purchases in a cafeteria. *Preventive Medicine, 23*, 788–792.

Jeffery, R.W., Drewnowski, A., Epstein, L.H., Stunkard, A.J., Wilson, T., and Hill, R. (2000). Long-term maintenance of weight loss: Current status. *Health Psychology, 19*, 5–16.

Jeffery, R.W., Forster, J.L., Dunn, B. V., French, S.A., McGovern, P.G., and Lando, H.A. (1993). Effects of work-site health promotion on illness-related absenteeism. *Journal of Occupational and Environmental Medicine, 35*, 1142–1146.

Jones, D.A. and West, R.R. (1996). Psychological rehabilitation after myocardial infarction: Multicentre randomised controlled trial. *British Medical Journal, 313*, 1517–1521.

Kaplan, R.M., Ries, A.L., Prewitt, L.M., and Eakin, E. (1994). Self-efficacy expectations predict survival for patients with chronic obstructive pulmonary disease. *Health Psychology, 13*, 366–368.

Kaslow, N.J. and Brown, F. (1995). Culturally sensitive family interventions for chronically ill youth: Sickle cell disease as an example. *Family Systems Medicine, 13*, 201–213.

Kaslow, N.J., Collins, M.H., Loundy, M.R., Brown, F., Hollins, L.D., and Eckman, J. (1997). Empirically-validated family interventions for pediatric psychology: Sickle cell disease as an exemplar. *Journal of Pediatric Psychology, 22*, 213–227.

Kazak, A.E., Penati, B., Brophy, P., and Himelstein, B. (1998). Pharmacologic and psychologic interventions for procedural pain. *Pediatrics, 102*, 59–66.

Kazak, A.E., Simms, S., Barakat, L., Hobbie, W., Foley, B., Golomb, V., and Best, M. (1999). Surviving cancer competently intervention program (SCCIP): A cognitive-behavioral and family therapy intervention for adolescent survivors of childhood cancer and their families. *Family Process, 38*, 175–191.

Kehoe, E.J. and Macrae, M. (1998). Classical conditioning. In W. O'Donohue (Ed.) *Learning and Behavior Therapy* (pp. 36–58). Boston: Allyn and Bacon.

Kelder, S.H., Perry, C.L., Klepp, K., and Lytle, L.L. (1994). Longitudinal tracking of adolescent smoking, physical activity, and food choice behaviors. *American Journal of Public Health, 84*, 1121–1126.

Keys, A. (1970). Coronary heart disease in seven countries. *Circulation, 41 (Suppl. 1)*, 1–211.

Kiecolt-Glaser, J.K. and Glaser, R. (1999) Psychoneuroimmunology and cancer: Fact or fiction? *European Journal of Cancer, 35*, 1603–1607.

Kiecolt-Glaser, J.K., Glaser, R., Cacioppo, J.T., MacCallum, R.C., Snydersmith, M., Kim, C., and Malarkey, W.B. (1997). Marital conflict in older adults: Endocrinological and immunological correlates. *Psychosomatic Medicine, 59*, 339–349.

Kiecolt-Glaser, J.K., Marucha, P.T., Malarkey, W.B., Mercado, A.M., Glaser, R. (1995). Slowing of wound healing by psychological stress. *Lancet, 346*, 1194–1196.

Kiecolt-Glaser, J.K., Page, G.G., Marucha, P.T., MacCallum, R.C., and Glaser, R. (1998). Psychological influences on surgical recovery. Perspectives from psychoneuro-immunology. *American Psychologist, 53*, 1209–1218.

Killen, J.D., Fortmann, S.P., Telch, M.J., and Newman, B. (1988). Are heavy smokers different from light smokers? A comparison after 48 hours without cigarettes. *Journal of the American Medical Association, 260*, 1581–1585.

Kleinman, A., Eisenberg, L., and Good, B. (1978). Culture, illness and care: Clinical lessons from anthropologic and cross-cultural research. *Annals of Internal Medicine, 88*, 251–258.

Knutsen, S. and Knutsen, R. (1991). The Tromso study: The family intervention study—the effect of intervention on some coronary risk factors and dietary habits, a 6-year follow-up. *Preventive Medicine, 20*, 197–212.

Kottke, T.E., Battista, R.N., DeFriese, G.H., and Brekke, M.L. (1988). Attributes of successful smoking cessation intervention in medical practice. A meta-analysis of 39 controlled trials. *Journal of the American Medical Association, 59*, 2883–2889.

Lang, E.V., Benotsch, E.G., Fick L.J., Lutgendorf, S., Berbaum, M.L., Berbaum, K.S., Logan, H., and Spiegel, D. (2000). Adjunctive non-pharmacological analgesia for invasive medical procedures: A randomised trial. *Lancet, 355*, 1486–1490.

Lang, E.V., Joyce, J.S., Spiegel, D., Hamilton, D., and Lee, K.K. (1996). Self-hypnotic relaxation during interventional radiological procedures: Effects on pain perception and intravenous drug use. *International Journal of Clinical and Experimental Hypnosis, 44*, 106–119.

Lask, B. and Matthew, D. (1979). Childhood asthma. A controlled trial of family psychotherapy. *Archives of Disease in Childhood, 54*, 116–119.

Leslie, E., Owen, N., and Fotheryham, M. (1998). *Campus-based Physical Activity Interventions: Process and Outcomes.* Sydney: Deakin University Press.

Levenson, R. and Gottman, J. (1983). Marital interaction: Physiological linkage and affective exchange. *Journal of Personality and Social Psychology, 45*, 587–597.

Levenson, R., Carstensen, L.L., and Gottman, J.M. (1994). The influence of age and gender on affect, physiology and their interrelations: A study of long term marriages. *Journal of Personality and Social Psychology, 67*, 56–58.

Lewis, C.E., Raczynski, J.M., Heath, G.W., Levinson, R., Hilyer, J.C., Jr., and Cutter, G.R. (1993). Promoting Physical Activity in Low-Income African-American Communities: The Parr Project. *Ethnicity and Disease, 3*, 106–118.

Linden, W., Stossel, C., and Maurice, J. (1996) Psychosocial interventions for patients with coronary artery disease: A meta-analysis. *Archives of Internal Medicine, 156*, 745–752.

Linn, M.W., Linn, B.S., and Harris, R. (1982). Effects of counseling for late stage cancer. *Cancer, 49*, 1048–1055.

Lipid Research Clinics Program. (1984a). The lipid research clinics coronary primary prevention trial results. II. The relationship of reduction in incidence of coronary heart disease to cholesterol lowering. *Journal of the American Medical Association, 251*, 365–374.

Lipid Research Clinics Program. (1984b). The lipid research clinics coronary primary prevention trial results. I. Reduction in incidence of coronary heart disease. *Journal of the American Medical Association, 251*, 351–364.

Luepker, R.V., Murray, D.M., Jacobs, D.R., Mittelmark, M.B., Bracht, N., Carlaw, R., Crow, R., Elmer, P., Finnegan, J., Folsom, A.R. et al. (1994). Community education for cardiovascular disease prevention: Risk factor changes in the Minnesota Heart Health Program. *American Journal of Public Health, 84*, 1383–1393.

Luepker, R.V., Perry, C.L., and McKinlay, S.M. (1996). Outcomes of a field trial to improve children's dietary patterns and physical activity: The Child and Adolescent Trial for Cardiovascular Health (CATCH). *Journal of the American Medical Association, 275*, 768–776.

Lustman, P.J., Anderson, R.J., Freedland, K.E., de Groot, M., Carney, R.M., and Clouse, R.E.. (2000). Depression and poor glycemic control: A meta-analytic review of the literature. *Diabetes Care, 23*, 934–942.

Lustman, P.J., Griffith, L.S., Gavard, J.A., and Clouse, R.E. (1992). Depression in adults with diabetes. *Diabetes Care, 15*, 1631–1639.

Maccoby, N. and Solomon, D. S. (1981). *Heart Disease Prevention: Community Studies.* Beverly Hills: Sage.

Magnan, S., Solberg, L.I., Kottke, T.E., Nelson, A.F., Amundson, G.M., Richards, S., and Reed, M.K. (1998). Improve: Bridge over troubled waters. *Joint Commission Journal on Quality Improvement, 24*, 566–578.

Manley, M., Lynn, W., Epps, R. P., Grande, D., Glynn, T., and Shopland, D. (1997a). The American Stop Smoking Intervention Study for cancer prevention: An overview. *Tobacco Control, 6*, S5–S11.

Manley, M.W., Pierce, J.P., Gilpin, E.A., Rosbrook, B., Berry, C., and Wun, L.-M. (1997b). Impact of the American stop smoking intervention study (ASSIST) on cigarette consumption. *Tobacco Control, 6*, S12–S16.

Manne, S.L., Girasek, D., and Ambrosino, J. (1994). An evaluation of the impact of a cosmetics class on breast cancer patients. *Journal of Psychosocial Oncology, 12*, 83–99.

Marlatt, G.A. and George, W.H. (1998). Relapse prevention and the maintenance of optimal health. In S.A. Schumaker et al. (Eds.) *The Handbook of Health Behavior Change, 2nd edition* (pp. 33–58). New York: Springer Publishing.

Marlatt, G.A. and Gordon, J.R. (Eds.) (1985) *Relapse Prevention*. New York: Guilford Press.

Marmot, M. (1994). Cardiovascular disease. *Journal of Epidemiology and Community Health, 48*, 2–4.

McBride, C.M., Curry, S.J., Taplin, S., Anderman, C., and Grothaus, L. (1993). Exploring environmental barriers to participation in mammography screening in an HMO. *Cancer Epidemiology, Biomarkers and Prevention, 2*, 599–605.

McDonald, C.J. (1976). Protocol-based computer reminders, the quality of care and the non-perfectibility of man. *New England Journal of Medicine, 295*, 1351–1355.

McEwen, B. (1998). Protective and damaging effects of stress mediators. *New England Journal of Medicine, 338*, 171–179.

McGinnis, M. (1993). 1992 national survey of worksite health promotion activities: Summary. *American Journal of Health Promotion, 7*, 452–464.

McKenzie, T.L., Nader, P.R., and Strikmiller, P.K. (1996). School physical education: Effect of the child and adolescent trial for cardiovascular health. *Preventive Medicine, 25*, 423–431.

McKinlay, J. (1995). The new public health approach to improving physical activity and autonomy in older populations. In E. Heikkinon (Ed.) *Preparation for Aging* (pp. 87–104). New York: Plenum Press.

McNabb, W.L., Quinn, M.T., Murphy, D.M., Thorp, F.K., and Cook, S. (1994). Increasing children's responsibility for diabetes self-care: The In Control study. *Diabetes Educator, 20*, 121–124.

Mendez, F. and Belendez, M. (1997). Effects of a behavioral intervention on treatment adherence and stress management in adolescents with IDDM. *Diabetes Care, 20*, 1370–1375.

Meyer, T.J. and Mark, M.M. (1995) Effects of psychosocial interventions with adult cancer patients: A meta-analysis of randomized experiments. *Health Psychology, 14*, 101–108.

Miller, W.L., Crabtree, B.F., McDaniel, R., and Stange, K. (1998). Understanding change in primary care practice using complexity theory. *Journal of Family Practice, 46*, 369–376.

Miller, W.R. and Rollnick, S. (1995). *Motivational Interviewing: Preparing People to Change Addictive Behavior*. New York: Guilford Press.

Mittleman, M.S., Ferris, S.H., Mackell, J.A., Ambinder, A., and Cohen, J. (1993). An intervention that delays institutionalization of Alzheimer's disease patients: Treatment of spouse caregivers. *The Gerontologist, 33*, 730–740.

Mittleman, M.S., Ferris, S.H., Shulman, E., Steinberg, G., Ambinder, A., Mackell, J.A., and Cohen, J. (1995). A comprehensive support program: Effect on depression in spouse caregivers of AD patients. *The Gerontologist, 35*, 792–802.

Mittleman, M.S., Ferris, S.H., Shulman, E., Steinberg, G., and Levin, B. (1996). A family intervention to delay nursing home placement of patients with Alzheimer's disease: A randomized controlled trial. *Journal of the American Medical Association, 276*, 1725–1731.

Mittman, B.S., Tonesk, X., and Jacobson, P.D. (1992). Implementing clinical practice guidelines: Social influence strategies and practitioner behavior change. *Quality Review Bulletin, 18*, 413–422.

Montazeri, A, Gillis, C.R., and McEwen, J. (1998). Quality of life in patients with lung cancer: A review of literature from 1970 to 1995. *Chest, 113*, 467–481.

Morgenstern, H., Gellert, G.A., Walter, S.D., Ostfeld, A.M., and Siegel, B.S. (1984). The impact of a psychosocial support program on survival with breast cancer: The importance of selection bias in program evaluation. *J. Chronic Disease, 37*, 273–282.

Morisky, D.E., DeMuth, N.M., Field-Fass, M., Green, L.W., and Levine, D.M. (1985). Evaluation of family health education to build social support for long-term control of high blood pressure. *Health Education Quarterly, 12*, 35–50.

Morisky, D.E., Levine, D.M., Green, L.W., Shapiro, S., Russell, R.P., and Smith, C.R. (1983). Five-year blood pressure control and mortality following health education for hypertensive patients. *American Journal of Public Health, 73*, 153–162.

Mosser, G., and Sakowski, J. (1996). Establishing a central structure for supporting guideline implementation. *Medical Interface, 9*, 136–139.

MRFIT Research Group. (1982). Multiple risk factor intervention trial. *Journal of the American Medical Association, 248*, 1465–1477.

Murray, D.M. (1995). Design and Analysis of Community Trials: Lessons from the Minnesota Heart Health Program. *American Journal of Epidemiology, 142*, 569–575.

Nader, P.R., Stone, E. J., Lyle, L.A., Perry, C.L., Osganian, S. K., Kelder, S., Webber, L.S., Elder, J. P., Montgomery, D., Feldman, H.A., Wu, M., Johnson, C., Parcel, G.S., and Leupker, R.V. (1999). Three-year maintenance of improved diet and physical activity: the CATCH cohort. *Archives of Pediatric and Adolescent Medicine, 153*, 695–704.

National Heart, Lung, and Blood Institute [NHLBI] (1998). *Behavioral Research in Cardiovascular, Lung, and Blood Health and Disease*, Department of Health and Human Services.

O'Donohue, W. (1998). Conditioning and third-generation behavior therapy. In W. O'Donohue (Ed.) *Learning and Behavior Therapy* (pp. 1–14). Boston: Allyn and Bacon.

Ockene, J.K., Emmons, K., Mermelstein, R., Perkins, K.A., Bonollo, D., Hollis, J.F., and Vorhees, C. (2000). Relapse and maintenance issues for smoking cessation. *Health Psychology, 19 (Suppl.)*, 17–31.

Ornish, D., Brown, S.E., Scherwitz, L.W., Billings, J.H.; Armstrong, W.T., and Ports, T.A. (1990). Can lifestyle changes reverse coronary heart disease? The Lifestyle Heart Trial. *Lancet, 336*, 129–133.

Oxman, A.D., Thomson, M.A., Davis, D.A., and Haynes, R.B. (1995). No magic bullets: A systematic review of 102 trials of interventions to improve professional practice. *Canadian Medical Association Journal, 153*, 1423–1431.

Padgett, D., Mumford, E., Hynes, M., and Carter, R. (1988). Meta-analysis of the effects of educational and psychosocial interventions on management of diabetes mellitus. *Journal of Clinical Epidemiology, 41*, 1007–1030.

Patti, R., and Resneck, H. (1972). Changing the agency from within. *Social Work, 17*, 48–57.

Pearce, J., LeBow, M., and Orchard, J. (1981). Role of spouse involvement in the behavioral treatment of overweight women. *Journal of Consulting and Clinical Psychology, 49*, 236–244.

Perri, M.G., Nezu, A.M., and Viegener, B.J. (1992). *Improving the Long-term Management of Obesity: Theory, Research, and Clinical Guidelines*. New York: John Wiley and Sons.

Perry, C.L., Kelder, S.H., Murray, D.M., and Klepp, K.I. (1992). Community-wide smoking prevention: Long-term outcomes of the Minnesota heart health program and the class of 1989 study. *American Journal of Public Health, 82*, 1210–1216.

Perry, C.L., Luepker, R.V., Murray, D.M., Hearn, M.D., Halper, A., Dudovitz, B., Maile, M.C., and Smyth, M. (1989). Parent involvement with children's health promotion: A one-year follow-up of the Minnesota home team. *Health Education Quarterly, 16*, 171–180.

Perry, C.L., Story, M., and Lytle, L.A. (1997). Promoting healthy dietary behaviors. In R.P. Weissberg, T.P. Gullotta, (Eds.), *Healthy Children 2010: Enhancing Children's Wellness. Issues in Children's and Families' Lives, Vol. 8* (pp. 214–249). Thousand Oaks, CA: Sage Publications.

Peterson, A.V. Jr., Kealey, K.A., Mann, S.L., Marek, P.M., and Sarason, I.G. (2000). Hutchinson smoking prevention project: long-term randomized trial in school-based tobacco use prevention—results on smoking. *Journal of the National Cancer Institute, 92*, 1979–1991.

Pierce, J.P., Farkas, A.J., and Gilpin, E.A. (1998). Beyond stages of change: The quitting continuum measures progress towards successful smoking cessation. *Addiction, 93*, 277–286.

Powell, L.H. and Thoresen, C.E. (1988) Effects of type A behavioral counseling and severity of prior acute myocardial infarction on survival. *American Journal of Cardiology, 62*, 1159–1163.

Primomo, J., Yates, B.C., and Woods, N.F. (1990). Social support for women during chronic illness: The relationship among sources and types of adjustment. *Research in Nursing and Health, 13*, 153–161.

Prochaska, J.O. and DiClemente, C.C. (1983). Stages and processes of self-change of smoking: Toward an integrative model of change. *Journal of Consulting and Clinical Psychology, 51*, 390–395.

Prochaska, J.O., Redding, C.A., and Evers, K.E. (1997). The trans theoretical model and stages of change. In K. Glanz, F.M. Lewis, and B.K. Rimer (Eds.) *Health Behavior and Health Education: Theory, Research, and Practice 2nd edition*. San Francisco: Jossey-Bass.

Prochaska, J.O., Velicer, W.F., Rossi, J.S., Goldstein, M.G., Marcus, B.H., Rakowski, W., Fiore, C., Harlow, L.L., Redding, C.A., Rosenbloom, D., and Rossi, S.R. (1994). Stages of change and decisional balance for 12 problem behaviors. *Health Psychology, 13*, 39–46.

Pronk, N.P. and O'Connor, P.J. (1997). Systems approach to population health improvement. *Journal of Ambulatory Care Management, 20*, 24–31.

Puska, P., Salonen, J.T., Nissinen, A., Tuomilehto, J., Vartiainen, E., Korhonen, H., Tanskanen, A., Ronnqvist, P., Koskela, K., and Huttunen, J. (1983). Change in risk factors for coronary heart disease during 10 years of a community intervention programme (North Karelia project). *British Medical Journal, 287*, 1840–1844.

Ransom, D.C. and Vandervoort, H.E. (1973). The development of family medicine: Problematic trends. *Journal of the American Medical Association, 225*, 1098–1102.

Redding, C.A., Armstrong, K.A., Prochaska, J.O., Grimley, D.M., Mahoney, W., LaForge, R., Velicer, W.F., Rossi, J.S., and Ruggiero, L. (1993). The transtheoretical model and cervical cancer prevention among minority female adolescents. *Proceedings of Psychooncology V: Psychosocial Factors in Cancer Risk and Survival* (p. 171). New York: Memorial Sloan-Kettering Cancer Center.

Reiss, D. (1981). *The family's construction of reality.* Cambridge: Harvard University Press.

Rescorla, R.A. (1988). Behavioral studies of Pavlovian conditioning. *Annual Review of Neuroscience, 11*, 329–352.

Richardson, J.L., Shelton, D.R., Krailo, M., and Levine, A.M. (1990) The effect of compliance with treatment on survival among patients with hematologic malignancies. *Journal of Clinical Oncology, 8*, 356–364.

Rimer, B.K. (1990). Perspectives on intrapersonal theories in health education and health behavior. In K. Glanz, F.M. Lewis, and B.K. Rimer (Eds.) *Health Behavior and Health Education: Theory, Research, and Practice* (pp. 140–157). San Francisco: Jossey-Bass.

Rogers, E.M. (1995). *Communication of innovations.* New York: The Free Press.

Rolland, J. (1984). Toward a psychosocial typology of chronic and life-threatening illness. *Family Systems Medicine, 2*, 245–262.

Rooney, B.L. and Murray, D.M. (1996). A meta-analysis of smoking prevention programs after adjustment for errors in the unit of analysis. *Health Education Quarterly, 23*, 48–64.

Rose, G.A. (1992). *The Strategy of Preventive Medicine.* New York: Oxford University Press.

Rosenstock, I.M. and Kirscht, J.P. (1974). The health belief model and personal health behavior. *Health Education Monographs, 2*, 470-473.

Rossi, J.S. (1992). *Stages of change for 15 health risk behaviors in an HMO population.* Paper presentation at 13th Meeting of the Society for Behavioral Medicine, New York, NY.

Roter, D.L., Hall, J.A., Merisca, R., Nordstrom, B., Cretin, D., and Svarstad, B. (1998). Effectiveness of interventions to improve patient compliance: A meta-analysis. *Medical Care, 36*, 1138–1161.

Rozanski, A., Blumenthal, J.A., and Kaplan, J. (1999) Impact of psychological factors on the pathogenesis of cardiovascular disease and implications for therapy. *Circulation, 99*, 2192–2217.

Ryden, O., Johnsson, P., Nevander, L., Sjoblad, S., and Westbom, L. (1993). Cooperation between parents in caring for diabetic children: Relations to metabolic control and parents' field-dependence-independence. *Diabetes Research and Clinical Practice, 20*, 223–229.

Saarni, C. and Crowley, M. (1990). The development of emotion regulation: Effects on emotional state and expression. In E. Blechman (Ed.) *Emotions and the Family: For Better or For Worse* (pp. 53–74). Hillsdale, NJ: Lawrence Erlbaum Associates.

Salina, D., Jason, L.A., Hedeker, D., Kaufman, J., Lesondak, L., McMahon, S.D., Taylor, S., and Kimball, P. (1994). A follow-up of a media-based worksite smoking cessation program. *American Journal of Community Psychology, 22,* 257–271.

Sallis, J.F., Calfas, K.J., Nichols, J.F., Sarkin, J.A., Johnson, M.F., Caparosa, S., Thompson, S., and Alcaraz, J.E. (1999). Evaluation of a university course to promote physical activity: Project GRAD. *Research Quarterly Exercise Sport, 70,* 1–10.

Sapolsky, R.M., Krey, L.C., and McEwen, B.S. (1986). The neuroendocrinology of stress and aging: The glucocorticoid cascade hypothesis. *Endocrinology Review, 7,* 284–301.

Satin, W., La Greca, A.M., Zigo, M.A., and Skyler, J.S. (1989). Diabetes in adolescence: Effects of multifamily group intervention parent simulation of diabetes. *Journal of Pediatric Psychology, 14,* 259–275.

Scheier, M.F., Matthews, K.A., Owens, J.F., Magovern, G.J., Lefebvre, R.C, Abbott, R.A, and Carver, C.S. (1989). Dispositional optimism and recovery from coronary artery bypass surgery: The beneficial effects on physical and psychological well-being. *Journal of Personality and Social Psychology, 57,* 1024–1040.

Schmoldt, R.A. (1989). Marital interaction and the health and well being of spouses. *Women and Health, 15,* 35–56.

Shumaker, S.A., Schron, E.B., Ockene, J.K., and McBee, W.L. (Eds.) (1998). *The Handbook of Behavior Change, 2nd edition.* New York: Springer.

Skinner, B.F. (1938). *The Behavior of Organisms.* Englewood Cliffs, NJ: Appleton-Century-Crofts.

Solberg, L.I., Isham, G.J., Kottke, T.E., Magnan, S., Nelson, A.F., Reed, M.K., and Richards, S. (1995). Competing HMOs collaborate to improve preventive services. *Joint Commission Journal on Quality Improvement, 21,* 600–610.

Solberg, L.I., Kottke, T.E., and Brekke, M.L. (1998). Will primary care clinics organize themselves to improve the delivery of preventive services? A randomized controlled trial. *Preventive Medicine, 27,* 623–631.

Solberg, L.I., Reger, L.A., Pearson, T.L., Cherney, L.M., O'Connor, P.J., Freeman, S.L., Lasch, S.L., and Bishop, D.B. (1997). Using continuous quality improvement to improve diabetes care in populations: The IDEAL model. Improving care for diabetics through improvement and active collaboration and leadership. *The Joint Commission Journal on Quality Improvement, 23,* 581–592.

Sorensen, G., Himmelstein, J., and Hunt, M. (1995). A model for worksite cancer prevention: Integration of health protection and health promotion in the WellWorks Project. *American Journal of Health Promotion, 10,* 55–62.

Sorensen, G., Lando, H., and Pechacek, T. F. (1993). Promoting smoking cessation at the workplace: Results of a randomized controlled intervention study. *Journal of Occupational Medicine, 35,* 121–126.

Sorensen, G., Morris, D. M., Hunt, M.K., Herbert, J.R., Harris, D.R., Stoddard, A., and Ockene, J.K. (1992). Work-Site nutrition intervention and employees' dietary habits: The Treatwell program. *American Journal of Public Health, 82,* 877–880.

Sorensen, G., Stoddard, A., Peterson, K., Cohen, N., Hunt, M. K., Stein, E., Palombo, R., and Lederman, R. (1999). Increasing fruit and vegetable consumption through worksites and families in the Treatwell 5-a-Day Study. *American Journal of Public Health*, 89, 54–60.

Sorensen, G., Thompson, B., Glanz, K., Feng, Z., Kinne, S., DiClemente, C., Emmons, K., Heimendinger, J., Probart, C., and Lichtenstein, E. (1996). Work site-based cancer prevention: Primary results from the Working well Trial. *American Journal of Public Health*, 86, 939–947.

Spiegel, D., and Classen, C. (1995) *Acute stress disorder: Treatment of psychiatric disorders: Anxiety, dissociative, and adjustment disorders.* Washington, DC: American Psychiatric Press.

Spiegel, D., Bloom, J.R., and Yalom, I. (1981) Group support for patients with metastatic cancer. A randomized outcome study. *Archives of General Psychiatry*, 38, 527–533.

Spiegel, D., Bloom, J.R., Kraemer, H.C., and Gottheil, E. (1989) Effect of psychosocial treatment on survival of patients with metastatic breast cancer. *Lancet*, 2 (8668), 888–891.

Spiegel, D., Frischholz, E.J., Fleiss, J.L., and Spiegel, H. (1993). Predictors of smoking abstinence following a single-session restructuring intervention with self-hypnosis. *American Journal of Psychiatry*, 150, 1090–1097.

Spiegel, D., Sephton, S.E., Terr, A.I., and Stites, D.P. (1998) Effects of psychosocial treatment in prolonging cancer survival may be mediated by neuroimmune pathways. *Annals of the New York Academy of Sciences*, 840, 674–683.

Stone, E. and Perry, C. (1990). United States: Perspectives in School Health. *Journal of School Health*, 60, 363–369.

Stone, E., Perry, C., and Luepker, R. (1989). Synthesis of cardiovascular behavioral research for youth health promotion. *Health Education Quarterly*, 16, 155–169.

Stone, E.J., McKenzie, T.L., Welk, G.J., and Booth, M.L. (1998). Effects of physical activity interventions in youth: review and synthesis. *American Journal of Preventive Medicine*, 15, 298–315.

Strecher, V.J. and Rosenstock, I.M. (1997). The Health Belief Model. In K. Glanz, F.M. Lewis, and B.K. Rimer (Eds.) *Health Behavior and Health Education: Theory, Research, and Practice, 2nd edition.* San Francisco: Jossey-Bass.

Strecher, V.J., De Vellis, B.M., Becker, M.H., and Rosenstock, I.M. (1986). The role of self-efficacy in achieving health behavior change. *Health Education Quarterly*, 13, 73–91.

Sundelin, J., Forsander, G., and Mattson, S.E. (1996). Family-oriented support at the onset of diabetes mellitus: A comparison of two group conditions during 2 years following diagnosis. *Acta Paediatrica*, 85, 49–55.

Sutton, S. (1996). Can "stages of change" provide guidance in the treatment of addictions? A critical examination of Prochaska and DiClemente's model. In G. Edwards and C. Dare (Eds.) *Psychotherapy, Psychological Treatments and the Addictions* (pp. 189–205). Cambridge: Cambridge University Press.

Sweeney, L. (1997). Weaving technology and policy together to maintain confidentiality. *Journal of Law, Medicine and Ethics*, 25, 98–110.

Tal, D., Gil-Spielberg, R., Antonovsky, H., Tal, A., and Moaz, B. (1990). Teaching families to cope with childhood asthma. *Family Systems Medicine*, 8, 135–144.

Tarlov, A., Kehrer, B., Hall, D., Samuels, S., Brown, G., Felix, M.R., and Ross, J.A. (1987). Foundation work: The health promotion program of the Henry J. Kaiser Family Foundation. *American Journal of Health Promotion, 2*, 74–80.

Telch, C.F. and Telch, M.J. (1986). Group coping skills instruction and supportive group therapy for cancer patients: A comparison of strategies. *Journal of Consulting and Clinical Psychology, 54*, 802–808.

Tell, G.S. and Vellar, O.K. (1987). Noncommunicable disease risk factor intervention in Norwegian adolescents: The Oslo youth study. In B. Hetzel and G. Berenson (Eds.) *Cardiovascular Risk Factors in Childhood: Epidemiology and Prevention* (pp. 203–217). Amsterdam: Elsevier Science Publishers.

Thomas-Dobersen, D., Butler-Simon, N., and Fleshner, M. (1993). Evaluation of a weight management intervention program in adolescents with IDDM. *Journal of the American Dietetic Association, 93*, 535–540.

Thomson O'Brien, M.A., Oxman, A.D., Davis, D.A., Haynes, R.B., Freemantle, N., and Harvey, E.L. (1999). Audit and feedback versus alternative strategies: Effects on professional practice and health care outcomes (Cochrane Review). In *The Cochrane Library, Issue 4*. Oxford: Update Software.

Tilley, B.C., Glanz, K., Kristal, A.R., Hirst, K., Li, S., Vernon, S.W., and Myers, R. (1999). Nutrition intervention for high-risk auto workers: Results of the next step trial. *Preventive Medicine, 28*, 284–292.

Uchino, B.N., Cacioppo, J.T., and Kiecolt-Glaser, J.K. (1996). The relationship between social support and psychological processes: A review with emphasis on underlying mechanisms and implications for health. *Psychological Bulletin, 119*, 488–531.

US Bureau of the Census (1998). Current Population Reports, Series P23-194, *Population Profile of the United States*, US Government Printing Office, Washington DC.

USDHHS (U.S. Department of Health and Human Services) (1985). *National Survey of Worksite Health Promotion Activities*. Washington, DC.

USDHHS (U.S. Department of Health and Human Services) (1992). *1992 National Survey of Worksite Health Promotion Activities*.Washington, DC.

Verschuren, W., Jacobs, D., Bloemberg, B., Bromhout, D., Menotti, A., Aravanis, C., Blackburn, H., Buzina, R., Dontas, A.S., and Fidanza, F., et al. (1995). Serum total cholesterol and long-term coronary heart disease mortality in different cultures. Twenty-five-year follow-up of the seven countries study. *Journal of the American Medical Association, 274*, 131–136.

Von Korff, M., Ormel, J., Katon, W., and Lin, E.H. (1992) Disability and depression among high utilizers of health care. A longitudinal analysis. *Archives of General Psychiatry 49*, 91–100.

Wadden, T.A., Sarwer, D.B., and Berkowitz, R.I. (1999). Behavioural treatment of the overweight patient. *Baillieres Best Practice and Research. Clinical Endocrinology and Metabolism, 13*, 93–107.

Wadden, T.A., Vogt, R.A., Foster, G.D., and Anderson, D.A. (1998). Exercise and the maintenance of weight loss: 1-year follow-up of a controlled clinical trial. *Journal of Consulting and Clinical Psychology, 66*, 429–433.

Wagner, E., Koepsell, T., Anderman, C., Cheadle, A., Curry, S., Psaty, B.M., Von Korff, M., Wickizer, T.M., Beery, W.L., Diehr, P.K., et al. (1991). The evaluation of the Henry J. Kaiser family foundation's community health promotion grant program: Design. *Journal of Clinical Epidemiology, 44*, 685–699.

Walsh, J.M.E. and McPhee, S.J. (1992). A systems model of clinical preventive care: An analysis of factors influencing patient and physician. *Health Education Quarterly, 19,* 157–175.

Wamboldt, M.Z. and Levin, L. (1995). Utility of multi-family psychoeducational groups for medically ill children and adolescents. *Family Systems Medicine, 13,* 151–161.

Weinstein, A.G., Faust, D.S., McKee, L., and Padman, R. (1992). Outcome of short-term hospitalization for children with severe asthma. *Journal of Allergy and Clinical Immunology, 90,* 66–75.

Wiedenfeld, S.A., O'Leary, A., Bandura, A., Brown, S., Levine, S., and Raska, K. (1990). Impact of perceived self-efficacy in coping with stressors on components of the immune system. *Journal of Personality and Social Psychology, 59,* 1082–1094.

Williams, R.B. and Littman, A.B. (1996) Psychosocial factors: Role in cardiac risk and treatment strategies. *Cardiol. Clin., 14,* 97–104.

Winkleby, M.A., Taylor, B., Jatulis, D., and Fortmann, S.P. (1996). The long-term effects of a cardiovascular disease prevention trial: The Stanford five-city project. *American Journal of Public Health, 86,* 1773–1779.

Woodward, B. (1997). Medical record confidentiality and data collection: current dilemma. *Journal of Law Medicine Ethics, 25,* 88-97.

Wyke, S. and Ford, G. (1992). Competing explanations for associations between marital status and health. *Social Science and Medicine, 34,* 523532.

6

Organizations, Communities, and Society: Models and Interventions

I ndividuals and families are embedded within social, political, and economic systems that shape behaviors and constrain access to resources necessary to maintain health (Brown, 1991; Gottlieb and McLeroy, 1994; Krieger, 1994; Krieger et al., 1993; Lantz et al., 1998; McKinlay, 1993; Sorensen et al., 1998a; Stokols, 1992, 1996; Susser and Susser, 1996a, b; Williams and Collins, 1995; WHO, 1986). The impact of social and environmental conditions is most visible in the growing gap between the health behaviors and health status of rich and poor, white and non-white (Krieger, 1994; Krieger et al., 1993; Lantz et al., 1998; Lillie-Blanton and LaVeist, 1996; Lynch et al., 1997; Williams and Collins, 1995). There is a need to better understand the role of organizational, community, and societal factors in determining health. This chapter continues to explore the ecologic framework, describing theoretical concepts and sample interventions at the organizational, community, and societal levels.

ORGANIZATIONS AND HEALTH

Formal and informal organizations constitute another framework for describing interactions between behavior and health. Organizations are important components of social and physical environments, and they exert considerable influence over the choices people make, the resources they have to aid them in those choices, and the factors in the workplace that could influence health status (e.g., work overload, exposure to toxic chemicals). As employees, consumers, customers, clients, and patients, people are influenced by the organizations to which they belong.

Porras (1987) and Porras and Robertson (1992) suggest four major categories of work settings that are targets for change: organizing arrangements, social factors, technology, and physical settings. Organizing arrangements include organizational goals and strategies for progressing toward them, organizational structure (e.g., formal division of labor, authority relationships, lines of communication), policies and procedures (the formal rules that govern the organization), and reward systems. Social factors include management style, informal social networks, and interaction processes (e.g., problem-solving, decision-making, conflict resolution). The technology category includes job design factors, work flow design, and technical systems. Physical settings include spatial configuration, interior design, and physical ambiance factors such as temperature, lighting, and noise. In their original typology, Porras and Robertson (1992) included individual attributes under the social factors umbrella. However, given the emphasis placed on individual beliefs, attitudes, and skills in health behavior research, those individual factors are suggested as a fifth category in the work setting for targeting change interventions.

Organizational Culture and Change

Organizational culture is the base upon which organizational and related individual behavior change occurs. The culture prescribes the "right way" to do things (Schein, 1990). An organizational culture that supports health is likely to adopt policies, procedures, and priorities that facilitate the healthy behaviors of employees; enhance employee health by reducing environmental risk factors; facilitate healthy behavior on the part of clients, customers, or members; and facilitate linkages to other organizations for health-enhancing purposes. The more health-enhancing policies an organization adopts, the more likely it is to be perceived as having a health-conscious culture (Basen-Enquist et al., 1998).

Organizational development (OD) is a set of behavioral-science-based theories, values, strategies, and techniques aimed at planned change in the organizational work setting (Porras and Robertson, 1992). Three important foundations are briefly described here: *systems theory*, employee *participation* in change efforts, and *action research*. *Systems theory* (Katz and Kahn, 1978) says that a change in one part of the system will influence other parts, and so there is a need to vigilantly monitor unexpected (and often undesired) changes. Increased *involvement and participation* of organizational members in decision-making and problem-solving processes enhances the quality of decisions and solutions, increases members' commitment to following through on plans, reduces organizational stress, and enhances employee well-being (Cotton et al., 1988; Ganster, 1995). The *action research* involves outside change agents working with organization members in a cyclical process of diagnosing problems, planning, implementing plans, monitoring, and evaluating progress (Argyris and Schon, 1989).

Planned-Change Models

Lewin (1951) developed an early and influential model for conceptualizing the change process. He posited three stages: first is unfreezing the old behavior, second is moving to a new behavior, and third is refreezing or stabilizing the new behavior. Thus, change was conceptualized as moving from one equilibrium point to another. To begin the process, the balance between opposing forces (those that facilitate and those that hinder change) must change. Lewin's "force field analysis" was instrumental in the development of subsequent models of change. For example, organizational theorists such as Lippitt and co-workers (1958) and Schein (1987) built on Lewin's three stages and linked them to psychological mechanisms for change and to action steps that change agents should take to facilitate progress through the stages.

INTERVENTIONS TARGETED AT ORGANIZATIONS

Organizational change is an integral component of a comprehensive ecologic approach to health behavior change that emphasizes how individual decisions and behaviors are influenced by the multiple layers of systems within which individuals are embedded (Stokols, 1996). As important components of the social and physical environments, organizations exert considerable influence over the choices people make, the resources they have to aid them in those choices, and the factors in the workplace that could affect health status (e.g., work overload, exposure to toxic chemicals). People are influenced by organizations as employees, consumers, customers, clients, and patients.

Changing Employee Health Behaviors

National surveys of work organizations clearly document a burgeon-ing interest in worksite health promotion programs (see McGinnis, 1993). These programs focus either on a single behavioral risk factor (e.g., smok-ing) or on multiple risk factors (e.g., behavioral risk factors associated with cardiovascular disease). Because many of these interventions are aimed primarily at individual behaviors, they are reviewed in Chapter 5. Here the organizational context for these programs is addressed.

In a review of 47 studies of health promotion programs that addressed multiple risk factors, Heaney and Goetzal (1997) found that almost all provided health education to employees. A smaller number of the pro-grams (25%) incorporated modifications in organizational policy or the work environment to facilitate employee behavior changes. Such modifi-cations included policies restricting or banning smoking on the premises, removing cigarette-vending machines, providing on-site exercise facili-ties, and providing healthier cafeteria food. A survey of health promotion programs funded by the Canadian Ministry of Health showed that more than half the programs reviewed reported modifications of health-com-promising aspects of the organization (Richard et al., 1996). Most of the organization-level interventions addressed organizing arrangements. With the exception of providing on-site fitness facilities, few programs at-tempted to change physical settings, social factors, or technologies. Pro-grams integrated into the culture of the organization were more likely to have multiple components and last longer than did those that had less support from top management and were less a part of the underlying fabric and culture of the organization (Heaney and Goetzal, 1997). Heaney and Goetzal (1997) concluded that providing opportunities for individual risk reduction counseling was necessary but not sufficient for effective worksite health promotion programs.

Studies of programs aimed at individual risk factors also provide some support for the importance of changing the organizational context to sup-port employee health behavior change (Glanz et al., 1996; Hennrikus and Jeffery, 1996). The example of smoking-control efforts at the workplace is illustrative. In their review, Eriksen and Gottlieb (1998) concluded that there is consistent evidence that smoking-control policies reduce ciga-rette consumption at work among smokers and reduce all employees' ex-posure to second-hand smoke. However, they found mixed evidence for policies aimed at prevalence of smoking and overall consumption of ciga-rettes (including during non-work hours). They also point out that many evaluation studies lacked the methodologic rigor necessary to permit confident causal inferences. And although several investigators have suggested the importance of looking at the degree of management support for smoking-control programs, the extent to which the organizational climate is consistent with control efforts, and the design and implementation of programs, few studies have done so.

Some worksite health promotion programs use organizational change theory to inform their strategies. More specifically, current standards of practice include employee participation in planning the efforts. This ranges from incorporating employee input into the assessment of employee health needs (e.g., through surveys or focus groups), to having employee advisory boards guide the planning process, to having employee groups take full responsibility for implementation. Although several large, randomized trials incorporated at least one strategy (Glasgow et al., 1995; Sorensen et al., 1996), a direct comparison of health promotion programs with and without planned employee involvement has not been made. In addition, results from randomized trials that incorporate employee involvement have been mixed.

Another strategy for incorporating organizational change into health promotion programming relies on training key figures in the organizations in methods for creating a supportive organizational culture and developing a comprehensive health promotion program. For example, Golaszewski and colleagues (1998) devised a seven-session curriculum for human resource managers who wanted to develop programs for employee heart health. The training addressed such issues as how to generate support among senior management; how to develop employee wellness committees; and how to conduct needs and resource assessments, diagnose organizational culture, and use employee benefits plans to support health promotion. Student interns were provided to the organizations, faculty from an academic medical center were available for consulting, and potential vendors for health promotion services were identified. Evaluated with a quasi-experimental design, the intervention organizations exhibited a significantly greater increase in organizational support for employee heart health than did the comparison organizations.

Reducing Environmental Risk Factors

Traditional worksite health promotion programs focus on individual change of personal risk factors. Occupational safety and health (OSH) programs address the influence of physical (e.g., noise, extreme temperatures), chemical, ergonomic, and psychosocial work hazards on employee health. According to Goldenhar and Schulte (1994), OSH programs can involve three strategies: engineering, administrative, and behavior change, used to address the different targets for organizational change presented in Figure 6-1. *Engineering strategies* modify technology or physical setting; *administrative strategies* modify the organizing arrangements or social factors; and *behavior change strategies* target beliefs, attitudes, and skills.

Examples of behavior change interventions in OSH include training to increase compliance with safety practices (Parkinson et al., 1989), use of personal protective equipment (Ewigman et al., 1990), and exercise to prevent occupationally related back injuries (Silverstein et al., 1988). Those interventions tend to focus almost exclusively on individual-level change (Goldenhar and Schulte, 1994). Strategies to enhance compliance with universal precautions among health care workers provide a case in point. Although descriptive research clearly indicates the influence of organizational safety climate and work task design on compliance rates, most interventions have targeted only individual employee knowledge, attitudes, and behaviors for change (DeJoy et al., 1995; Gershon et al., 1995).

Few OSH interventions address more than a single type of environmental exposure or use more than a single intervention strategy. However, no matter the exposure or strategy used, organizational change principles are needed to initiate, implement, and maintain OSH programs. Programs oriented to reducing adverse psychosocial work exposures illustrate that point. A voluminous literature documents the consequences of occupational psychosocial stressors such as work overload, role conflict, job insecurity, unpredictability, ambiguity, responsibility for the work of others, and poor relationships with supervisors and co-workers (Hurrell and Murphy, 1992). Much research supports the benefits of psychosocial resources, such as social support and control or decision latitude over how one's job is done (Baker et al., 1996; House, 1981; Israel et al., 1989; Karasek and Theorell, 1990). These psychosocial resources can directly affect employee well-being, and they can buffer employees from the negative effects of stress. Baker et al. (1996) give a comprehensive presentation of the stress process in occupational settings.

Strategies for reducing the harm caused by psychosocial stressors most often entail individual behavior change strategies or administrative change strategies. Those efforts focus either on developing personal strat-

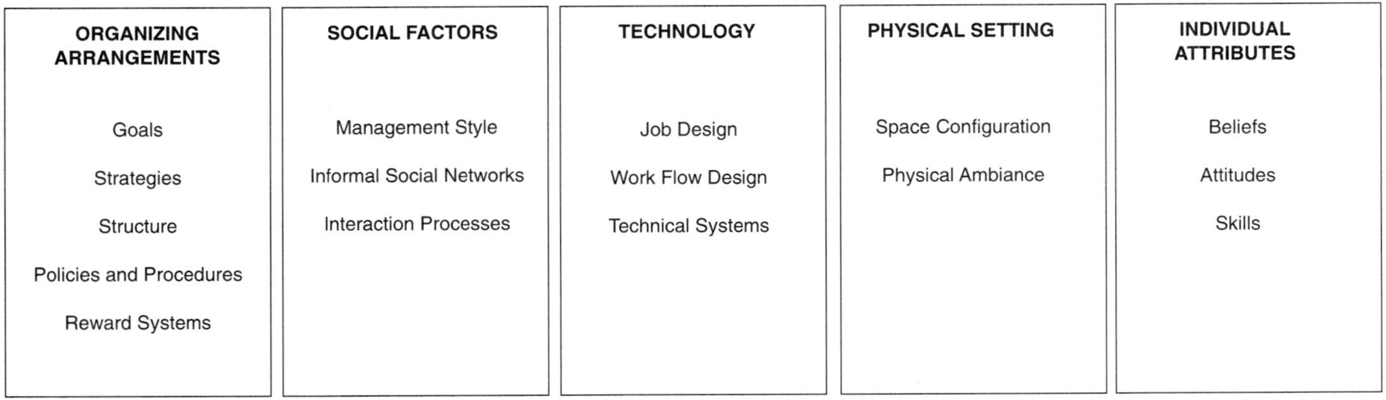

ORGANIZING ARRANGEMENTS	SOCIAL FACTORS	TECHNOLOGY	PHYSICAL SETTING	INDIVIDUAL ATTRIBUTES
Goals	Management Style	Job Design	Space Configuration	Beliefs
Strategies	Informal Social Networks	Work Flow Design	Physical Ambiance	Attitudes
Structure	Interaction Processes	Technical Systems		Skills
Policies and Procedures				
Reward Systems				

FIGURE 6-1 Potential Targets for Organizational Change Interventions. SOURCE: Modified and reproduced by special permission of the Publisher, Cnsulting Psychologists Press, Inc., Palo Alto, CA 94303 from *Handbook of Industrial & Organizational Psychology*, 2nd ed., vol. 3, by Marvin D. Dunnette and Leatta M. Hough (Eds.). Copyright 1992 by Consulting Psychologists Press, Inc. All rights reserved. Further reproduction is prohibited without the Publisher's written consent.

egies for alleviating stress-related symptoms (e.g., relaxation techniques, biofeedback, exercise) or on increasing employees' coping capacity (e.g., cognitive restructuring, problem-solving skill building, stressor recognition). (See Murphy [1996] for a review of these strategies.) Administrative strategies involve changing the way work is organized, distributed, supervised, and rewarded, for example by using clear job descriptions (to reduce uncertainty or unnecessary conflict), providing for flexible scheduling, and holding regular work team meetings so that employees can voice concerns and engage in group problem solving. Members of work teams that meet regularly or that have leaders trained in facilitating group problem solving report receiving more social support from their supervisors and experiencing less role ambiguity and higher job satisfaction (Heaney, 1991; Jackson, 1983).

In addition to these behavior change and administrative strategies, environmental psychologists suggest that changes in the physical setting can reduce occupational stressors and enhance psychosocial resources (Sundstrom and Altman, 1989). For example, the physical proximity of employee work stations and the presence of "gathering places," such as mailrooms or lunchrooms, have been associated with the quantity and quality of employee social interactions.

Behavior change strategies are usually "expert guided" (Karasek, 1992) in that they depend on health professionals or other outside consultants to counsel, train, or educate employees. The administrative strategies described here either were expert guided or were guided by the employees themselves. An example of the latter was the formation of an agency-wide labor/management stress committee in a study of stress among social workers in a child protective services agency (Cahill, 1992; Cahill and Feldman, 1993). Working with outside researchers, this committee developed goals to reduce sources of worksite stress, such as poor communication, and strengthen psychosocial resources, such as decision-making latitude over job tasks. Workers, management, and researchers then collaborated to develop, implement, and evaluate different interventions. For example, a computerized information system was introduced to reduce the workload and frustration associated with intake and tracking of clients. Ergonomically correct computer workstations were provided. All employees were trained to use the new system and had easy access to technical assistance. Evaluation of the project suggested that the staff who were most involved in the intervention experienced gains in job decision latitude, productivity, and job satisfaction.

Karasek (1992) reviewed 19 case studies of occupational stress reduction programs gathered from countries around the world. He concluded that the programs that focused solely on individual-level coping enhancement—even when they involved substantial resources—were not effective. Programs that attempted to change work organization, task structure, or communication patterns in worksites were more likely to be effective. Karasek (1992) concluded that this was particularly true when participatory strategies (e.g., worker discussions in quality circles or "health circles" to identify stressors and develop plans to reduce them) were used.

Several intervention studies attempting to increase employee participation in and influence over work-related decisions have shown positive effects on employee stress and well-being (e.g., Israel et al., 1992; Jackson, 1983; Landsbergis and Vivona-Vaughan, 1995; Schurman and Israel, 1995; Terra, 1995; Wall and Clegg, 1981). Participatory action research (PAR) has been proposed as a promising approach to occupational health interventions (see Israel et al., 1992; Schurman, 1996; Schurman and Israel, 1995). PAR entails collaboration between researchers and members of an organization in a data-guided, problem-solving approach to enhance an organization's ability to provide a safe and healthy work environment. PAR builds on many of the tenets of organizational development and it has been used as a stress reduction intervention with some success, particularly in Scandinavia (DiMartino, 1992; Israel et al., 1992; Lindstrom, 1995; Schurman and Israel, 1995; Terra, 1995).

No direct empirical comparisons of individual behavior change approaches with organizational-level change approaches to stress reduction have been conducted. Indeed, an either/or approach is not likely to enhance understanding of the stress reduction process. The ecologic approach, models of the stress process, systems theory, and the organizational development literature suggest that stress reduction approaches that use several points of intervention are likely to be most effective. Thus, comprehensive programs that address both changing the organizational processes that are causing stress and strengthening employees' skills and resources for coping with stress could be most promoting of employee health. Some efforts along these lines are promising (see Monroy et al., 1998), but more research is needed to elucidate fully the potential of these interventions.

Lessons From Organizational Change Interventions

In 1988, the observation was made that the "most striking feature" of studies examining the effects of organizational-level interventions to enhance worker control is "the sheer lack of them" (Murphy, 1988). This observation still applies today to the broader arena of organizational change strategies intended to enhance health. Although more studies are being done now, the scarcity of well-evaluated interventions is still apparent.

A few recurring themes emerge from the findings of existing studies. First, they address a relatively narrow set of organizational targets. Few interventions attempt to modify social factors, technology, or physical setting. The results of studies that do address these factors (see, e.g., Cahill, 1992; Heaney, 1991; Sundstrom and Altman, 1989) have been encouraging. Second, many studies did not consider the organizational culture of their participants. Given the potential importance of organizational culture to the success of change efforts (Schein, 1990), future studies should routinely assess and diagnose this factor. Several validated instruments for measuring organizational climate (the more superficial manifestation of organizational culture) and its receptivity to health innovations are available (Basen-Engquist et al., 1998; Steckler et al., 1992). Third, many studies found that when the external change agents terminated their involvement with the target organizations, intervention benefits quickly dissipated. Efforts to build capacity for sustaining organizational changes among organization members can address this problem.

The same critique applies to the areas of worksite health promotion and occupational health and safety programs. Over the past decade, it has become clear that generic programs are not likely to be optimally effective because they do not consider organizational culture or the beliefs, attitudes, needs, and resources of organization members. The prescription for this challenge is two-fold: strong formative research, and participation of all relevant stakeholders in the planning and conduct of health-promoting activities. Careful formative research is likely to illuminate important local issues and challenges, and stakeholders' participation is likely to enhance the program quality and increase commitment to follow through with the program activities.

COMMUNITIES AND HEALTH

Individual-level risk factors, families, and organizations influence health behavior and health status, and so do social and environmental conditions. This phenomenon is most visible in the growing gap between the health behaviors and health status of rich and poor, White and non-White (Krieger, 1994; Krieger et al., 1993; Lantz et al., 1998; Lillie-Blanton and LaVeist, 1996; Lynch et al., 1997; Williams and Collins, 1995). There is a need to better explain how the broader community and societal factors help determine the health status of individuals and groups. Some important conceptual constructs regarding the nature of communities as they relate to health outcomes are discussed below.

Communities of Identity

There are numerous definitions for and considerable confusion about what is meant by "community" (Heller, 1989; Klein, 1968; Rogers-Warren and Warren, 1977; Sarason, 1984; Steuart, 1993; Warren, 1975). Particularly important for this discussion of community-level change is the recognition that a "catchment area" or "population" is not a community but a geographic entity (e.g., city, county) that has a population aggregate with numerical but not a functional meaning (Steuart, 1993). Here, community means "unit of identity" created and recreated through social interactions (Hatch et al., 1993; Steckler et al., 1993; Steuart, 1993). A community in this sense is characterized by the following elements (Israel et al., 1994):

- Its membership has a sense of identity and belonging.
- It has common symbol systems: similar language, rituals, and ceremonies.
- It has shared values and norms.
- It offers mutual influence—community members have influence and are influenced by one another.
- It has shared needs and a shared commitment to meeting them.
- It has a shared emotional connection—members share common history, experiences, and support.

Thus, a community of identity can exist within a defined geographic neighborhood or as a geographically dispersed group among whose members there is a sense of common identity. A city or catchment area might not be a community as defined here, or it might include numerous different and overlapping communities of identity (Israel et al., 1998).

Community-Level Constructs

Communities as units of identity are also indigenous "units of solution" that include members with the knowledge, skills, and expertise necessary to solve problems at the community level (Steuart, 1993). Community-level change can reduce the numerous social, structural, and environmental stressors that affect health but that are beyond the ability of any one person to control or change (e.g., poverty, discrimination, income inequalities, crime, inadequate housing). Community-level change also can strengthen the situational factors (e.g., social support, community empowerment, community capacity, community cohesion) that protect against the effects of stress on health. Community-level change involves bringing together the skills and resources within a community to collectively identify stressors and protective factors and implement ways to promote good health. Although it often is possible to affect the stressors and protective factors within a given community of identity, it also is frequently necessary to bring together several communities of identity to extend the units of solution to address more complex issues (Steuart, 1993).

Geography versus Identity and Action

It is important to recognize the distinction between population-based, community-wide interventions (which have for the most part defined community as a geographic place within which to carry out interventions that usually are focused on individual behavior change) and community-level change interventions (in which the emphasis is on working with and strengthening communities of identity to foster social and structural changes that are associated with the health status of the community as a whole).

There are numerous community-level constructs to help inform the role of the community as a unit of identity and solution, such as "sense of community" (Parker et al., in press; McMillan and Chavis, 1986), "community competence" (Cottrell, 1976; Eng and Parker, 1994), "community capacity" (Goodman et al., 1998), and "community empowerment" (Israel et al., 1994; Wallerstein, 1992).

Theories of Change for Community-Level Interventions

Interventions at the community level pose many challenges. Unlike clinical trials, it is usually impossible to have randomized control groups;

even finding comparison communities is frequently unrealistic. Interventions at the community level are often dynamic and change with the interactions. The interventions can be complex, working toward change in social, economic, physical, and/or political factors among individuals, organizations, families, as well as the community itself (Kubisch et al., 1998). A number of useful conceptual constructs and typologies provide frameworks for thinking about community-level interventions, as described below.

Chin and Benne (1969) explicate three different theoretical assumptions regarding changes in human systems, each of which has different implications for conducting community-level interventions. First, the "rational-empirical" construct assumes that humans are rational and that they will follow their self-interest once it is made clear to them, and that a person or community will adopt a proposed change if it is rationally justified. Second, the "normative-re-educative" construct assumes that actions are supported by socio-cultural norms, values, attitudes, and significant relationships, and the commitments on the part of individuals and communities to these norms; and that change will occur only as those involved are brought to change their normative orientations. This is similar to Lewin's (1951) model, presented earlier, for conceptualizing change as a continuous process that involves an unfreezing, a changing, and a refreezing phase. Third, the "power-coercive" construct assumes that the change or influence process will either occur through compliance of those with less power to the ideas, direction and leadership of those with greater power (i.e., power over); or when that power is questioned or in conflict that there is collective power (i.e., power with) in which change occurs when those with less power come together to transform power relations from one group to another (Minkler and Wallerstein, 1997).

Warren (1975) conceptualizes purposive change in communities as being based on different configurations with respect to the agreement–disagreement dimensions of an issue, as well as other intervening variables. He posits three situations on a continuum that have different implications for community-level purposive change: (1) "issue consensus"—where there is basic agreement within the community on an issue and how it should be resolved; (2) "issue difference"—where no agreement yet exists on the issue, but there is the possibility that the community will reach issue consensus; and (3) "issue dissensus"—where members of the community either refuse to recognize the issue or are in strong disagreement with the change being proposed and there is little likelihood of achieving issue consensus.

Minkler and Wallerstein (1997), in their typology of community organization and community building, posit a two-by-two figure that is anchored on the horizontal axis by the constructs of "consensus" and "conflict," and on the vertical axis the constructs of "needs-based" and "strengths-based". Thus, different models or approaches to community change are based on different assumptions regarding the issues being addressed and the relationships that exist within the community (i.e., consensus or conflict), and the assessment of the community that drives the change process (i.e., needs-based or strengths-based).

Recently, Weiss (1995) proposed "theory-based evaluation," or the theory of change, challenging program planners to assess "how and why the program will work." In the theory of change approach, the first step is to articulate clearly the goals of the intervention and specific pathways to attain them (hypotheses). Consensus among the key participants about the goals is important. Agreement on the desired final outcome provides clarity on what to measure in the beginning and over the long term. Evidence from previous interventions is useful in identifying any weak assumptions in the hypotheses that might need rethinking. The pathways are likely to be a sequence of activities and their expected outcomes that lay out the key steps to the anticipated change. Specific interim outcomes provide options for measurements that can be used to see if the changes are occurring according to the original hypotheses. In this way, theory of change can help to guide decisions about what to measure and when to expect the change. Multiple theories of change can be applied simultaneously within a program with multiple pathways leading to the goal of the intervention (Weiss, 1995). Effective implementation of the theory of change approach does not ensure that the goals will be attained, but does provide the framework for evaluating the success of the intervention. Furthermore, by tracking progress with interim goals, it can help to distinguish problems with the hypotheses from problems with the implementation of the intervention and thereby allow midcourse corrections in the interventions (Milligan et al., 1998).

COMMUNITY-LEVEL INTERVENTIONS

It is beyond the scope of this chapter to provide an exhaustive review of the various approaches to community change interventions. Within the community-organizing literature there is extensive discussion of change models, such as community development, social action, community building, and empowerment-oriented social action. There is also a long history of community organizing for health (see Clark and Gakuru, 1982; el-Askari et al., 1998; Eng and Parker, 1994; Friedman, 1997; Freudenberg, 1984; Fullilove, 1998; Gibbs, 1983; Hofrichter, 1993; Kass and Freudenberg, 1997; Medoff and Sklar, 1994; Minkler, 1997; Minkler and Wallerstein, 1997; Nash, 1993; Newman, 1993; Wallerstein et al., 1997; Young and Padilla, 1990). However, as discussed throughout this report, within the field of public health per se, considerably less emphasis and fewer resources have been placed on conducting and evaluating community-level interventions in the United States (Israel et al., 1998; Lomas, 1998). The very nature of these interventions—with their emphasis on the social, cultural, economic, and political context of communities of identity, and on the role of community involvement in and control of an evolving process for which full specification of goals and objectives is not possible at the beginning—and the necessary commitment to the long time frame required to bring about major community-level changes preclude application of traditional evaluation designs and methods to assess effectiveness (Israel et al., 1998; Minkler and Wallerstein, 1997; Patrick and Wickizer, 1995; Wallerstein and Sanchez-Merki, 1994). Therefore, for the purposes of this section, a brief description is provided of two key studies of community-level interventions. In keeping with an ecologic framework, it is important to recognize that these interventions also targeted individual-level factors, although they are not discussed here.

Tenderloin Senior Organizing Project

Over a 16-year period, the Tenderloin Senior Organizing Project (TSOP) involved community members in the Tenderloin district of San Francisco, focusing on low-income elderly residents in single-room occupancy hotels. TSOP was established in 1979 by faculty and graduate students at the School of Public Health, University of California, Berkeley, with the initial goals of enhancing mental and physical health by reducing social isolation and providing health education, and of bringing together local residents to identify common problems and solutions for addressing those shared concerns (Minkler, 1992, 1997).

TSOP drew on four conceptual domains—social support, critical consciousness, social action, and democratic citizenship—to foster community empowerment and competence (Minkler, 1997). TSOP's intervention strategies evolved, including problem-posing discussions, support groups, leadership training, organizing tenants' associations, and the formation of interhotel groups and coalitions. Its accomplishments included establishment of hotel-based minimarkets, reduction of the neighborhood crime rate, improved pest control, upgrading of substandard plumbing and wiring, agreements for the removal of lead-based paint, cleanup of a vacant lot used as an illegal dump, recognition by hotel management of the tenants' associations as the organized voice of residents in the buildings, and the successful diffusion and replication of the TSOP model in other cities (Minkler, 1997).

Minkler (1997) offers several lessons from the TSOP experience for those interested in community organizing in the health field:

- the importance of the community, rather than an outside organizer, in defining needs and priorities;
- the need for an initial and continuing community diagnosis and assessment to identify and build on community strengths and resources;
- the flexible implementation of theories and methodologies, tailoring them to a particular community context;
- the importance of using participatory and empowering approaches to evaluate community-level change interventions;
- the necessity of long-range planning and developing diversified bases of funding.

East Side Village Health Worker Partnership

The East Side Village Health Worker Partnership (ESVHWP) is a project of the Detroit Community-Academic Urban Research Center, funded in 1995 through a cooperative agreement with the Centers for Disease Control and Prevention (Parker et al., 1998; Schulz et al., 1998). The project is a partnership between the University of Michigan School of Public Health, the Detroit Health Department, seven community-based organizations (Butzel Family Center, Friends of Parkside, Kettering Butzel Health Initiative, Warren/Conner Development Coalition, Islandview Development Coalition, V.I.S.I.O.N., East Side Parish Nurse Network), and the Henry Ford Health System. The partnership involves community-based participatory research with two broad goals: identifying and explaining the intrapersonal, interpersonal, organizational, community, and public policy factors in the stress model associated with poor health outcomes on Detroit's east side; and designing, implementing, and evaluating a collaborative lay health advisor intervention aimed at reducing stressors and strengthening protective factors associated with health, as identified by members of the community.

The objectives of this intervention incorporate change at several levels. Of particular importance is having lay health advisors (Village Health Workers [VHWs]) assist community residents in identifying and solving problems that affect the health of the community. More than 40 VHWs have completed an initial eight-session training program. They meet monthly to share experiences and skills and to participate in additional training in grant writing and community organizing, for example. The results of a random-sample community survey and in-depth interviews and focus group discussions with VHWs, steering committee members (representatives from each partner organization) and key community members identified four priority areas: parenting, support of women, crime and relationships with the police, and community organizing (Parker et al., 1998; Schulz et al., 1998). VHWs participated in monthly meetings at the police precincts, assisted in arson prevention (Maciak et al., 1998), organized neighborhood block clubs, established a fresh fruit and vegetable minimarket for neighborhood residents, and developed support mechanisms for women who have child care responsibilities.

The ESVHWP is using quantitative and qualitative data collection methods for several purposes. For example, a group interview with the Steering Committee developed a local stress model and guided the design of items on a community survey (Parker et al., 1998; Schulz et al., 1998). The survey is being used for basic research (e.g., to test the relationships of the variables in the stress model, see Schulz et al., 2000a,b; Parker et al., 2001) and evaluation purposes (e.g., to examine the effect of the intervention on reducing such stressors as crime and on strengthening such protective factors as social support and perceived control). One aim of the evaluation is to assess the extent to which the intervention has changed community-level factors, including the community's sense of competence, empowerment, and cohesion (Eng and Parker, 1994; Fullilove, 1998; Goodman et al., 1998; Israel et al., 1994; Lomas, 1998).

Lessons from Community Change Interventions

Many social, economic, and environmental factors that affect health are disproportionately represented in minority communities and among women. Therefore, greater emphasis is needed on public health interventions that involve communities of identity with the goal of collectively identifying resources, needs, and solutions that can influence community-level variables. There are several challenges and barriers to this approach and several factors that facilitate intervention effectiveness (e.g., Israel et al., 1998; Patrick and Wickizer, 1995). More resources are needed to support such community change efforts, as is an expanded set of methodologic tools to evaluate program success (Chapter 7). The Theory of Change for communities may help in developing evaluation approaches. In addition, the limits of community change interventions and the need to engage in broader policy programs that can affect social and structural factors must be recognized.

SOCIETY AND HEALTH

Research consistently reveals an inverse relationship between social class and a variety of diseases (Feinleib, 1996; Haan et al., 1987; Kaplan, 1989; Kitagawa and Hauser, 1973; Tomatis, 1992). In addition, these differentials are also increasingly prominent in the prevalence of health behaviors (Moss, in press; Winkleby et al., 1990). Studies have similarly reported that people with low incomes or minimal education levels are especially likely to exhibit multiple risk-related behaviors (Emmons et al., 1994). Interventions are needed to address the "pockets of prevalence" of risk-related behaviors to reduce the social inequalities of risk. The structure and function of society per se thus constitute the final framework within which interactions between behavior and health should be considered.

Interventions designed for low-income populations also must consider the social context that influences health behaviors and health status. Socioeconomic class affects the availability of an array of social and material resources that ultimately have profound effects on health (Aday, 1993; Graham, 1994a; Kaplan, 1995). For example, the Alameda County (California) Study (Berkman and Syme, 1979) identified multiple risk factors associated with low income, including smoking, obesity, unmet needs for food and medical care, unsafe neighborhoods, and lack of social supports (Kaplan, 1995). Graham (1994a,b) demonstrated the relevance of these socioeconomic factors for one risk-related behavior, smoking. Based on a qualitative study, she found that low-income women used smoking as a means of coping with economic pressure and the resulting demands placed on them to care for others. Indeed, spending on cigarettes appears to be protected because it is viewed as a necessary luxury. Using survey data, Graham (1994b) found that, compared with their nonsmoking counterparts, working-class mothers who smoke generally care for more children and for children in poorer health, and are more likely to be providing that care alone. A larger proportion of smokers had insufficient resources to meet the basic needs of their families, and they lived in less desirable neighborhoods than did women with higher incomes. She concluded that smoking among working-class women was linked to the caring responsibilities and material circumstances that shape their lives (Graham, 1994b). Similarly, Romano and colleagues (1991) found that African American individuals who reported experiencing high levels of stress associated with their socioeconomic circumstances—such as being out of work or not having enough money to meet basic needs—were more likely to smoke than were those reporting better circumstances.

Even beyond the stressors associated with low income, social structure clearly shapes people's daily lives (Amick et al., 1995; Kaplan, 1995; Wilkinson, 1996). For example, there are many ways the effects of income extend beyond purchasing power to influence daily life. Middle-class neighborhoods have proportionally more pharmacies, restaurants, banks, and specialty stores; low-income areas have more fast food restaurants, check cashing stores, liquor stores, and laundromats. Typical food purchases cost approximately 15% more in poor neighborhoods, and fresh produce can cost as much as 22% more than in higher income areas. In addition, the quality of the food on average is poorer in low-income areas (Trout, 1993). Relatively higher food costs in low-income neighborhoods could be associated with their relatively fewer supermarkets and with greater reliance on small and medium-sized stores (Crockett et al., 1992) in which the quality, quantity, and variety of fresh fruits and vegetables and meats is limited (Morris et al., 1992). As a result, people living in low-income areas often are much less able to meet their needs for healthful foods.

The public health response to social class differences in health behaviors must extend to changes in social structure to improve the day-to-day realities of low-income populations—factors that clearly shape health behaviors and health status. Broad-based policy initiatives designed to reduce social inequalities are likely to contribute to improved health at the individual and community levels (Amick et al., 1995; Anderson and Armstead, 1995; Kaplan, 1995; Minkler, 1989).

The constellation of factors operating at the society level constitutes an extremely complex system with multiple interactions and feedback mechanisms. It is beyond the scope of this report to address the full range of issues that function at this level or their ramifications for the health status of individuals and populations. Therefore, a brief description of several important factors is presented to illustrate the importance of considering them at the society level and of assessing some of their interactions with those that function elsewhere.

Government and Societal Constraints on Health

Many social, economic, political, and cultural factors are associated with health and disease for which changes in individual health behaviors alone are not likely to result in improved health and quality of life. Public health law has been defined as the legal powers and duties of government to assure the conditions for people to be healthy (Gostin, 2000; IOM, 1988). Government uses a number of means to prevent injury and disease and to promote the population's health. Laws and regulations, like other prevention strategies, can intervene at each level discussed in this chapter in several ways to secure safer behavior among the population (Haddon et al., 1964; IOM, 1999). Finally, public policy interventions undertaken by government are given particular emphasis, but an analogous role can be served by other large components of civil society: employers, unions, health care organizations, citizens' groups, or public interest foundations. Similarly, the distinctions between levels of government (nation, state, county, etc.) are beyond the scope of this report. For the purposes of discussing behavior and health, government is treated as a single component.

SOCIETY-LEVEL INTERVENTIONS

Health Targets

In 1979, the Surgeon General's report *Healthy People* (USDHHS, 1979) presented national goals for reducing premature deaths. Soon afterwards, *Objectives for the Nation* (USDHHS, 1980) provided health objectives for the following 10 years in the United States. These targets proved to be an effective approach to setting priorities and evaluating progress in health promotion and disease prevention. Subsequently, *Healthy People*

2000 (USDHHS, 1990) and *Healthy People 2010* (USDHHS, 2000) carried on the tradition with updated goals for the coming decade. Health targets have also become part of the strategies for health policy in the United Kingdom, Australia, and the World Health Organization. The advantages and drawbacks to this approach are reviewed by van Herten and Gunner-Schepers (2000). On the positive side, the process of formulating the targets provides insights, reveals gaps, and stimulates debate. By helping to establish realistic goals, it improves resource management and provides benchmarks for progress. The objections to this approach include the concerns that it oversimplifies the health issues and that some objectives that are more difficult to quantify will be ignored. Using health targets incorporates a variety of approaches used at the government-level; national health campaigns and legislation are discussed briefly below.

Health Communication Campaigns

Interventions can be aimed at individual behavior—providing education or incentives for healthier choices. Government health messages can be highly important in advancing the public's health by informing people about hidden risks and by providing guidance about safer alternatives. The effectiveness of national campaigns is extensively reviewed and analyzed in an IOM report (2001). One example, the National 5-A-Day Campaign, is described here to illustrate the scope of this type of intervention (Stables, 2000; Heimendinger et al., 1996). This campaign was initiated by the National Cancer Institute in partnership with the Produce for Better Health Foundation, to increase the dietary intake of fruits and vegetables to the recommended five servings each day. The intervention has multiple components. Mass media marketing is used to increase public awareness through newsletters, websites, television, publications, special events, and promotional items. Consumers are targeted at time of purchase with brochures, recipes, advertising, coupons, etc. The food industry and retail stores are provided with training and promotional kits, and they agree to display materials and hold special events that advance the message. At the community level, programs are designed to meet the specific needs of the community members. Interventions are aimed at schools, worksites, clinics, religious centers, etc. Activities include such events as garden projects, wellness seminars, booths at state fairs, and local media events. The 5-A-Day Campaign also provides funding for evaluation to assess the impact of the various programs and the effectiveness of the advertising. Media campaigns regarding the use of tobacco provide an interesting example for both government and the tobacco industry, which are described in Chapter 8.

Regulatory Approaches

The government can exercise its legislative powers to deter risk behaviors by imposing civil and criminal penalties (e.g., seatbelt and motorcycle helmet laws). This kind of regulation prescribes specific behavior either for the entire population (e.g., speed limits) or for segments of it (e.g., age-restricted tobacco and alcoholic beverage sales). The government also can create incentives for individual behavior change. For example, it can exercise its taxation authority to discourage unhealthy activities, such as tobacco use or excessive consumption of alcohol, or encourage healthy ones, for example, by providing tax deductions for health care expenditures. The effect of taxation on tobacco use is described in Chapter 8.

The law also can regulate the agents of behavior change, for example by requiring safer product design. Government can regulate unsafe products directly (e.g., passive restraints in cars, trigger locks on handguns, or childproof caps on medicines) or indirectly through the tort system (e.g., tobacco, automobile, or firearms litigation). Government also can help provide the means for safer behavior by removing legal impediments to behavior change (e.g., dismantling drug paraphernalia or needle prescription laws that impede access to sterile injection equipment).

Furthermore, the law can change the informational, physical, social, or economic environment to facilitate safer behavior. Government can demand accurate labeling and instructions (e.g., on foods, pharmaceutical products, nutritional supplements) or restrict commercial advertising of hazardous products and activities (e.g., tobacco, alcoholic beverages, gambling); enact housing and building codes to prevent injury and disease (e.g., sanitation, lead paint); and make environments safer (e.g., guards on upper-level apartment windows, median barriers on highways, regulations for safe disposal of toxic substances).

Addressing Socioeconomic Status and Health

The role of socioeconomic status in health (Chapter 4) is an issue that can only be handled at a societal level. The international scope of this issue is reflected in the concerns it has raised from the World Health Organization (WHO), the World Bank, and the European Community (Whitehead, 1998; Gwatkin, 2000). Many efforts have been implemented to review the evidence and to search for solutions to the problem (see Gwatkin, 2000). The concern goes beyond providing equitable access to health care to addressing the basic links between social inequality and health.

In 1992, WHO set the following target: "By the year 2000, the differences in health status between countries and between groups within countries should be reduced by at least 25%, by improving the level of health of disadvantaged nations and groups" (Dahlgren and Whitehead, 1992). Approaches were aimed at reducing poverty (e.g., compressed income scales or progressive tax systems), decreasing unhealthy living conditions (e.g., urban renewal programs), improving working conditions (e.g., legislation to eliminate physical health hazards at work or organizational reforms for less stressful working arrangements), decreasing unemployment (e.g., creation of new jobs or minimizing the impact through increased public awareness of available assistance), improving lifestyle (e.g., targeting the most disadvantaged groups for smoking or nutrition education or interventions), and providing access to health care (e.g., availability of insurance and culturally appropriate training for health care providers).

More recently, an Independent Inquiry (Acheson et al., 1998) examined the health inequalities in England and put forward several recommendations. Three areas were considered critical: improving the health of families with children, reducing disparity in income while improving the living conditions of the poor, and assessing all relevant public policies for their effect on health inequalities. The report pointed out that many areas not normally associated with health have an impact on the social inequities that influence health; these include poverty, income, tax and benefits, education, employment, housing and environment, transportation, pollution, and nutrition.

Others in the international community have participated in the discussions concerning how to address the problem of health inequities. Gwatkin (2000) suggested directing efforts toward reducing differences between the rich and the poor rather than improving societal averages. Barzach (2000) recommended a focus on prevention and control of certain priority pathologies with the expectation that these efforts would later provide a framework that could be generalized to broader issues. Dahlgren (2000) emphasized progressive financial strategies for health insurance with access to services based on need rather than on ability to pay. Tarlov (1999) proposed a framework for thinking about interventions classed as either ameliorative or corrective and directed toward five objectives: enhancing child development, strengthening community cohesion, providing opportunities for self-fulfillment, increasing socioeconomic well-being, and modulating hierarchical structuring. This is just a sampling of the perspectives from the international community. While there seems to be no consensus on the optimal approaches to rectify the health impact of disparities in socioeconomic status, there does seem to be agreement that the issue deserves attention.

REFERENCES

Acheson, D., Barker, D., Chambers, J., Graham, H., Marmot, M., and Whitehead, M. (1998). *Independent Inquiry into Inequalities in Health Report*. London: The Stationery Office. Accessed on line January 16, 2001. http://www.official-documents.co.uk/document/doh/ih/contents.htm

Aday, L. (1993). *At Risk in America: The Health Care Needs of Vulnerable Populations in the United States*. San Francisco: Jossey-Bass.

Amick, B.C., Levine, S., Tarlov, A.R., and Walsh, D.C. (Eds.) (1995). *Introduction to Society and Health*. Oxford: Oxford University Press.

Anderson, N. and Armstead, C. (1995). Toward understanding the association of socioeconomic status and health: A new challenge for the biopsychosocial approach. *Psychosomatic Medicine*, 57, 213–225.

Argyris, C. and Schon, D.A. (1989). Participatory action research and action science compared. *American Behavioral Scientist*, 9, 612–623.

Baker, E., Israel, B., and Schurman, S. (1996). The integrated model: Implications for worksite health promotion and occupational health and safety practice. *Health Education Quarterly*, 23, 175–188.

Barzach, M. (2000). Overcoming inequity means finding approaches that work. *Bulletin of the World Health Organization*, 78, 77–78.

Basen-Engquist, K, Hudmon. K, Tripp. M, and Chamberlain, R. (1998). Worksite health and safety climate: Scale development and effects of a health promotion intervention. *Preventive Medicine*, 27, 111–119.

Berkman, L.F. and Syme, S.L. (1979) Social networks, host resistance, and mortality: A nine-year follow-up study of Alameda County residents. *American Journal of Epidemiology*, 109, 186–204.

Brown, E.R. (1991). Community action for health promotion: A strategy to empower individuals and communities. *International Journal of Health Services*, 21, 441–456.

Cahill, J. (1992). Computers and stress reduction on social service workers in New Jersey. *Conditions of Work Digest*, 11, 197–203.

Cahill, J. and Feldman, L.H. (1993). Computers in child welfare: Planning for a more serviceable work environment. *Child Welfare*, 72, 3–12.

Chin, R. and Benne, K.D. (1969). General strategies for effecting change in human systems. In W.G. Bennis, K.D. Benne, and R. Chin (Eds.) *The Planning of Change* (pp. 32–59). New York: Holt, Rinehart & Winston.

Clark, N.M. and Gakuru, O.N. (1982). The effect on health and self-confidence of participation in collaborative learning activities. *Hygiene, 1(2)*, 47–56.

Cotton, J.L., Vollrath, D.A., Froggatt, K.L., Lengnick-Hall, M.L., and Jennings, K.R. (1988). Employee participation: Diverse forms and different outcomes. *Academy of Management Review, 13*, 8–22.

Cottrell, L.S. (1976). The competent community, In B.H. Kaplan, R.N. Wilson, and A.H. Lighton (Eds.) *Further Explorations in Social Psychiatry*. New York: Basic Books.

Crockett, E., Clancy, K., and Bowering, J. (1992). Comparing the cost of a thrifty food plan market basket in three areas of New York state. *Journal of Nutrition Education, 24*, 72S–79S.

Dahlgren, G. (2000). Efficient equity-oriented strategies for health. *Bulletin of the World Health Organization, 78*, 79–81.

Dahlgren, G. and Whitehead, M. (1992). *Policies and Strategies to Promote Equity in Health*. Copenhagen: World Health Organization.

Dannenberg, A.L., Gielen, A.C., Beilenson, P.L., Wilson, M.H., and Joffe, A. (1993). Bicycle helmet laws and educational campaigns: An evaluation of strategies to increase children's helmet use. *American Journal of Public Health, 83*, 667–674.

DeJong, W. and Hingson, R. (1998). Strategies to reduce driving under the influence of alcohol. *Annual Review of Public Health, 19*, 359–378.

DeJoy, D.M., Murphy, L.R., and Gershon, R.M. (1995). Safety climate in health care settings. In A.C. Bittner and P.C. Champney (Eds.) *Advances in Industrial Ergonomics and Safety VII* (pp. 923–929). New York: Taylor and Francis.

DiMartino, V. (Ed.) (1992). *Preventing Stress at Work: Conditions of Work Digest (Vol II)*. Geneva, Switzerland: International Labour Office.

el-Askari, G., Freestone, J., Irizarry, C., Kraut, K.L., Mashiyama, S.T., Morgan, M.A., and Walton, S. (1998). The Healthy Neighborhoods Project: A local health department's role in catalyzing community development. *Health Education and Behavior, 25*, 146–159.

Emmons, K.M., Marcus, B.H., Linnan, L., Rossi, J.S., and Abrams, D.B. (1994) Mechanisms in multiple risk factor interventions: Smoking, physical activity, and dietary fat intake among manufacturing workers. *Preventive Medicine, 23*, 481–489.

Eng, E. and Parker, E. (1994). Measuring community competency and the Mississippi Delta: Interface between program evaluation and empowerment. *Health Education Quarterly, 21*, 199–220.

Erdmann, T.C., Feldman, K.W., Rivara, F.P., Heimbach, D.M., and Wall, H.A. (1991). Tap water burn prevention: The effect of legislation. *Pediatrics, 88*, 572–577.

Eriksen, M.P. and Gottlieb, N.H. (1998). A review of the health impact of smoking control at the workplace. *American Journal of Health Promotion, 13*, 83–105.

Ewigman, B.G., Kivlahan, C.H., Hosokawa, M.C., and Horman, D. (1990). Efficacy of an intervention to promote use of hearing protection devices by firefighters. *Public Health Reports, 105*, 53–59.

Feinleib, M. (1996). Editorial: New directions for community intervention studies. *American Journal of Public Health, 86*, 1696–1697.

Freudenberg, N. (1984). *Not in our Backyards! Community Action for Health and the Environ*ment. New York: Monthly Review Press.

Friedman, W. (1997). Research, organizing, and the campaign for community policing in Chicago. In P. Nyden, A. Figert, M. Shibley, and D. Burrows (Eds.) *Building Community: Social Science in Action* (pp. 202–209). Thousand Oaks, CA: Pine Forge Press.

Fullilove, M.T. (1998). Promoting social cohesion to improve health. *Journal of the American Medical Womens Association, 53,* 72–76.

Ganster, D.C. (1995). Interventions for building healthy organizations: Suggestions from the stress research literature. In L.R. Murphy, J.J. Hurrell, S.L. Sauter, and G.P. Keita (Eds.) *Job Stress Interventions* (pp. 323–336). Washington, DC: American Psychological Association.

Gershon, R., Vlahov, D., Felknor, S.A, Vesley, D., Johnson, P.C, Delclos, G.L., and Murphy, L.R. (1995). Compliance with universal precautions among health care workers at three regional hospitals. *American Journal of Infection Control, 23,* 225–236.

Gibbs, L.M. (1983). Community response to an emergency situation: Psychological destruction and the Love Canal. *American Journal of Community Psychology, 11,* 116–125.

Glanz, K., Sorensen, G., and Farmer, A. (1996). The health impact of worksite nutrition and cholesterol intervention programs. *American Journal of Health Promotion, 10,* 453–470.

Glasgow, R.E., Terborg, J.R., Hollis, J.F., Severson, H.H., and Boles, S.M. (1995). Take Heart: Results from the initial phase of a work-site wellness program. *American Journal of Public Health, 85,* 209–216.

Golaszewski, T., Barr, D., and Cochran, S. (1998). An organization-based intervention to improve support for employee heart health. *American Journal of Health Promotion, 13,* 26–35.

Goldenhar, L.M. and Schulte, P.A. (1994). Intervention research in occupational health and safety. *Journal of Occupational Medicine, 36,* 763–775.

Goodman, R.M., Speers, M.A., McLeroy, K., Fawcett, S., Kegler, M., Parker, E., Smith, S.R., Sterling, T.D., and Wallerstein, N. (1998). Identifying and defining the dimensions of community capacity to provide a basis for measurement. *Health Education and Behavior, 25,* 258–278.

Gostin, L.O. (2000). Public law in a new century. 1. Law as a tool to advance the community's health. *Journal of the American Medical Association 83,* 2837–2841.

Gottlieb, N.H. and McLeroy, K.R. (1994). Social health. In M.P. O'Donnell and J.S Harris (Eds.) *Health Promotion in the Workplace,* 2nd Edition (pp. 459–493). Albany, NY: Delmar.

Graham, H. (1994a). Gender and class as dimensions of smoking behavior in Britain: Insights from a survey of mothers. *Social Science and Medicine, 38,* 691–698.

Graham, H. (1994b). *When Life's a Drag: Women, Smoking and Disadvantage.* London: University of Warwick, Department of Health.

Gwatkin, D.R. (2000). Health inequalities and the health of the poor: What do we know? What can we do? *Bulletin of the World Health Organization, 78,* 3–17.

Haan, M., Kaplan, G., and Camacho, T. (1987). Poverty and health: Prospective evidence from the Alameda County Study. *American Journal of Epidemiology, 125,* 989–998.

Haddon, W., Jr., Sussman, E.A., and Klein, D. (1964). *Accident Research: Methods and Approaches*. New York: Harper and Row.

Hatch, J., Moss, N., Saran, A., Presley-Cantrell, L., and Mallory, C. (1993). Community research: Partnership in Black communities. *American Journal of Preventive Medicine*, 9 *(Suppl.)*, 27–31.

Heaney, C.A and Goetzal, R.Z (1997). A review of health-related outcomes of multi-component worksite health promotion programs. *American Journal of Health Promotion*, 11, 290–308.

Heaney, C.A. (1991). Enhancing social support at the workplace: Assessing the effects of the caregiver support program. *Health Education Quarterly*, 18, 477–494.

Heimendinger, J., Van Duyn, M.A., Chapelsky, D., Foerster, S., and Stables, G. (1996). The national 5 A Day for Better Health Program: A large-scale nutrition intervention. *Journal of Public Health Management and Practice*, 2, 27–35

Heller, K. (1989). Ethical dilemmas in community intervention. *American Journal of Community Psychology*, 17, 367–378.

Hennrikus, D.J. and Jeffery, R.W. (1996). Worksite intervention for weight control: A review of the literature. *American Journal of Health Promotion*, 10, 471–498.

Hofrichter, R. (Ed.) (1993). *Toxic Struggles: The Theory and Practice of Environmental Justice*. Philadelphia: New Society Publishers.

House, J.S. (1981). *Work, Stress and Social Support*. Reading, MA: Addison-Wesley.

Hurrell, J.J., Jr. and Murphy, L.R. (1992). An overview of occupational stress and health. In W. Rom (Ed.) *Environmental and Occupational Medicine*, 2nd edition (pp. 675–684). Boston: Little Brown.

IOM (Institute of Medicine) (1988). *The Future of Public Health*. Washington, DC: National Academy Press.

IOM (Institute of Medicine) (1999). *Reducing the Burden of Injury: Advancing Prevention and Treatment*. Washington, DC: National Academy Press.

IOM (Institute of Medicine) (2001). *Speaking of Health: Assessing Health Communication. Strategies for Diverse Populations*. In C. Chrvala and S. Scrimshaw (Eds.). Washington, DC: National Academy Press.

Israel, B.A., Checkoway, B., Schulz, A.J. and Zimmerman, M.A. (1994). Health education and community empowerment: Conceptualizing and measuring perceptions of individual, organizational, and community control. *Health Education Quarterly*, 21, 149–170.

Israel, B.A., House, J.S., Schurman, S.J., Heaney, C.A., and Mero, R.P. (1989). The relation of personal resources, participation, influence, interpersonal relationships and coping strategies to occupational stress, job strains and health: A multivariate analysis. *Work and Stress*, 3, 163–194.

Israel, B.A., Schulz, A.J., Parker, E.A., and Becker, A.B. (1998). Review of community-based research: Assessing partnership approaches to improve public health. *Annual Review of Public Health*, 19, 173–202.

Israel, B.A., Schurman, S.J., Hugentobler, M.K. and House, J.S. (1992). A participatory action research approach to reducing occupational stress in the United States. *Conditions of Work Digest: Preventing Stress at Work*, 11, 152–163.

Jackson, S. (1983). Participation in decision-making as a strategy for reducing job-related strain. *Journal of Applied Psychology*, 68, 3–19.

Kaplan, G. (1989). *Health Disease, and the Social Structure*. Englewood Cliffs, NJ: Prentice-Hall.

Kaplan, G. (1995). Where do shared pathways lead? Some reflections on a research agenda. *Psychosomatic Medicine, 57*, 208–212.

Karasek, R. (1992). Stress prevention through work organization. *Conditions of Work Digest*, 11. Geneva: ILO.

Karasek, R. and Theorell, T. (1990). *Healthy Work: Stress, Productivity and the Reconstruction of Working Life*. New York: Basic Books.

Kass, D. and Freudenberg, N. (1997). Coalition building to prevent childhood lead poisoning: A case study from New York City. In M. Minkler (Ed.) *Community Organizing and Community Building for Health* (pp. 278–288). New Brunswick, NJ: Rutgers University Press.

Katz, D. and Kahn, R.L. (1978). *The Social Psychology of Organizations* New York: Wiley.

Kitagawa, E. and Hauser, P. (1973). *Differential Mortality in the United States: A Study in Socioeconomic Epidemiology*. Cambridge, MA: Harvard University Press.

Klein, D.C. (1968). *Community Dynamics and Mental Health*. New York: Wiley.

Krieger, N. (1994). Epidemiology and the web of causation: Has anyone seen the spider. *Social Science and Medicine, 39*, 887–903.

Krieger, N., Rowley, D.L, Herman, A.A., Avery, B., and Phillips, M.T. (1993). Racism, sexism and social class: Implications for studies of health, disease and well-being. *American Journal of Preventive Medicine, 9*, 82–122.

Kubisch, A.C., Fulbright-Anderson, K., and Connell, J.P. (1998). Evaluating community initiatives: a progress report. In K. Fulbright-Anderson, A.C. Kubisch, and J.P. Connell (Eds.) *New Approaches to Evaluating Community Initiatives Volume 2 Theory, Measurement, and Analysis* Washington, DC: Aspen Institute. Accessed online February 23, 2001. http://www.aspenroundtable.org/vol2/kubisch.htm

Landsbergis, P. and Vivona-Vaughan, E. (1995). Evaluation of an occupational stress intervention in a public agency. *Journal of Organizational Behavior, 16*, 29–48.

Lantz, P.M., House, J.S., Lepkowski, J.M., Williams, D.R., Mero, R.P., and Chen, J. (1998). Socioeconomic factors, health behaviors, and mortality. *Journal of the American Medical Association, 279*, 1703–1708.

Lewin, K. (1951) *Field Theory in Social Science*. New York: Harper.

Lillie-Blanton, M. and LaVeist. T. (1996). Race/ethnicity, the social environment, and health. *Social Science and Medicine, 43*, 83–92.

Lindstrom, K. (1995). Finnish research in organizational development and job redesign. In G. Keita, J. Hurrell, and L. Murphy (Eds.) *Job Stress Interventions: Current Practices and New Directions* (pp. 283–294). Washington, DC: American Psychological Association.

Lippitt, R., Watson, J., and Westley, B. (1958). *Dynamics of Planned Change*. New York: Harcourt and Brace.

Lomas, J. (1998). Social capital and health: Implications for public health and epidemiology. *Social Science and Medicine, 47*, 1181–1188.

Lynch, J.W., Kaplan, G.A, and Salonen, J.T. (1997). Why do poor people behave poorly? Variation in adult health behaviours and psychosocial characteristics by stages of the socioeconomic lifecourse. *Social Science and Medicine, 44*, 809–819.

Maciak, B.J., Moore, M.T., Leviton, L.C., and Guinan, M.E. (1998). Preventing Halloween arson in an urban setting: a model for multisectoral planning and community participation. *Health Education and Behavior, 25*, 194–211.

McGinnis, M. (1993). 1992 National survey of worksite health promotion activities: Summary. *American Journal of Health Promotion, 7*, 452–464.

McKinlay, J.B. (1993). The promotion of health through planned sociopolitical change: Challenges for research and policy. *Social Science and Medicine, 36*, 109–117.

McMillan, D. and Chavis, D. (1986). Sense of community: A definition and theory. *Journal of Community Psychology, 14*, 6–23.

Medoff, P. and Sklar, H. (1994). *Streets of Hope: The Fall and Rise of an Urban Neighborhood.* Boston: South End Press.

Milligan, S., Coulton, C., York, P., and Register R. (1998) Implementing a theory of change evaluation in the Cleveland community-building initiative: A case study. In K. Fulbright-Anderson, A.C. Kubisch, and J.P. Connell (Eds.) *New Approaches to Evaluating Community Initiatives. Volume 2. Theory, Measurement, and Analysis.* Washington, DC: Aspen Institute. Accessed online February 23, 2001. http://www.aspenroundtable.org/vol2/milligan.htm

Minkler, M. (1989). Health education, health promotion and the open society: An historical perspective. *Health Education Quarterly, 16*, 17–30.

Minkler, M. (1992). Community organizing among the elderly poor in the United States: A case study. *International Journal of Health Services, 22*, 303–316.

Minkler, M. (1997). Scapegoating the elderly: New voices, old theme. *Journal of Public Health Policy, 18*, 8–12.

Minkler, M. and Wallerstein, N. (1997). Improving health through community organization and community building. In K. Glanz, F.M. Lewis, and B.K. Rimer (Eds.) *Health Behavior and Health Education: Theory, Research and Practice, 2nd edition* (pp. 241–269). San Francisco: Jossey-Bass.

Monroy, J., Jonas, H., Mathey, J., and Murphy, L. (1998). Holistic stress management at Corning, Incorporated. In M.K. Gowing, J.D. Kraft, and J.C. Quick (Eds.) *The New Organizational Reality* (pp. 239–256). Washington, DC: American Psychological Association.

Morris, P., Neuhauser, L., and Campbell, C. (1992). Food security in rural America: A study of the availability and costs of food. *Journal of Nutrition Education, 24 (Suppl.),* S52–S58.

Moss, N.E. (in press). Socio-economic inequalities in women's health. *Women and Health.*

Murphy, L.R. (1988). Workplace interventions for stress reduction and prevention. In C.L. Cooper and R. Payne (Eds.) *Causes, Coping and Consequences of Stress at Work* (pp. 301–339). Chichester: John Wiley and Sons.

Murphy, L.R. (1996). Stress management in work settings: A critical review of the health effects. *American Journal of Health Promotion, 11*, 112–135.

Nash, F. (1993). Church-based organizing as participatory research: The northwest community organization and the Pilsen resurrection project. *American Sociologist, Spring*, 38–55.

Newman, P. (1993). The grassroots movement for environmental justice: Fighting for our lives. *New Solutions, Summer*, 87–95.

Ni, H., Sacks, J.J., Curtis, L., Cieslak, P.R., and Hedberg, K. 1997. Evaluation of a statewide bicycle helmet law via multiple measures of helmet use. *Archives of Pediatric and Adolescent Medicine*, *151*, 59–65.

Parker, E.A., Liechtenstein, R.L., Shultz, A.J., Israel, B.A., Schork, M.A., Steinman, K.J., and James, S.A. (2001). Disentangling measures of individual perceptions of community social dynamics: Results of a community survey. *Health Education and Behavior*, *28*, in press.

Parker, E.A., Schulz, A.J., Israel, B.A., and Hollis, R. (1998). Detroit's East Side Village Health Worker Partnership: Community-based lay health advisor intervention in an urban area. *Health Education and Behavior*, *25*, 24–45.

Parkinson, D.K, Bromet, E.J, Dew, M.A, Dunn, L.O., Barkman, M., and Wright, M. (1989). Effectiveness of the United Steel Workers of America coke oven intervention program. *Journal of Occupational Medicine*, *31*, 464–472.

Patrick, D.L. and Wickizer, T.M. (1995). Community and health. In B.C. Amick, S. Levine, A.R. Tarlov, and D. Chapman Walsh (Eds.) *Society and Health* (pp. 46–91). New York: Oxford University Press.

Porras, J.I. (1987). *Stream Analysis: A Powerful Way to Diagnose and Manage Organizational Change*. Reading, MA: Addition-Wesley.

Porras, J.I. and Robertson, P.J. (1992). Organizational development: theory practice, and research. In M.D. Dunnette and L.M. Hough (Eds.) *Handbook of Industrial and Organizational Psychology*, *2nd Edition Vol. 3* (pp. 719–822). Palo Alto, CA: Consulting Psychologist Press.

Richard, L., Potvin, L., Kishchuk, N., Prlic, H., and Green, L.W. (1996). Assessment of the integration of the ecological approach in health promotion programs. *American Journal of Health Promotion*, *10*, 318–328.

Rogers-Warren, A. and Warren, S.F. (Eds.) (1977). *Ecological Perspectives in Behavior Analysis*. Baltimore, MD: University Park Press.

Romano, P.S., Bloom, J., and Syme, S.L. (1991). Smoking, social support, and hassles in an urban African-American community. *American Journal of Pubic Health*, *81*, 1415–1422.

Sarason, S.B. (1984). *The Psychological Sense of Community: Prospects for a Community Psychology*. San Francisco: Jossey-Bass.

Schein, E.H. (1987). *Process Consulting*. Reading, MA: Addition Wesley.

Schein, E.H. (1990). Organization culture. *American Psychologist*, *45*, 109–119.

Schulz, A.J., Israel, B.A., Williams, D.R. Parker, E.A., Becker, A. B., and James, S.A. (2000a). Social Inequalities, stressors and indicators of health status among women living in Detroit. *Social Science and Medicine*, *51*, 1639–1653.

Schulz, A.J., Parker, E.A., Israel, B.A., Becker, A.B., Maciak, B.J., and Hollis, R. (1998). Conducting a participatory community-based survey for a community health intervention on Detroit's east side. *Journal of Public Health Management and Practice*, *4*, 10–24.

Schulz, A.J., Williams, D.R., Israel, B.A., Becker, A.B., Parker, E.A., James, S.A. and Jackson, J. (2000b). Unfair treatment, neighborhood effects, and mental health in the Detroit metropolitan area. *Journal of Health and Social Behavior*, *41*, 314–332.

Schurman, S.J. (1996). Making the "new American workplace" safe and healthy: A joint labor-management-researcher approach. *American Journal of Industrial Medicine*, *29*, 373–377.

Schurman, S.J. and Israel, B.A. (1995). Redesigning work systems to reduce stress: a participatory action research approach to organizational change. In G. Keita, J. Hurrell, and L. Murphy (Eds.) *Job Stress Interventions: Current Practices and New Directions* (pp. 235–264). Washington, DC: American Psychological Association.

Silverstein, B.A, Armstrong, T.J., Longmate, A., and Woody, D. (1988). Can in-plant exercise control musculoskeletal symptoms? *Journal of Occupational Medicine, 30,* 922–927.

Sorensen, G., Emmons, K., Hunt, M.K. and Johnston, D. (1998). Implications of the results of community intervention trials. *Annual Review of Public Health, 19,* 379–416.

Sorensen, G., Thompson, B., Glanz, K., Feng, Z., Kinne, S., DiClemente, C., Emmons, K., Heimendinger, J., Probart, C., and Lichtenstein, E. (1996). Work site-based cancer prevention: Primary results from the Working well Trial. *American Journal of Public Health, 86,* 939–947.

Stables, G. (2000) The US 5 A Day Program: A model for increasing fruit and vegetable consumption. I. The role of the US National Cancer Institute and public partners. In G. Stables and M. Farrell (Eds.) *5 A Day International Symposium Proceedings.* New York: CABI Publishing. Accessed on line February 27, 2001. http://5aday.gov/proceedings.htm

Steckler, A., Goodman, R.M., McLeroy, K.R., Davis, S., and Koch, G. (1992). Measuring the diffusion of innovative health promotion programs. *American Journal of Health Promotion, 6,* 214–224.

Steckler, A.B., Dawson, L., Israel, B.A., and Eng, E. (1993). Community health development: An overview of the works of Guy W. Steuart. *Health Education Quarterly, Supplement 1,* S3–S20.

Steuart, G.W. (1993). Social and cultural perspectives: Community intervention and mental health. *Health Education Quarterly, Supplement 1,* S99–S111.

Stokols, D. (1992). Establishing and maintaining healthy environments: Toward a social ecology of health promotion. *American Psychologist, 47,* 6–22.

Stokols, D. (1996). Translating social ecological theory into guidelines for community health promotion. *American Journal of Health Promotion, 10,* 282–298.

Sundstrom, E. and Altman, I. (1989). Physical environments and work-group effectiveness. In L.L. Cummings and B. Staw (Eds.) *Research in Organizational Behavior Vol. II* (pp. 175-209). Greenwich, CT: JAI Press.

Susser, M. and Susser, E. (1996a). Choosing a future for epidemiology. I. Eras and paradigms. *American Journal of Public Health, 86,* 668–673.

Susser, M. and Susser, E. (1996b). From black box to Chinese boxes and eco-epidemiology. *American Journal of Public Health, 86,* 674–677.

Tarlov, A.R. (1999) Public policy frameworks for improving population health. *Annals of the New York Academy of Sciences, 896,* 281–293.

Terra, N. (1995). The prevention of job stress by redesigning jobs and implementing self-regulating teams. In L.R. Murphy, J.J. Hurrell, S.L. Sauter, and G.P. Keita (Eds.) *Job Stress Interventions* (pp. 265–281). Washington, DC: American Psychological Association..

Tomatis, L. (1992). Poverty and cancer. *Cancer Epidemiology, Biomarkers and Prevention, 1,* 167–175.

Trout, D. (1993). *The Thin Red Line: How the Poor Still Pay More*. San Francisco, CA: Consumers Union of the United States.

USDHHS (U.S. Department of Health and Human Services) (1979). *Promoting Health/ Preventing Disease: Objectives for the Nation*. Washington, DC: U.S. Department of Health and Human Services.

USDHHS (U.S. Department of Health and Human Services) (1980). *Healthy People: The Surgeon General's Report on Health Promotion and Disease Prevention*. Washington, DC: U.S. Department of Health and Human Services.

USDHHS (U.S. Department of Health and Human Services) (1990). *Healthy People 2000: National Health Promotion and Disease Prevention Objectives*. Washington, DC: U.S. Department of Health and Human Services.

USDHHS (U.S. Department of Health and Human Services) (2000). *Healthy People 2010: Understanding and improving health*. Washington, DC: U.S. Department of Health and Human Services.

Van Herten, L.M. and Gunning-Schepers, L.J. (2000) Targets as a tool in health policy. Part I. Lessons learned. *Health Policy, 52*, 1–11.

Wall, T.D. and Clegg, C.W. (1981). A longitudinal study of group work redesign. *Journal of Occupational Behavior, 2*, 31–49.

Wallerstein N. (1992). Powerlessness, empowerment, and health: Implications for health promotion programs. *American Journal of Health Promotion, 6*, 197–205.

Wallerstein, N. and Sanchez-Merki, V. (1994). Freirian praxis in health education: Research results from an adolescent prevention program. *Health Education Research, 9*, 105–118.

Wallerstein, N., Sanchez-Merki, V. and Dow, L. (1997). Freirian praxis in health education and community organizing. In M. Minkler (Ed.) *Community Organizing and Community Building for Health* (pp. 195–211). New Brunswick, NJ: Rutgers University Press.

Warren, B.S. (1975). Public Health Reports, December 5, 1919: Coordination and expansion of Federal health activities. *Public Health Reports, 90*, 270–277.

Warren, R.L. (1975). Types of purposive social change at the community level. In R.M. Kramer and H. Specht (Eds.) *Readings in Community Organization Practice*, 2nd edition (pp. 134–149). Englewood Cliffs, NJ: Prentice-Hall.

Weiss, C.H. (1995). Nothing as practical as good theory: Exploring theory-based evaluation for comprehensive community initiatives for children and families. In J. Connell, A.C. Kubisch, L.B. Schorr, and C.H. Weiss (Eds.) *New Approaches to Evaluating Community Initiatives: Concepts, Methods, and Contexts*. Washington, DC: Aspen Institute. Accessed online February 23, 2001. http://www.aspenroundtable.org/ vol1/weiss.htm

Whitehead, M. (1998). Diffusion of ideas on social inequalities in health: A European perspective. *The Millbank Quarterly, 76*, 469–492

Wilkinson, R. (1996). *Unhealthy Societies: The Afflictions of Inequality*. London: Routledge.

Williams, D.R. and Collins, C. (1995). US socioeconomic and racial differences in health: Patterns and explanations. *Annual Review of Sociology, 21*, 349–386.

Winkleby, M.A., Fortmann, S.P., and Barrett, D.C. (1990). Social class disparities in risk factors for disease: Eight-year prevalence patterns by level of education. *Preventive Medicine, 19*, 1–12.

World Health Organization (WHO). (1986). *Ottawa Charter for Health Promotion.* Copenhagen: WHO.

Young, E. and Padilla, M. (1990). Mujeres Unidas en Accion: A popular education process. *Harvard Educational Review, 60,* 1–18.

7

Evaluating and Disseminating Intervention Research

E fforts to change health behaviors should be guided by clear criteria of efficacy and effectiveness of the interventions. However, this has proved surprisingly complex and is the source of considerable debate.

The principles of science-based interventions cannot be overemphasized. Medical practices and community-based programs are often based on professional consensus rather than evidence. The efficacy of interventions can only be determined by appropriately designed empirical studies. Randomized clinical trials provide the most convincing evidence, but may not be suitable for examining all of the factors and interactions addressed in this report.

Information about efficacious interventions needs to be disseminated to practitioners. Furthermore, feedback is needed from practitioners to determine the overall effectiveness of interventions in real-life settings. Information from physicians, community leaders, public health officials, and patients are all-important for determining the overall effectiveness of interventions.

The preceding chapters review contemporary research on health and behavior from the broad perspectives of the biological, behavioral, and social sciences. A recurrent theme is that continued multidisciplinary and interdisciplinary efforts are needed. Enough research evidence has accumulated to warrant wider application of this information. To extend its use, however, existing knowledge must be evaluated and disseminated. This chapter addresses the complex relationship between research and application. The challenge of bridging research and practice is discussed with respect to clinical interventions, communities, public agencies, systems of health care delivery, and patients.

During the early 1980s, the National Heart, Lung, and Blood Institute (NHLBI) and the National Cancer Institute (NCI) suggested a sequence of research phases for the development of programs that were effective in modifying behavior (Greenwald, 1984; Greenwald and Cullen, 1984; NHLBI, 1983): hypothesis generation (phase I), intervention methods development (phase II), controlled intervention trials (phase III), studies in defined populations (phase IV), and demonstration research (phase V). Those phases reflect the importance of methods development in providing a basis for large-scale trials and the need for studies of the dissemination and diffusion process as a means of identifying effective application strategies. A range of research and evaluation methods are required to address diverse needs for scientific rigor, appropriateness and benefit to the communities involved, relevance to research questions, and flexibility in cost and setting. Inclusion of the full range of phases from hypothesis generation to demonstration research should facilitate development of a more balanced perspective on the value of behavioral and psychosocial interventions.

EVALUATING INTERVENTIONS

Assessing Outcomes

Choice of Outcome Measures

The goals of health care are to increase life expectancy and improve health-related quality of life. Major clinical trials in medicine have evolved toward the documentation of those outcomes. As more trials documented effects on total mortality, some surprising results emerged. For example, studies commonly report that, compared with placebo, lipid-lowering agents reduce total cholesterol and low-density lipoprotein cholesterol, and might increase high-density lipoprotein cholesterol, thereby reducing the risk of death from coronary heart disease (Frick et al., 1987; Lipid Research Clinics Program, 1984). Those trials usually were not associated with reductions in death from all causes (Golomb, 1998; Muldoon et al., 1990). Similarly, He et al. (1999) demonstrated that intake of dietary sodium in overweight people was not related to the incidence of coronary heart disease but was associated with mortality form coronary heart disease. Another example can be found in the treatment of cardiac arrhythmia. Among adults who previously suffered a myocardial infarction, symptomatic cardiac arrhythmia is a risk factor for sudden death (Bigger, 1984). However, a randomized drug trial in 1455 post-infarction patients demonstrated that those who were randomly assigned to take an anti-arrhythmia drug showed reduced arrhythmia, but were significantly more likely to die from arrhythmia and from all causes than those assigned to take a placebo. If investigators had measured only heart rhythm changes, they would have concluded that the drug was beneficial. Only when primary health outcomes were considered was it established that the drug was dangerous (Cardiac Arrhythmia Suppression Trial (CAST) Investigators, 1989).

Many behavioral intervention trials document the capacity of interventions to modify risk factors (NHLBI, 1998), but relatively few Level I studies measured outcomes of life expectancy and quality of life. As the examples above point out, assessing risk factors may not be adequate. Ramifications of interventions are not always apparent until they are fully evaluated. It is possible that a recommendation for a behavioral change could increase mortality through unforeseen consequences. For example, a recommendation of increased exercise might heighten the incidence of roadside auto fatalities. Although risk factor modification is expected to improve outcomes, assessment of increased longevity is essential. Measurement of mortality as an endpoint does necessitate long-duration trials that can incur greater costs.

Outcome Measurement

One approach to representing outcomes comprehensively is the quality-adjusted life year (QALY). QALY is a measure of life expectancy (Gold et al., 1996; Kaplan and Anderson, 1996) that integrates mortality and morbidity in terms of equivalents of well-years of life. If a woman expected to live to age 75 dies of lung cancer at 50, the disease caused 25 lost life-years. If 100 women with life expectancies of 75 die at age 50, 2,500 (100 × 25 years) life-years would be lost. But death is not the only outcome of concern. Many adults suffer from diseases that leave them more or less disabled for long periods. Although still alive, their quality of life is diminished. QALYs account for the quality-of-life consequences of ill-nesses. For example, a disease that reduces quality by one-half reduces QALY by 0.5 during each year the patient suffers. If the disease affects 2 people, it will reduce QALY by 1 (2 × 0.5) each year. A pharmaceutical treatment that improves life by 0.2 QALYs for 5 people will result in the equivalent of 1 QALY if the benefit is maintained over a 1-year period. The basic assumption is that 2 years scored as 0.5 each add to the equiva-lent of 1 year of complete wellness. Similarly, 4 years scored as 0.25 each are equivalent to 1 year of complete wellness. A treatment that boosts a patient's health from 0.50 to 0.75 on a scale ranging from 0.0 (for death) to 1.0 (for the highest level of wellness) adds the equivalent of 0.25 QALY. If the treatment is applied to 4 patients, and the duration of its effect is 1 year, the effect of the treatment would be equivalent to 1 year of complete wellness. This approach has the advantage of considering benefits and side-effects of treatment programs in a common term. Although QALYs typically are used to assess effects on patients, they also can be used as a measure of effect on others, including caregivers who are placed at risk because their experience is stressful. Most important, QALYs are required for many methods of cost-effectiveness analysis. The most controversial aspect of the methodology is the method for assigning values along the scale. Three methods are commonly used: standard reference gamble, time-tradeoff, and rating scales. Economists and psychologists differ on their preferred approach to preference assessment. Economists typically prefer the standard gamble because it is consistent with the axioms of choice outlined in decision theory (Torrence, 1976). Economists also ac-cept time-tradeoff because it represents choice even though it is not ex-actly consistent with the axioms derived from theory (Bennett and Torrence, 1996). However, evidence from experimental studies questions many of the assumptions that underlie economic models of choice. In particular, human evaluators do poorly at integrating complex probability information when making decisions involving risk (Tversky and Fox, 1995). Economic models often assume that choice is rational. However, psychological experiments suggest that methods commonly used for choice studies do not represent the true underlying preference continuum (Zhu and Anderson, 1991). Some evidence supports the use of simple rating scales (Anderson and Zalinski, 1990). Recently, research by economists has attempted to integrate studies from cognitive science, while psycho-gists have begun investigations of choice and decision-making (Tversky and Shafir, 1992). A significant body of studies demonstrates that different methods for estimating preferences will produce different values (Lenert and Kaplan, 2000). This happens because the methods ask different questions. More research is needed to clarify the best method for valuing health states.

The weighting used for quality adjustment comes from surveys of patient or population groups, an aspect of the method that has generated considerable discussion among methodologists and ethicists (Kaplan, 1994). Preference weights are typically obtained by asking patients or people randomly selected from a community to rate cases that describe people in various states of wellness. The cases usually describe level of functioning and symptoms. Although some studies show small but significant differences in preference ratings between demographic groups (Kaplan, 1998), most studies have shown a high degree of similarity in preferences (see Kaplan, 1994, for review). A panel convened by the U.S. Department of Health and Human Services reviewed methodologic issues relevant to cost and utility analysis (the formal name for this approach) in health care. The panel concluded that population averages rather than patient group preference weights are more appropriate for policy analysis (Gold et al., 1996).

Several authors have argued that resource allocation on the basis of QALYs is unethical (see La Puma and Lawlor, 1990). Those who reject the use of QALY suggest that QALY cannot be measured. However, the reliability and validity of quality-of-life measures are well documented (Spilker, 1996). Another ethical challenge to QALYs is that they force health care providers to make decisions based on cost-effectiveness rather than on the health of the individual patient.

Another common criticism of QALYs is that they discriminate against the elderly and the disabled. Older people and those with disabilities have lower QALYs, so it is assumed that fewer services will be provided to them. However, QALYs consider the increment in benefit, not the starting point. Programs that prevent the decline of health status or programs that prevent deterioration and functioning among the disabled do perform well in QALY outcome analysis. It is likely that QALYs will not reveal benefits for heroic care at the very end of life. However, most people prefer not to take treatment that is unlikely to increase life expectancy or improve quality of life (Schneiderman et al., 1992). Ethical issues relevant to the use of cost-effectiveness analysis are considered in detail in the report of the Panel on Cost-Effectiveness in Health and Medicine (Gold et al., 1996).

Evaluating Clinical Interventions

Behavioral interventions have been used to modify behaviors that put people at risk for disease, to manage disease processes, and to help patients cope with their health conditions. Behavioral and psychosocial interventions take many forms. Some provide knowledge or persuasive information; others involve individual, family, group, or community programs to change or support changes in health behaviors (such as in tobacco use, physical activity, or diet); still others involve patient or health care provider education to stimulate behavior change or risk-avoidance. Behavioral and psychosocial interventions are not without consequence for patients and their families, friends, and acquaintances; interventions cost money, take time, and are not always enjoyable. Justification for interventions requires assurance that the changes advocated are valuable. The kinds of evidence required to evaluate the benefits of interventions are discussed below.

Evidence-Based Medicine

Evidence-based medicine uses the best available scientific evidence to inform decisions about what treatments individual patients should receive (Sackett et al., 1997). Not all studies are equally credible. Last (1995) offered a hierarchy of clinical research evidence, shown in Table 7-1. Level I, the most rigorous, is reserved for the randomized clinical trials (RCT), in which participants are randomly assigned to the experimental condition or to a meaningful comparison condition—the most widely accepted standard for evaluating interventions. Such trials involve

TABLE 7-1 Research Evidence Hierarchy

Level	Element
I.	Randomized controlled trial
II.	Controlled trial without randomization
	Cohort or case control analytic study
	Multiple time series
	Uncontrolled experiment with dramatic results
III.	Case study
	Expert opinion

SOURCE: Last, 1995, by permission of Lancet Ltd. All rights reserved.

either "single blinding" (investigators know which participants are assigned to the treatment and groups but participants do not) or "double blinding" (neither the investigators nor the participants know the group assignments) (Friedman et al., 1985). Double blinding is difficult in behavioral intervention trials, but there are some good examples of single-blind experiments. Reviews of the literature often grade studies according to levels of evidence. Level I evidence is considered more credible than Level II evidence; Level III evidence is given little weight.

There has been concern about the generalizability of RCTs (Feinstien and Horwitz, 1997; Horwitz, 1987a,b; Horwitz and Daniels, 1996; Horwitz et al., 1996, 1990; Rabeneck et al., 1992), specifically because the recruitment of participants can result in samples that are not representative of the population (Seligman, 1996). There is a trend toward increased heterogeneity of the patient population in RCTs. Even so, RCTs often include stringent criteria for participation that can exclude participants on the basis of comorbid conditions or other characteristics that occur frequently in the population. Furthermore, RCTs are often conducted in specialized settings, such as university-based teaching hospitals, that do not draw representative population samples. Trials sometimes exhibit large dropout rates, which further undermine the generalizability of their findings.

Oldenburg and colleagues (1999) reviewed all papers published in 1994 in 12 selected journals on public health, preventive medicine, health behavior, and health promotion and education. They graded the studies according to evidence level: 2% were Level I RCTs and 48% were Level II. The authors expressed concern that behavioral research might not be credible when evaluated against systematic experimental trials, which are more common in other fields of medicine. Studies with more rigorous experimental designs are less likely to demonstrate treatment effectiveness (Heaney and Goetzel, 1997; Mosteller and Colditz, 1996). Although there have been relatively few behavioral intervention trials, those that have been published have supported the efficacy of behavioral interventions in a variety of circumstances, including smoking, chronic pain, cancer care, and bulimia nervosa (Compas et al., 1998).

Efficacy and Effectiveness

Efficacy is the capacity of an intervention to work under controlled conditions. Randomized clinical trials are essential in establishing the effects of a clinical intervention (Chambless and Hollon, 1998) and in determining that an intervention *can* work. However, demonstration of efficacy in an RCT does not guarantee that the treatment will be effective in actual practice settings. For example, some reviews suggest that behavioral interventions in psychotherapy are generally beneficial (Matt and Navarro, 1997), others suggest that interventions are less effective in clinical settings than in the laboratory (Weisz et al., 1992), and others find particular interventions equally effective in experimental and clinical settings (Shadish et al., 1997).

The Division of Clinical Psychology of the American Psychological Association recently established criteria for "empirically supported" psychological treatments (Chambless and Hollon, 1998). In an effort to establish a level of excellence in validating the efficacy of psychological interventions the criteria are relatively stringent. A treatment is considered empirically supported if it is found to be more effective than either an alternative form of treatment or a credible control condition in at least two RCTs. The effects must be replicated by at least two independent laboratories or investigative teams to ensure that the effects are not attributable to special characteristics of a specific investigator or setting. Several health-related behavior change interventions meeting those criteria have been identified, including interventions for management of chronic pain, smoking cessation, adaptation to cancer, and treatment of eating disorders (Compas et al., 1998).

An intervention that has failed to meet the criteria still has potential value and might represent important or even landmark progress in the field of health-related behavior change. As in many fields of health care, there historically has been little effort to set standards for psychological treatments for health-related problems or disease. Recently, however, managed-care and health maintenance organizations have begun to monitor and regulate both the type and the duration of psychological treatments that are reimbursed. A common set of criteria for making coverage decisions has not been articulated, so decisions are made in the absence of appropriate scientific data to support them. It is in the best interest of the public and those involved in the development and delivery of health-related behavior change interventions to establish criteria that are based on the best available scientific evidence. Criteria for empirically supported treatments are an important part of that effort.

Evaluating Community-Level Interventions

Evaluating the effectiveness of interventions in the communities requires different methods. Developing and testing interventions that take a more comprehensive, ecologic approach, and that are effective in reducing risk-related behaviors and influencing the social factors associated with health status, require many levels and types of research (Flay, 1986; Green et al., 1995; Greenwald and Cullen, 1984). Questions have been raised about the appropriateness of RCTs for addressing research questions when the unit of analysis is larger than the individual, such as a group, organization, or community (McKinlay, 1993; Susser, 1995). While this discussion uses the community as the unit of analysis, similar principles apply to interventions aimed at groups, families, or organizations.

Review criteria of community interventions have been suggested by Hancock and colleagues (Hancock et al., 1997). Their criteria for rigorous scientific evaluation of community intervention trials include four domains: (1) design, including the randomization of communities to condition, and the use of sampling methods that assure representativeness of the entire population; (2) measures, including the use of outcome measures with demonstrated validity and reliability and process measures that describe the extent to which the intervention was delivered to the target audience; (3) analysis, including consideration of both individual variation within each community and community-level variation within each treatment condition; and (4) specification of the intervention in enough detail to allow replication.

Randomization of communities to various conditions raises challenges for intervention research in terms of expense and statistical power (Koepsell et al., 1995; Murray, 1995). The restricted hypotheses that RCTs test cannot adequately consider the complexities and multiple causes of human behavior and health status embedded within communities (Israel et al., 1995; Klitzner, 1993; McKinlay, 1993; Susser, 1995). A randomized controlled trial might actually alter the interaction between an intervention and a community and result in an attenuation of the effectiveness of the intervention (Fisher, 1995; McKinlay, 1993). At the level of community interventions, experimental control might not be possible, especially when change is unplanned. That is, given the different sociopolitical structures, cultures, and histories of communities and the numerous factors that are beyond a researcher's ability to control, it might be impossible to identify and maintain a commensurate comparison community (Green et al., 1996; Hollister and Hill, 1995; Israel et al., 1995; Klitzner, 1993;

Mittelmark et al., 1993; Susser, 1995). Using a control community does not completely solve the problem of comparison, however, because one "cannot assume that a control community will remain static or free of influence by national campaigns or events occurring in the experimental communities" (Green et al., 1996, p. 274).

Clear specification of the conceptual model guiding a community intervention is needed to clarify how an intervention is expected to work (Koepsell, 1998; Koepsell et al., 1992). This is the contribution of the Theory of Change model for communities described in Chapter 6. A theoretical framework is necessary to specify mediating mechanisms and modifying conditions. Mediating mechanisms are pathways, such as social support, by which the intervention induces the outcomes; modifying conditions, such as social class, are not affected by the intervention but can influence outcomes independently. Such an approach offers numerous advantages, including the ability to identify pertinent variables and how, when, and in whom they should be measured; the ability to evaluate and control for sources of extraneous variance; and the ability to develop a cumulative knowledge base about how and when programs work (Bickman, 1987; Donaldson et al., 1994; Lipsey, 1993; Lipsey and Polard, 1989). When an intervention is unsuccessful at stimulating change, data on mediating mechanisms can allow investigators to determine whether the failure is due to the inability of the program to activate the causal processes that the theory predicts or to an invalid program theory (Donaldson et al., 1994).

Small-scale, targeted studies sometimes provide a basis for refining large-scale intervention designs and enhance understanding of methods for influencing group behavior and social change (Fisher, 1995; Susser, 1995; Winkleby, 1994). For example, more in-depth, comparative, multiple-case-study evaluations are needed to explain and identify lessons learned regarding the context, process, impacts, and outcomes of community-based participatory research (Israel et al., 1998).

Community-Based Participatory Research and Evaluation

As reviewed in Chapter 4, broad social and societal influences have an impact on health. This concept points to the importance of an approach that recognizes individuals as embedded within social, political, and economic systems that shape their behaviors and constrain their access to resources necessary to maintain their health (Brown, 1991;

Gottlieb and McLeroy, 1994; Krieger, 1994; Krieger et al., 1993; Lalonde, 1974; Lantz et al., 1998; McKinlay, 1993; Sorensen et al., 1998a, b; Stokols, 1992, 1996; Susser and Susser, 1996a,b; Williams and Collins, 1995; World Health Organization [WHO], 1986). It also points to the importance of expanding the evaluation of interventions to incorporate such factors (Fisher, 1995; Green et al., 1995; Hatch et al., 1993; Israel et al., 1995; James, 1993; Pearce, 1996; Sorensen et al., 1998a,b; Steckler et al., 1992; Susser, 1995).

This is exemplified by community-based participatory programs, which are collaborative efforts among community members, organization representatives, a wide range of researchers and program evaluators, and others (Israel et al., 1998). The partners contribute "unique strengths and shared responsibilities" (Green et al., 1995, p. 12) to enhance understanding of a given phenomenon, and they integrate the knowledge gained from interventions to improve the health and well-being of community members (Dressler, 1993; Eng and Blanchard, 1990-1; Hatch et al., 1993; Israel et al., 1998; Schulz et al., 1998a). It provides "the opportunity…for communities and science to work in tandem to ensure a more balanced set of political, social, economic, and cultural priorities, which satisfy the demands of both scientific research and communities at higher risk" (Hatch et al., 1993, p. 31). The advantages and rationale of community-based participatory research are summarized in Table 7-2 (Israel et al., 1998). The term "community-based participatory research," is used here to clearly differentiate from "community-based research," which is often used in reference to research that is placed in the community but in which community members are not actively involved.

Table 7-3 presents a set of principles, or characteristics, that capture the important components of community-based participatory research and evaluation (Israel et al., 1998). Each principle constitutes a continuum and represents a goal, for example, equitable participation and shared control over all phases of the research process (Cornwall, 1996; Dockery, 1996; Green et al., 1995). Although the principles are presented here as distinct items, community-based participatory research integrates them.

There are four major foci of evaluation with implications for research design: *context, process, impact,* and *outcome* (Israel, 1994; Israel et al., 1995; Simons-Morton et al., 1995). A comprehensive community-based participatory evaluation would include all types, but it is often financially practical to pursue only one or two. Evaluation design is extensively reviewed in the literature (Campbell and Stanley, 1963; Cook and

TABLE 7-2 Rationale for Community-Based Participatory Research

Rationale	Reference
Enhances the relevance and usefulness of research data for all partners involved	Brown 1995; Cousins and Earl 1995; Schulz et al. 1998b
Joins partners with diverse skills, knowledge, expertise, and sensitivities to address complex problems	Butterfoss et al., 1993; Hall 1992; Himmelman 1992; Israel et al. 1989; Schensul et al. 1987
Improves quality and validity of research by engaging local knowledge and local theory based on experience of people involved	Altman 1995; Bishop 1996; deKoning and Martin 1996; Dressler 1993; Elden and Levin 1991; Gaventa 1993; Hall 1992; Maguire 1987; Schensul et al. 1987; Vega 1992
Recognizes limitations of concept of "value-free" science (Denzin 1994) and encourages self-reflexive, engaged, and self-critical role of researchers	Denzin, 1994; Reason 1994; Zich and Temoshok 1986
Acknowledges that knowledge is power, thus knowledge gained can be used by all partners involved to direct resources and influence policies that will benefit community	deKoning and Martin 1996; Dressler 1993; Hall 1992; Himmelman 1992; Maguire 1987; Tandon 1981
Strengthens research and program development capacity of partners	Altman 1995; Green et al. 1995; Schensul et al. 1987; Schulz, et al. 1998a; Singer 1993, 1994
Creates theory grounded in social experience and creates better informed and more effective practice guided by such theories	Altman 1995; Schensul 1985
Increases possibility of overcoming understandable distrust of research on part of communities that have historically been subjects of such research	Hatch et al. 1993; Schulz, et al. 1998b
Has potential to "bridge the cultural gaps that may exist" (Brown, 1995, p. 211) between partners involved	Bishop 1994, 1996; Hatch et al. 1993; Schulz et al. 1998b; Vega 1992

continued on next page

TABLE 7-2 Continued

Rationale	Reference
Overcomes fragmentation and separation of individual from culture and context that are often evident in more narrowly defined, categorical approaches	Green et al. 1995; Israel et al. 1994; Reason 1994; Stokols 1996
Is consistent with implications or principles of practice that emanate from conceptual framework of stress process, for example, context-specific, comprehensive approach, and multiple outcomes	Israel et al., 1996
Provides additional funds and possible employment opportunities for community partners	Altman 1995; Nyden and Wiewel 1992; Schulz et al. 1998b
Aims to improve health and well-being of communities involved, both directly through examining and addressing identified needs and indirectly through increasing power and control over research process	Durie 1996; Green et al. 1995; Hatch et al. 1993; Schulz et al. 1998a, deKoning and Martin 1996; Israel and Schurman 1990; Israel et al. 1994; Wallerstein 1992
Involves communities that have been marginalized on basis of race, ethnicity, class, gender, sexual orientation in examining consequences of marginalization and attempting to reduce and eliminate it	deKoning and Martin 1996; Gaventa 1993; Hatch et al. 1993; Krieger 1994; Maguire 1987; Vega 1992; Williams and Collins 1995

SOURCE: Israel et al., 1998. Reprinted with permission of Pergaus Books Publishers, a member of Perseus Books, L.L.C.

Reichardt, 1979; Dignan, 1989; Green, 1977; Green and Gordon, 1982; Green and Lewis, 1986; Guba and Lincoln, 1989; House, 1980; Israel et al., 1995; Patton, 1987, 1990; Rossi and Freeman, 1989; Shadish et al., 1991; Stone et al., 1994; Thomas and Morgan, 1991; Windsor et al., 1994; Yin, 1993).

Context encompasses the events, influences, and changes that occur naturally in the project setting or environment during the intervention

TABLE 7-3 Principles of Community-Based Participatory Research and Evaluation

Principle	Reference
Recognizes community as unit of identity	Hatch et al. 1993; Israel et al. 1994; Klein 1968; Sarason 1984; Steckler et al., 1993; Steuart 1993; Stringer 1996
Builds on strengths and resources within community	Berger and Neuhaus, 1977; CDC/ATSDR 1997; Israel and Schurman, 1990; McKnight 1987, 1994; Minkler 1989; Putnam, 1993; Steuart 1993
Facilitates collaborative partnerships in all phases of research	Bishop 1994; 1996; CDC/ATSDR 1997; Cornwall and Jewkes 1995; deKoning and Martin 1996; Durie 1996; Fawcett 1991; Gaventa 1993; Goodman 1999; Green et al. 1995; Hatch et al. 1993; Israel et al. 1992a, b; Levine et al. 1992; Lillie-Blanton and Hoffman 1995; Maguire 1996; Mittelmark et al. 1993; Nyden and Wiewel 1992; Park et al. 1993; Schulz, et al. 1998a; Singer 1993; Stringer 1996
Integrates knowledge and action for benefit of all partners	Cornwall and Jewkes 1995; deKoning and Martin 1996; Fawcett 1991; Green et al. 1995; Israel et al. 1994; Lather, 1986; Lincoln and Reason 1996; Maguire 1987; Park et al. 1993; Reason 1988; Schulz, et al. 1998a; Singer 1993; Stringer 1996
Promotes a colearning and empowering process that attends to social inequalities	Bishop 1994, 1996; CDC/ATSDR 1997; Cornwall and Jewkes 1995; deKoning and Martin 1996; Elden and Levin, 1991; Eng and Parker 1994; Freire 1987; Israel et al. 1994; Labonte 1994; Lillie-Blanton and Hoffman 1995; Maguire, 1987; Nyden and Wiewel 1992; Robertson and Minkler 1994; Schulz, et al. 1998a; Singer 1993; Stringer 1996; Yeich and Levine, 1992

continued on next page

TABLE 7-3 Continued

Principle	Reference
Involves cyclic and iterative process	Altman 1995; Cornwall and Jewkes 1995; Fawcett et al. 1996; Hatch et al. 1993; Israel et al. 1994; Levine et al. 1992; Reason 1994; Smithies and Adams 1993; Stringer 1996; Tandon 1981
Addresses health from both positive and ecological perspectives	Antonovsky 1985; Baker and Brownson 1999; Brown 1991; Durie 1996; Goodman 1999; Gottlieb and McLeroy 1994; Hancock 1993; Israel et al. 1994; Krieger 1994; McKinlay 1993; Schulz, et al. 1998a; Stokols 1992, 1996; WHO 1986
Disseminates findings and knowledge gained to all partners	Bishop 1996; Dressler 1993; Fawcett 1991; Fawcett et al. 1996; Francisco et al. 1993; Gaventa 1993; Hall 1992; Israel et al, 1992a; Lillie-Blanton and Hoffman 1995; Maguire 1987; Schulz et al. 1998a; Singer 1994; Whitehead 1993
Involves long-term commitment of all partners	CDC/ATSDR 1997; Hatch et al. 1993; Israel et al., 1992a; Mittelmark et al. 1993; Schulz et al. 1998a,b

SOURCE: Israel et al., 1998. Reprinted with permission of Pergaus Books Publishers, a member of Perseus Books, L.L.C.

that might affect the outcomes (Israel et al., 1995). Context data provide information about how particular settings facilitate or impede program success. Decisions must be made about which of the many factors in the context of an intervention might have the greatest effect on project success.

Evaluation of process assesses the extent, fidelity, and quality of the implementation of interventions (McGraw et al., 1994). It describes the actual activities of the intervention and the extent of participant exposure, provides quality assurance, describes participants, and identifies the internal dynamics of program operations (Israel et al., 1995).

A distinction is often made in the evaluation of interventions between *impact* and *outcome* (Green and Lewis, 1986; Israel et al., 1995;

Simons-Morton et al., 1995; Windsor et al., 1994). Impact evaluation assesses the effectiveness of the intervention in achieving desired changes in targeted mediators. These include the knowledge, attitudes, beliefs, and behavior of participants. Outcome evaluation examines the effects of the intervention on health status, morbidity, and mortality. Impact evaluation focuses on what the intervention is specifically trying to change, and it precedes an outcome evaluation. It is proposed that if the intervention can effect change in some intermediate outcome ("impact"), the "final" outcome will follow.

Although the association between impact and outcome may not always be substantiated (as discussed earlier in this chapter), impact may be a necessary measure. In some instances, the outcome goals are too far in the future to be evaluated. For example, childhood cardiovascular risk factor intervention studies typically measure intermediate gains in knowledge (Parcel et al., 1989) and changes in diet or physical activity (Simons-Morton et al., 1991). They sometimes assess cholesterol and blood pressure, but they do not usually measure heart disease because that would not be expected to occur for many years.

Given the aims and the dynamic context within which community-based participatory research and evaluation are conducted, methodologic flexibility is essential. Methods must be tailored to the purpose of the research and evaluation and to the context and interests of the community (Beery and Nelson, 1998; deKoning and Martin, 1996; Dockery, 1996; Dressler, 1993; Green et al., 1995; Hall, 1992; Hatch et al., 1993; Israel et al., 1998; Marin and Marin, 1991; Nyden and Wiewel, 1992; Schulz et al., 1998b; Singer, 1993; Stringer, 1996). Numerous researchers have suggested greater use of qualitative data, from in-depth interviews and observational studies, for evaluating the context, process, impact, and outcome of community-based participatory research interventions (Fortmann et al., 1995; Goodman, 1999; Hugentobler et al., 1992; Israel et al., 1995, 1998; Koepsell et al., 1992; Mittelmark et al., 1993; Parker et al., 1998; Sorensen et al., 1998a; Susser, 1995). Triangulation is the use of multiple methods and sources of data to overcome limitations inherent in each method and to improve the accuracy of the information collected, thereby increasing the validity and credibility of the results (Denzin, 1970; Israel et al., 1995; Reichardt and Cook, 1980; Steckler et al., 1992). For examples of the integration of qualitative and quantitative methods in research and evaluation of public-health interventions, see Steckler et al. (1992) and Parker et al. (1998).

Assessing Government Interventions

Despite the importance of legislation and regulation to promote public health, the effectiveness of government interventions are poorly understood. In particular, policymakers often cannot answer important empirical questions: do legal interventions work and at what economic and social cost? In particular, policymakers need to know whether legal interventions achieve their intended goals (e.g., reducing risk behavior). If so, do legal interventions unintentionally increase other risks (risk/risk tradeoff)? Finally, what are the adverse effects of regulation on personal or economic liberties and general prosperity in society? This is an important question not only because freedom has an intrinsic value in democracy, but also because activities that dampen economic development can have health effects. For example, research demonstrates the positive correlation between socioeconomic status and health (Chapter 4).

Legal interventions often are not subjected to rigorous research evaluation. The research that has been done, moreover, has faced challenges in methodology. There are so many variables that can affect behavior and health status (e.g., differences in informational, physical, social, and cultural environments) that it can be extraordinarily difficult to demonstrate a causal relationship between an intervention and a perceived health effect. Consider the methodologic constraints in identifying the effects of specific drunk-driving laws. Several kinds of laws can be enacted within a short period, so it is difficult to isolate the effect of each law. Publicity about the problem and the legal response can cross state borders, making state comparisons more difficult. Because people who drive under the influence of alcohol also could engage in other risky driving behaviors (e.g., speeding, failing to wear safety belts, running red lights), researchers need to control for changes in other highway safety laws and traffic law enforcement. Subtle differences between comparison communities can have unanticipated effects on the impact of legal interventions (DeJong and Hingson, 1998; Hingson, 1996).

Despite such methodologic challenges, social science researchers have studied legal interventions, often with encouraging results. The social science, medical, and behavioral literature contains evaluations of interventions in several public health areas, particularly in relation to injury prevention (IOM, 1999; Rivara et al., 1997a,b). For example, studies have evaluated the effectiveness of regulations to prevent head injuries (bicycle helmets: Dannenberg et al., 1993; Kraus et al., 1994; Lund et al., 1991; Ni et al., 1997; Thompson et al., 1996a,b), choking and suffocation (refrigerator disposal and warning labels on thin plastic bags: Kraus, 1985), child poisoning (childproof packaging: Rogers, 1996), and burns (tap water: Erdmann et al., 1991). One regulatory measure that has received a great deal of research attention relates to reductions in cigarette-smoking (Chapter 6).

Legal interventions can be an important part of strategies to change behaviors. In considering them, government and other public health agencies face difficult and complex tradeoffs between population health and individual rights (e.g., autonomy, privacy, liberty, property). One example is the controversy over laws that require motorcyclists to wear helmets. Ethical concerns accompany the use of legal interventions to mandate behavior change and must be part of the deliberation process.

COST-EFFECTIVENESS EVALUATION

It is not enough to demonstrate that a treatment benefits some patients or community members. The demand for health programs exceeds the resources available to pay for them so that treatments provide clinical benefit and value for money. Investigators, clinicians, and program planners must demonstrate that their interventions constitute a good use of resources.

Well over $1 trillion is spent on health care each year in the United States. Current estimates suggest that expenditures on health care exceed $4000 per person (Health Care Financing Administration, 1998). Investments are made in health care to produce good health status for the population, and it is usually assumed that more investment will lead to greater health. Some expenditures in health care produce relatively little benefit; others produce substantial benefits. Cost-effectiveness analysis (CEA) can help guide the use of resources to achieve the greatest improvement in health status for a given expenditure.

Consider the medical interventions in Table 7-4, all of which are well-known, generally accepted, and widely used. Some are traditional medical care and some are preventive programs. To emphasize the focus on increasing good health, the table presents the data in units of health bought for $1 million rather than in dollars per unit of health, the usual approach in CEA. The life-year is the most comprehensive unit measure of health. Table 7-4 reveals several important points about resource allocation. There is tremendous variation among the interventions in what can be accomplished for $1 million; which nets 7,750 life-years if used for influenza vaccinations for the elderly, 217 life-years if applied to smoking-cessation

TABLE 7-4 Life-Years Yielded by Selected Interventions per $1 Million, 1997 Dollars

Intervention	Life Years/$1 Million
Antihypertensive medication, U.S. population	
Propranolol	51
Captopril	8
Influenza vaccine, persons 65+ years old	7750
Tetanus booster every 10 years	4
Pap smear	
Every 3 years	36
Every 2 years	1
Every year	< 0.5
Thyroid screening every 5 years	
Women	98
Men	40
Lovastatin at 20 milligrams per day, primary prevention in men with total cholesterol 300+ milligrams per decaliter	
Age 55-64 years, high risk	42
Age 35-44 years, low risk	2
Smoking-cessation programs	217

Based on cost-effectiveness ratios from the original articles, which were updated to 1997 dollars by using the medical care component of the Consumer Price Index.

SOURCES, in order from top: Edelson et al., 1990; Office of Technology Assessment, 1981; Balestra and Littenberg, 1993; Eddy, 1990; Danese et al., 1996; Goldman et al., 1991; Cromwell et al., 1997.

programs, but only 2 life-years if used to supply Lovastatin to men aged 35–44 who have high total cholesterol but no heart disease and no other risk factors for heart disease.

How effectively an intervention contributes to good health depends not only on the intervention, but also on the details of its use. Antihypertensive medication is effective, but Propranolol is more cost-effective than Captopril. Thyroid screening is more cost-effective in women than in men. Lovastatin produces more good health when targeted at older high-risk men than at younger low-risk men. Screening for cervical cancer at 3-year intervals with the Pap smear yields 36 life-years per $1 million (compared with no screening), but each $1 million spent to increase the frequency of screening to 2 years brings only 1 additional life-year.

The numbers in Table 7-4 illustrate a central concept in resource allocation: opportunity cost. The true cost of choosing to use a particular intervention or to use it in a particular way is not the monetary cost per se, but the health benefits that could have been achieved if the money had been spent on another service instead. Thus, the opportunity cost of providing annual Pap smears ($1 million) rather than smoking-cessation programs is the 217 life-years that could have been achieved through smoking cessation.

The term cost-effectiveness is commonly used but widely misunderstood. Some people confuse cost-effectiveness with cost minimization. Cost minimization aims to reduce health care costs regardless of health outcomes. CEA does not have cost-reduction per se as a goal but is designed to obtain the most improvement in health for a given expenditure. CEA also is often confused with cost/benefit analysis (CBA), which compares investments with returns. CBA ranks the amount of improved health associated with different expenditures with the aim of identifying the appropriate level of investment. CEA indicates which intervention is preferable given a specific expenditure.

Usually, costs are represented by the net or difference between the total costs of the intervention and the total costs of the alternative to that intervention. Typically, the measure of health is the QALY. The net health effect of the intervention is the difference between the QALYs produced by an intervention and the QALYs produced by an alternative or other comparative base.

Comprehensive as it is, CEA does not include everything that might be relevant to a particular decision—so it should never be used mechanically. Decision-makers can have legitimate reasons to emphasize particular groups, benefits, or costs more heavily than others. Furthermore, some decisions require information that cannot be captured easily in a CEA, such as the effect of an intervention on individual privacy or liberty.

CEA is an analytical framework that arises from the question of which ways of promoting good health—procedures, tests, medications, educational programs, regulations, taxes or subsidies, and combinations and variations of these—provide the most effective use of resources. Specific recommendations about behavioral and psychosocial interventions will contribute the most to good health if they are set in this larger context and based on information that demonstrates that they are in the public interest. However, comparing behavioral and psychosocial interventions with other ways of promoting health on the basis of cost-effectiveness requires additional research. Currently there are too few studies that meet this standard to support such recommendations.

DISSEMINATION

A basic assumption underlying intervention research is that tested interventions found to be effective are disseminated to and implemented in clinics, communities, schools, and worksites. However, there is a sizable gap between science and practice (Anderson, 1998; Price, 1989, 1998). Researchers and practitioners need to ensure that an intervention is effective, and that the community or organization is prepared to adopt, implement, disseminate, and institutionalize it. There also is a need for demonstration research (phase V) to explain more about the process of dissemination itself.

Dissemination to Consumers

Biomedical research results are commonly reported in the mass media. Nearly every day people are given information about the risks of disease, the benefits of treatment, and the potential health hazards in their environments. They regularly make health decisions on the basis of their understanding of such information. Some evidence shows that lay people often misinterpret health risk information (Berger and Hendee, 1989; Fischhoff, 1999a) as do their doctors (Kalet et al., 1994; Kong et al., 1986). On the question of such a widely publicized issue as mammography, for example, evidence suggests that women overestimate their risk of getting breast cancer by a factor of at least 20 and that they overestimate the benefits of mammography by a factor of 100 (Black et al., 1995). In a study of 500 female veterans (Schwartz et al., 1997), half the women overestimated their risk of death from breast cancer by a factor of 8. This did not appear to be because the subjects thought that they were more at risk than other women; only 10% reported that they were at higher risk than the average woman of their age. The topic of communication of health messages to the public is discussed at length in an IOM report, *Speaking of Health: Assessing Health Communication. Strategies for Diverse Populations* (IOM, 2001).

Communicating Risk Information

Improving communication requires understanding what information the public needs. That necessitates both descriptive and normative analyses, which consider what the public believes and what the public should know, respectively. Juxtaposing normative and descriptive analyses might provide guidance for reducing misunderstanding (Fischhoff and Downs, 1997). Formal normative analysis of decisions involves the creation of decision trees, showing the available options and the probabilities of various outcomes of each, whose relative attractiveness (or aversiveness) must be evaluated by people. Although full analyses of decision problems can be quite complex, they often reveal ways to drastically simplify individuals' decision-making problems—in the sense that they reveal a small number of issues of fact or value that really merit serious attention (Clemen, 1991; Merz et al., 1993; Raiffa, 1968). Those few issues can still pose significant challenges for decision makers. The actual probabilities can differ from people's subjective probabilities (which govern their behavior). For example, a woman who overestimates the value of a mammogram might insist on tests that are of little benefit to her and mistrust the political/medical system that seeks to deny such care (Woloshin et al., 2000). Obtaining estimates of subjective probabilities is difficult. Although eliciting probabilities has been studied in other contexts over the past two generations (vonWinterfeldt and Edwards, 1986; Yates, 1990), it has received much less attention in medical contexts, where it can pose questions that people are unwilling or unable to confront (Fischhoff and Bruine de Bruin, 1999).

In addition to such quantitative beliefs, people often need a qualitative understanding of the processes by which risks are created and controlled. This allows them to get an intuitive feeling for the quantitative estimates, to feel competent to make decisions in their own behalf, to monitor their own experience, and to know when they need help (Fischhoff, 1999b; Leventhal and Cameron, 1987). Not seeing the world in the same way as scientists do also can lead lay people to misinterpret communications directed at them. One common (and some might argue, essential) strategy for evaluating any public health communication or research instrument is to ask people to think aloud as they answer draft versions of questions (Ericsson and Simon, 1994; Schriver, 1989). For example, subjects might be asked about the probability of getting HIV from unprotected sexual activity. Reasons for their assessments might be explored as they elaborate on their impressions and the assumptions they use (Fischhoff, 1999b; McIntyre and West, 1992). The result should both reveal their intuitive theories and improve the communication process.

When people must evaluate their options, the way in which information is framed can have a substantial effect on how it is used (Kahneman and Tversky, 1983; Schwartz, 1999; Tversky and Kahneman, 1988). The fairest presentation of risk information might be one in which multiple perspectives are used (Kahneman and Tversky, 1983, 1996). For example, one common situation involves small risks that add up over the course of time, through repeated exposures. The chances of being injured in an automobile crash are very small for any one outing, whether or not the driver wears a seatbelt. However, driving over a lifetime creates a substantial risk—and a substantial benefit for seatbelt use. One way to communicate that perspective is to do the arithmetic explicitly, so that subjects understand it (Linville et al., 1993). Another method that helps people to understand complex information involves presenting ranges rather than best estimates. Science is uncertain, and it should be helpful for people to understand the intervals within which their risks are likely to fall (Lipkus and Hollands, 1999).

Risk communication can be improved. For example, many members of the public have been fearful that proximity to electromagnetic fields and power lines can increase the risk of cancer. Studies revealed that many people knew very little about properties of electricity. In particular, they usually were unaware that exposure decreases as a function of the cube root of distance from the lines. After studying mental models of this risk, Morgan (1995) developed a tiered brochure that presented the problem at a variety of risks. The brochure addressed common misconceptions and explained why scientists disagree about the risks posed by electromagnetic fields. Participants on each side of the debate reviewed the brochure for fairness. Several hundred thousand copies of the brochure have now been distributed. This approach to communication requires that the public listen to experts, but it also requires that the experts listen to the public. Providing information is not enough; it is necessary to take the next step to demonstrate that the information is presented in an unbiased fashion and that the public accurately processes what is offered (Edworthy and Adams, 1997; Hadden, 1986; Morgan et al., 2001; National Research Council, 1989).

The electromagnetic field brochure is an example of a general approach in cognitive psychology, in which communications are designed to create coherent mental models of the domain being considered (Ericsson and Simon, 1994; Fischhoff, 1999b; Gentner and Stevens, 1983; Johnson-Laird, 1980). The bases of these communications are formal models of the domain. In the case of the complex processes creating and controlling risks, the appropriate representation is often an influence diagram, a directed graph that captures the uncertain relationships among the factors involved (Clemen, 1991; Morgan et al., 2001). Creating such a diagram requires pooling the knowledge of diverse disciplines, rather than letting each tell its own part of the story. Identifying the critical messages requires considering both the science of the risk and recipients' intuitive conceptualizations.

Presentation of Clinical Research Findings

Research results are commonly misinterpreted. When a study shows that the effect of a treatment is statistically significant, it is often assumed that the treatment works for every patient or at least for a high percentage of those treated. In fact, large experimental trials, often with considerable publicity, promote treatments that have only minor effects in most patients. For example, contemporary care for high blood serum cholesterol has been greatly influenced by results of the Coronary Primary Prevention Trial or CPPT Lipid Research Clinics Program, 1984, in which men were randomly assigned to take a placebo or cholestyramine. Cholestyramine can significantly lower serum cholesterol and, in this trial, reduced it by an average of 8.5%. Men in the treatment group experienced 24% fewer heart attack deaths and 19% fewer heart attacks than did men who took the placebo.

The CPPT showed a 24% reduction in cardiovascular mortality in the treated group. However, the absolute proportions of patients who died of cardiovascular disease were similar in the 2 groups: there were 38 deaths among 1900 participants (2%) in the placebo group and 30 deaths among 1906 participants (1.6%) in the cholestyramine group. In other words, taking the medication for 6 years reduced the chance of dying from cardiovascular disease from 2% to 1.6%.

Because of the difficulties in communicating risk ratio information, the use of simple statistics, such as the number needed to treat (NNT), has been suggested (Sackett et al., 1997). NNT is the number of people that must be treated to avoid one bad outcome. Statistically, NNT is defined as the reciprocal of the absolute-risk reduction. In the cholesterol example, if 2% (0.020) of the patients died in the control arm of an experiment and 1.6% (0.016) died in the experimental arm, the absolute risk reduction is 0.020 − 0.016 = 0.004. The reciprocal of 0.004 is 250. In this case, 250 people would have to be treated for 6 years to avoid 1 death from coronary heart disease. Treatments can harm as well as benefit, so in addition to calculating the NNT, it is valuable to calculate the number needed to harm (NNH). This is the number of people a clinician would need to treat to produce one adverse event. NNT and NNH can be modified for those in particular risk groups. The advantage of these simple numbers is that they allow much clearer communication of the magnitude of treatment effectiveness.

Shared Decision Making

Once patients understand the complex information about outcomes, they can fully participate in the decision-making process. The final step in disseminating information to patients involves an interactive process that allows patients to make informed choices about their own health-care.

Despite a growing consensus that they should be involved, evidence suggests that patients are rarely consulted. Wennberg (1995) outlined a variety of common medical decisions in which there is uncertainty. In each, treatment selection involves profiles of risks and benefits for patients. Thiazide medications can be effective at controlling blood pressure, they also can be associated with increased serum cholesterol; the benefit of blood pressure reduction must be balanced against such side effects as dizziness and impotence.

Factors that affect patient decision making and use of health services are not well understood. It is usually assumed that use of medical services is driven primarily by need, that those who are sickest or most disabled use services the most (Aday, 1998). Although illness is clearly the major reason for service use, the literature on small-area variation demonstrates that there can be substantial variability in service use among communities that have comparable illness burdens and comparable insurance coverage (Wennberg, 1998). Therefore, social, cultural, and system variables also contribute to service use.

The role of patients in medical decision making has undergone substantial recent change. In the early 1950s, Parsons (1951) suggested that patients were excluded from medical decision making unless they assumed the "sick role," in which patients submit to a physician's judgment, and it is assumed that physicians understand the patients' preferences. Through a variety of changes, patients have become more active. More information is now available, and many patients demand a greater role (Sharf, 1997). The Internet offers vast amounts of information to patients; some of it misleading or inaccurate (Impicciatore et al., 1997). One difficulty is that many patients are not sophisticated consumers of technical medical information (Strum, 1997).

Another important issue is whether patients want a role. The literature is contradictory on this point; at least eight studies have addressed the issue. Several suggest that most patients express little interest in participating (Cassileth et al., 1980; Ende et al., 1989; Mazur and Hickam, 1997; Pendleton and House, 1984; Strull et al., 1984; Waterworth and Luker, 1990). Those studies challenge the basis of shared medical decision making. Is it realistic to engage patients in the process if they are not interested? Deber (Deber, 1994; Deber et al., 1996) has drawn an important distinction between problem solving and decision making. Medical problem solving requires technical skill to make an appropriate diagnosis and select treatment. Most patients prefer to leave those judgments in the hands of experts (Ende et al., 1989). Studies challenging the notion that patients want to make decisions typically asked questions about problem solving (Ende et al., 1989; Pendleton and House, 1984; Strull et al., 1984).

Shared decision making requires patients to express personal preferences for desired outcomes, and many decisions involve very personal choices. Wennberg (1998) offers examples of variation in health care practices that are dominated by physician choice. One is the choice between mastectomy and lumpectomy for women with well-defined breast cancer. Systematic clinical trials have shown that the probability of surviving breast cancer is about equal after mastectomy and after lumpectomy followed by radiation (Lichter et al., 1992). But in some areas of the United States, nearly half of women with breast cancer have mastectomies (for example, Provo, Utah); in other areas less than 2% do (for example, New Jersey; Wennberg, 1998). Such differences are determined largely by surgeon choice; patient preference is not considered. In the breast cancer example, interviews suggest that some women have a high preference for maintaining the breast, and others feel more comfortable having more breast tissue removed. The choices are highly personal and reflect variations in comfort with the idea of life with and without a breast. Patients might not want to engage in technical medical problem solving, but they are the only source of information about preferences for potential outcomes.

The process by which patients exercise choice can be difficult. There have been several evaluations of efforts to involve patients in decision making. Greenfield and colleagues (1985) taught patients how to read their own medical records and offered coaching on what questions to ask during encounters with physicians. In this randomized trial involving patients with peptic ulcer disease, those assigned to a 20-minute treatment had fewer functional limitations and were more satisfied with their care than were patients in the control group. A similar experiment involving patients treated for diabetes showed that patients randomly assigned to receive visit preparation scored significantly better than controls on three dimensions of health-related quality of life (mobility, role performance, physical activity). Furthermore, there were significant improvements for biochemical measures of diabetes control (Greenfield et al., 1988).

Many medical decisions are more complex than those studied by Greenfield and colleagues. There are usually several treatment alternatives, and the outcomes for each choice are uncertain. Also, the importance of the outcomes might be valued differently by different people. Shared decision-making programs have been proposed to address those concerns (Kasper et al., 1992). The programs usually use electronic media. Some involve interactive technologies in which a patient becomes familiar with the probabilities of various outcomes. With some technologies, the patient also has the opportunity to witness others who have embarked on different treatments. Video allows a patient to witness the outcomes of others who have made each treatment choice. A variety of interactive programs have been systematically evaluated. In one study (Barry et al., 1995), patients with benign prostatic hyperplasia were given the opportunity to use an interactive video. The video was generally well received, and the authors reported that there was a significant reduction in the rate of surgery and an increase in the proportion who chose "watchful waiting" after using the decision aid. Flood et al. (1996) reported similar results with an interactive program.

Not all evaluations of decision aids have been positive. In one evaluation of an impartial video for patients with ischemic heart disease, (Liao et al., 1996) 44% of the patients found it helpful for making treatment choices but more than 40% reported that it increased their anxiety (Liao et al., 1996). Most of the patients had received advice from their physicians before watching the video.

Despite enthusiasm for shared medical decision making, little systematic research has evaluated interventions to promote it (Frosch and Kaplan, 1999). Systematic experimental trials are needed to determine whether the use of shared decision aids enhances patient outcomes. Although decision aids appear to enhance patient satisfaction, it is unclear whether they result in reductions in surgery, as suggested by Wennberg (1998), or in improved patient outcomes (Frosch and Kaplan, 1999).

Dissemination Through Organizations

The effect of any preventive intervention depends both on its ability to influence health behavior change or reduce health risks and on the extent to which the target population has access to and participates in the program. Few preventive interventions are free-standing in the community. Rather, organizations serve as "hosts" for health promotion and disease prevention programs. Once a program has proven successful in demonstration projects and efficacy trials, it must be adopted and implemented by new organizations. Unfortunately, diffusion to new organizations often proceeds very slowly (Murray, 1986; Parcel et al., 1990).

A staged change process has been proposed for optimal diffusion of preventive interventions to new organizations. Although different researchers have offered a variety of approaches, there is consensus on the importance of at least four stages (Goodman et al., 1997):

- dissemination, during which organizations are made aware of the programs and their benefits;
- adoption, during which the organization commits to initiating the program;
- implementation, during which the organization offers the program or services;
- maintenance or institutionalization, during which the organization makes the program part of its routines and standard offerings.

Research investigating the diffusion of health behavior change programs to new organizations can be seen, for example, in adoption of prevention curricula by schools and of preventive services by medical care practices.

Schools

Schools are important because they allow consistent contact with children over their developmental trajectory and they provide a place where acquisition of new information and skills is normative (Orlandi, 1996b). Although much emphasis has been placed on developing effective health behavior change curricula for students throughout their school years, the literature is replete with evaluations of school-based curricula that suggest that such programs have been less than successful (Bush et al., 1989; Parcel et al., 1990; Rohrbach et al., 1996; Walter, 1989). Challenges or barriers to effective diffusion of the programs include organizational issues, such as limited time and resources, few incentives for the organization to give priority to health issues, pressure to focus on academic curricula to improve student performance on proficiency tests, and unclear role delineation in terms of responsibility for the program; extra-organizational issues or "environmental turbulence," such as restructuring of schools, changing school schedules or enrollments, uncertainties in public funding; and characteristics of the programs that make them incompatible with the potential host organizations, such as being too long, costly, and complex (Rohrbach et al., 1996; Smith et al., 1995).

Initial or traditional efforts to enhance diffusion focused on the characteristics of the intervention program, but more recent studies have focused on the change process itself. Two NCI-funded studies to diffuse tobacco prevention programs throughout schools in North Carolina and Texas targeted the four stages of change and were evaluated through randomized, controlled trials (Goodman et al., 1997; Parcel et al., 1989, 1995; Smith et al., 1995; Steckler et al., 1992). Teacher-training interventions appeared to enhance the likelihood of implementation in each study (an effect that has been replicated in other investigations; see Perry et al., 1990). However, other strategies (e.g., process consultation, newsletters, self-paced instructional video) were less successful at enhancing adoption and institutionalization. None of the strategies attempted to change the organizing arrangements (such as reward systems or role responsibilities) of the school districts to support continued implementation of the program.

These results suggest that further reliance on organizational change theory might greatly enhance the diffusion of programs more rapidly and thoroughly. For example, Rohrbach et al. (1996, pp. 927–928) suggest that "change agents and school personnel should work as a team to diagnose any problems that may impede program implementation and develop action plans to address them [and that] . . . change agents need to promote the involvement of teachers, as well as that of key administrators, in decisions about program adoption and implementation." These suggestions are clearly consistent with an organizational development approach. Goodman and colleagues (1997) suggest that the North Carolina intervention might have been more effective had it included more participative problem diagnosis and action planning, and had consultation been less directive and more oriented toward increasing the fit between the host organization and the program.

Medical Practices

Primary care medical practices have long been regarded as organizational settings that provide opportunities for health behavior interventions. With the growth of managed care and its financial incentives for prevention, these opportunities are even greater (Gordon et al., 1996). Much effort has been invested in the development of effective programs and processes for clinical practices to accomplish health behavior change. However, the diffusion of such programs to medical practices has been slow (e.g., Anderson and May, 1995; Lewis, 1988).

Most systemic programs encourage physicians, nurses, health educators, and other members of the health-professional team to provide more consistent change-related statements and behavioral support for health-enhancing behaviors in patients (Chapter 5). There might be fundamental aspects of a medical practice that support or inhibit efforts to improve health-related patient behavior (Walsh and McPhee, 1992). Visual reminders to stay up-to-date on immunizations, to stop smoking cigarettes, to use bicycle helmets, and to eat a healthy diet are examples of systemic support for patient activation and self-care (Lando et al., 1995). Internet support for improved self-management of diabetes has shown promise (McKay et al., 1998). Automated chart reminders to ask about smoking status, update immunizations, and ensure timely cancer-screening examinations—such as Pap smears, mammography, and prostate screening—are systematic practice-based improvements that increase the rate of success in reaching stated goals on health process and health behavior measures (Cummings et al., 1997). Prescription forms for specific telephone call-back support can enhance access to telephone-based counseling for weight loss, smoking cessation, and exercise and can make such behavioral teaching and counseling more accessible (Pronk and O'Connor, 1997). Those and other structural characteristics of clinical practices are being used and evaluated as systematic practice-based changes that can improve treatment for, and prevention of, various chronic illnesses (O'Connor et al., 1998).

Barriers to diffusion include physician factors, such as lack of training, lack of time, and lack of confidence in one's prevention skills; health-care system factors, such as lack of health-care coverage and inadequate reimbursement for preventive services in fee-for-service systems; and office organization factors, such as inflexible office routines, lack of reminder systems, and unclear assignment of role responsibilities (Thompson et al., 1995; Wagner et al., 1996).

The capitated financing of many managed-care organizations greatly reduces system barriers. Interventions that have focused solely on physician knowledge and behavior have not been very effective. Interventions that also addressed office organization factors have been more effective (Solberg et al., 1998b; Thompson et al., 1995). For example, the diffusion of the Put Prevention Into Practice (PPIP) program (Griffith et al., 1995), a comprehensive federal effort, was recommended by the U.S. Preventive Services Task Force and is distributed by federal agencies and through professional associations. Using a case study approach, McVea and colleagues (1996) studied the implementation of the program in family practice settings. They found that PPIP was "used not at all or only sporadically by the practices that had ordered the kit" (p. 363). The authors suggested that the practices that provided selected preventive services did not adopt the PPIP because they did not have the organizational skills and resources to incorporate the prevention systems into their office routines without external assistance.

Summary

Descriptive research clearly indicates a need for well-conceived and methodologically-rigorous diffusion research. Many of the barriers to more rapid and effective diffusion are clearly "systems problems" (Solberg et al., 1998b). Thus, even though the results are somewhat mixed, recent work applying systems approaches and organizational development strategies to the diffusion dilemma is encouraging. In particular, the emphasis on building internal capacity for diffusion of the preventive interventions—for example, continuous quality improvement teams (Solberg et al., 1998a) and the identification and training of "program champions" within the adopting systems (Smith et al., 1995)—seems crucial for institutionalization of the programs.

Dissemination to Community-Based Groups

This section examines three aspects of dissemination: the need for dissemination of effective community interventions, community readiness for interventions, and the role of dissemination research.

Dissemination of Effective Community Interventions

Dissemination requires the identification of core and adaptive elements of an intervention (Pentz et al., 1990; Pentz and Trebow, 1997;

Price, 1989). Core elements are features of an intervention program or policy that *must* be replicated to maintain the integrity of the interventions as they are transferred to new settings. They include theoretically based behavior change strategies, targeting of multiple levels of influence, and the involvement of empowered community leaders (Florin and Wandersman, 1990; Pentz, 1998). Practitioners need training in specific strategies for the transfer of core elements (Bero et al., 1998; Orlandi, 1986). In addition, the amount of intervention delivered and its reach into the targeted population might have to be unaltered to replicate behavior change in a new setting. Research has not established a quantitative "dose" of intervention or a quantitative guide for the percentage of core elements that must be implemented to achieve behavior change. Process evaluation can provide guidance regarding the desired intensity and fidelity to intervention protocol. Botvin and colleagues (1995), for example, found that at least half the prevention program sessions needed to be delivered to achieve the targeted effects in a youth drug abuse prevention program. They also found that increased prevention effects were associated with fidelity to the intervention protocol, which included standardized training of those implementing the program, implementation within 2 weeks of that training, and delivery of at least two program sessions or activities per week (Botvin et al., 1995).

Adaptive elements are features of an intervention that can be tailored to local community, organizational, social, and economic realities of a new setting without diluting the effectiveness of the intervention (Price, 1989). Adaptations might include timing and scheduling or culturally meaningful themes through which the educational and behavior change strategies are delivered.

Community and Organizational Readiness

Community and organizational factors might facilitate or hinder the adoption, implementation, and maintenance of innovative interventions. Diffusion theory assumes that the unique characteristics of the adopter (such as community, school, or worksite) interact with the specific attributes of the innovation (risk factor targets) to determine whether and when an innovation is adopted and implemented (Emmons et al., 2000; Rogers, 1983, 1995). Rogers (1983, 1995) has identified characteristics that predict the adoption of innovations in communities and organizations. For example, an innovation that has a *relative advantage* over the idea or activity that it supersedes is more likely to be adopted. In the case of health promotion, organizations might see smoke-free worksites as having a relative advantage not only for employee health, but also for the reduction of absenteeism. An innovation that is seen as *compatible* with adopters' sociocultural values and beliefs, with previously introduced ideas, or with adopters' perceived needs for innovation is more likely to be implemented. The less *complex* and clearer the innovation, the more likely it is to be adopted. For example, potential adopters are more likely to change their health behaviors when educators provide clear specification of the skills needed to change the behaviors. *Trialability* is the degree to which an innovation can be experimented with on a limited basis. In nutrition education, adopters are more likely to prepare low-fat recipes at home if they have an opportunity to taste the results in a class or supermarket and are given clear, simple directions for preparing them. Finally, *observability* is the degree to which the results of an innovation are visible to others. In health behavior change, an example of observability might be attention given to a health promotion program by the popular press (Pentz, 1998; Rogers, 1983).

Dissemination Research

The ability to identify effective interventions and explain the characteristics of communities and organizations that support dissemination of those interventions provides the basic building blocks for dissemination. It is necessary, however, to learn more about how dissemination occurs to increase its effectiveness (Pentz, 1998). What are the core elements of interventions, and how can they be adapted (Price, 1989)? How do the predictors of diffusion function in the dissemination process (Pentz, 1998)? What characteristics of community leaders are associated with dissemination of prevention programs? What personnel and material resources are needed to implement and maintain prevention programs? How can written materials and training in program implementation be provided to preserve fidelity to core elements (Price, 1989)?

Dissemination research could help identify alternatives to conceptualizing transfer of intervention technology from research to the practice setting. Rather than disseminating an exact replication of specific tested interventions, program transfer might be based on core and adaptive intervention components at both the individual and community organizational levels (Blaine et al., 1997; Perry 1999). Dissemination might also be viewed as replicating a community-based participatory research process, or as a planning process that incorporates core components (Perry 1999), rather than exact duplication of all aspects of intervention activities.

The principles of community-based participatory research presented here could be operationalized and used as criteria for examining the extent to which these dimensions were disseminated to other projects. The guidelines developed by Green and colleagues (1995) for classifying participatory research projects also could be used. Similarly, based on her research and experience with children and adolescents in school health behavior change programs, Perry (1999) developed a guidebook that outlines a 10-step process for developing communitywide health behavior programs for children and adolescents.

Facilitating Interorganizational Linkages

To address complex health issues effectively, organizations increasingly form links with one another to form either dyadic connections (pairs) or networks (Alter and Hage, 1992). The potential benefits of these interorganizational collaborations include access to new information, ideas, materials, and skills; minimization of duplication of effort and services; shared responsibility for complex or controversial programs; increased power and influence through joint action; and increased options for intervention (e.g., one organization might not experience the political constraints that hamper the activities of another; Butterfoss et al., 1993). However, interorganizational linkages have costs. Time and resources must be devoted to the formation and maintenance of relationships. Negotiating the assessment and planning processes can take a longer time. And sometimes an organization can find that the policies and procedures of other organizations are incompatible with its own (Alter and Hage, 1992; Butterfoss et al., 1993).

One way a dyadic linkage between organizations can serve health-promoting goals grows out of the diffusion of innovations through organizations. An organization can serve as a "linking agent" (Monahan and Scheirer, 1988), facilitating the adoption of a health innovation by organizations that are potential implementors. For example, the National Institute for Dental Research (NIDR) developed a school-based program to encourage children to use a fluoride mouth rinse to prevent caries. Rather than marketing the program directly to the schools, NIDR worked with state agencies to promote the program. In a national study, Monahan and Scheirer (1988) found that when state agencies devoted more staff to the program and located a moderate proportion of their staff in regional offices (rather than in a central office) there was likely to be a larger proportion of school districts implementing the program. Other programs, such as the Heart Partners program of the American Heart Association (Roberts-Gray et al., 1998), have used the concept of linking agents to diffuse preventive interventions. Studies of these approaches attempt to identify the organizational policies, procedures, and priorities that permit the linking agent to successfully reach a large proportion of the organizations that might implement the health behavior program. However, the research in this area does not allow general conclusions or guidelines to be drawn.

Interorganizational networks are commonly used in community-wide health initiatives. Such networks might be composed of similar organizations that coordinate service delivery (often called consortia) or organizations from different sectors that bring their respective resources and expertise to bear on a complex health problem (often called coalitions). Multihospital systems or linkages among managed-care organizations and local health departments for treating sexually transmitted diseases (Rutherford, 1998) are examples of consortia. The interorganizational networks used in Project ASSIST and COMMIT, major NCI initiatives to reduce the prevalence of smoking, are examples of coalitions (U.S. Department of Health and Human Services, 1990).

Stage theory has been applied to the formation and performance of interorganizational networks (Alter and Hage, 1992; Goodman and Wandersman, 1994). Various authors have posited somewhat different stages of development, but they all include: initial actions, to form the coalition; the formalization of the mission, structure, and processes of the coalition; planning, development, and implementation of programmatic activities; and accomplishment of the coalition's health goals. Stage theory suggests that different strategies are likely to facilitate success at different stages of development (Lewin, 1951; Schein, 1987). The complexity, formalization, staffing patterns, communication and decision-making patterns, and leadership styles of the interorganizational network will affect its ability to progress toward its goals (Alter and Hage, 1992; Butterfoss et al., 1993; Kegler et al., 1998a,b).

In 1993, Butterfoss and colleagues reviewed the literature on community coalitions and found "relatively little empirical evidence" (p. 315) to bring to bear on the assessment of their effectiveness. Although the use of coalitions in community-wide health promotion continues, the accumulation of evidence supporting their effectiveness is still slim. Several case studies suggest that coalitions and consortia can be successful in bringing about changes in health behaviors, health systems, and health status (e.g., Butterfoss et al., 1998; Fawcett et al., 1997; Kass and Freudenberg, 1997; Myers et al., 1994; Plough and Olafson, 1994). However, the conditions under which coalitions are most likely to thrive and the strategies and processes that are most likely to result in effective functioning of a coalition have not been consistently identified empirically.

Evaluation models, such as the FORECAST model (Goodman and Wandersman, 1994) and the model proposed by the Work Group on Health Promotion and Community Development at the University of Kansas (Fawcett et al., 1997), address the lack of systematic and rigorous evaluation of coalitions. These models provide strategies and tools for assessing coalition functioning at all stages of development, from initial formation to ultimate influence on the coalition's health goals and objectives. They are predicated on the assumption that the successful passage through each stage is necessary, but not sufficient, to ensure successful passage through the next stage. Widespread use of these and other evaluation frameworks and tools can increase the number and quality of the empirical studies of the effects of interorganizational linkages.

Orlandi (1996a) states that diffusion failures often result from a lack of fit between the proposed host organization and the intervention program. Thus, he suggests that if the purpose is to diffuse an existing program, the design of the program and the process of diffusion need to be flexible enough to adapt to the needs and resources of the organization. If the purpose is to develop and disseminate a new program, innovation development and transfer process should be integrated. Those conclusions are consistent with some of the studies reviewed above. For example, McVea et al. (1996) concluded that a "one size fits all" approach to clinical preventive systems was not likely to diffuse effectively.

REFERENCES

Aday, L.A. (1998). Evaluating the Healthcare System: Effectiveness, Efficiency, and Equity. Chicago: Health Administration Press.

Alter, C. and Hage, J. (1992). *Organizations Working Together*. Newbury Park, CA: Sage.

Altman, D.G. (1995). Sustaining interventions in community systems: On the relationship between researchers and communities. *Health Psychology*, 14, 526–536.

Anderson, L.M. and May, D.S. (1995). Has the use of cervical, breast, and colorectal cancer screening increased in the United States? *American Journal of Public Health*, 85, 840–842.

Anderson, N.B. (1998). *After the discoveries, then what? A new approach to advancing evidence-based prevention practice* (pp. 74–75). Programs and abstracts from NIH Conference, Preventive Intervention Research at the Crossroads, Bethesda, MD.

Anderson, N.H., and Zalinski, J. (1990). Functional measurement approach to self-estimation in multiattribute evaluation. In N.H. Anderson (Ed.), *Contributions to Information Integration Theory, Vol. 1: Cognition; Vol. 2: Social; Vol. 3: Developmental.* (pp. 145–185): Hillsdale, NJ: Erlbaum Press.

Antonovsky, A. (1985). The life cycle, mental health and the sense of coherence. *Israel Journal of Psychiatry and Related Sciences, 22 (4)*, 273–280.

Baker, E.A. and Brownson, C.A. (1999). Defining characteristics of community-based health promotion programs. In R.C. Brownson, E.A. Baker, and L.F. Novick (Eds.) *Community-Based Prevention Programs that Work* (pp. 7–19). Gaithersburg, MD: Aspen.

Balestra, D.J. and Littenberg, B. (1993). Should adult tetanus immunization be given as a single vaccination at age 65? A cost-effectiveness analysis. *Journal of General Internal Medicine*, 8, 405–412.

Barry, M.J., Fowler, F.J., Mulley, A.G., Henderson, J.V., and Wennberg, J.E. (1995). Patient reactions to a program designed to facilitate patient participation in treatment decisions for benign prostatic hyperplasia. *Medical Care, 33*, 771–782.

Beery, B. and Nelson, G. (1998). Evaluating community-based health initiatives: Dilemmas, puzzles, innovations and promising directions. Making outcomes matter. Seattle: Group Health/Kaiser Permanente Community Foundation.

Bennett, K.J. and Torrance, G.W. (1996). Measuring health preferences and utilities: Rating scale, time trade-off and standard gamble methods. In B. Spliker (Ed.) *Quality of Life and Pharmacoeconomics in Clinical Trials* (pp. 235–265). Philadelphia: Lippincott-Raven.:

Berger, E.S. and Hendee, W.R. (1989). The expression of health risk information. *Archives of Internal Medicine, 149*, 1507–1508.

Berger, P.L. and Neuhaus, R.J. (1977). To empower people: The role of mediating structures in public policy. Washington, DC: American Enterprise Institute for Public Policy Research.

Bero, L.A., Grilli, R., Grimshaw, J.M., Harvey, E., Oxman, A.D., and Thomson, M.A. (1998). Closing the gap between research and practice: An overview of systematic reviews of interventions to promote the implementation of research findings. *British Medical Journal, 317*, 465–468.

Bickman, L. (1987). The functions of program theory. *New Directions in Program Evaluation, 33*, 5–18.

Bigger, J.T.J. (1984). Antiarrhythmic treatment: An overview. *American Journal of Cardiology, 53*, 8B–16B.

Bishop, R. (1994). Initiating empowering research? *New Zealand Journal of Educational Studies, 29*, 175–188.

Bishop, R. (1996). Addressing issues of self-determination and legitimation in Kaupapa Maori research. In B. Webber (Ed.) *Research Perspectives in Maori Education* (pp. 143–160). Wellington, New Zealand: Council for Educational Research.

Black, W.C., Nease, R.F.J., and Tosteson, A.N. (1995). Perceptions of breast cancer risk and screening effectiveness in women younger than 50 years of age. *Journal of the National Cancer Institute, 87*, 720–731.

Blaine, T.M., Forster, J.L., Hennrikus, D., O'Neil, S., Wolfson, M., and Pham, H. (1997). Creating tobacco control policy at the local level: Implementation of a direct action organizing approach. *Health Education and Behavior, 24*, 640–651.

Botvin, G.J., Baker, E., Dusenbury, L., Botvin, E.M., and Diaz, T. (1995). Long-term follow-up results of a randomized drug abuse prevention trial in a white middle-class population. *Journal of the American Medical Association, 273*, 1106–1112.

Brown, E.R. (1991). Community action for health promotion: A strategy to empower individuals and communities. *International Journal of Health Services, 21*, 441–456.

Brown, P. (1995). The role of the evaluator in comprehensive community initiatives. In J.P. Connell, A.C. Kubisch, L.B. Schorr, and C.H. Weiss (Eds.) *New Approaches to Evaluating Community Initiatives* (pp. 201–225). Washington, DC: Aspen.

Bush, P.J, Zuckerman, A.E, Taggart, V.S, Theiss, P.K, Peleg, E.O, and Smith, S.A (1989). Cardiovascular risk factor prevention in black school children: The Know Your Body: Evaluation Project. *Health Education Quarterly, 16*, 215–228.

Butterfoss, F.D, Morrow, A.L., Rosenthal, J., Dini, E., Crews, R.C., Webster, J.D., and Louis, P. (1998). CINCH: An urban coalition for empowerment and action. *Health Education and Behavior, 25*, 212–225.

Butterfoss, F.D, Goodman, R.M., and Wandersman, A. (1993). Community coalitions for prevention and health promotion. *Health Education Research, 8*, 315–330.

Campbell, D.T. and Stanley, J.C. (1963). *Experimental and Quasi-Experimental Designs for Research*. Chicago: Rand McNally.

Cardiac Arrhythmia Suppression Trial (CAST) Investigators. (1989). Preliminary report: Effect of encainide and flecainide on mortality in a randomized trial of arrhythmia suppression after myocardial infarction. The Cardiac Arrhythmia Suppression Trial (CAST) Investigators. *New England Journal of Medicine, 321*, 406–412.

Cassileth, B.R., Zupkis, R.V., Sutton-Smith, K., and March, V. (1980). Information and participation preferences among cancer patients. *Annals of Internal Medicine, 92*, 832–836.

Centers for Disease Control, Agency for Toxic Substances and Disease Registry (CDC/ATSDR). (1997). *Principles of Community Engagement*. Atlanta: CDC Public Health Practice Program Office.

Chambless, D.L. and Hollon, S.D. (1998). Defining empirically supported therapies. *Journal of Consulting and Clinical Psychology, 66*, 7–18.

Clemen, R.T. (1991). *Making Hard Decisions*. Boston: PWS-Kent.

Compas, B.E., Haaga, D.F., Keefe, F.J., Leitenberg, H., and Williams, D.A. (1998). Sampling of empirically supported psychological treatments from health psychology: Smoking, chronic pain, cancer, and bulimia nervosa. *Journal of Consulting and Clinical Psychology, 66*, 89–112.

Cook, T.D. and Reichardt, C.S. (1979). *Qualitative and Quantitative Methods in Evaluation Research*. Beverly Hills, CA: Sage.

Cornwall, A. (1996). Towards participatory practice: Participatory rural appraisal (PRA) and the participatory process. In K. deKoning, and M. Martin (Eds.) *Participatory Research in Health: Issues and Experiences* (pp. 94–107). London: Zed Books.

Cornwall, A. and Jewkes, R. (1995). What is participatory research? *Social Science and Medicine, 41*, 1667–1676.

Cousins, J.B. and Earl, L.M. (Eds.) (1995). *Participatory Evaluation: Studies in Evaluation Use and Organizational Learning.* London: Falmer.

Cromwell, J., Bartosch, W.J., Fiore, M.C., Hasselblad, V., and Baker, T. (1997). Cost-effectiveness of the clinical practice recommendations in the AHCPR guideline for smoking cessation. *Journal of the American Medical Association, 278*, 1759–1766.

Cummings, N.A., Cummings, J.L., and Johnson, J.N. (Eds.). (1997). *Behavioral Health in Primary Care: A Guide for Clinical Integration.* Madison, CT: Psychosocial Press.

Danese, M.D., Powe, N.R., Sawin, C.T., and Ladenson, P.W. (1996). Screening for mild thyroid failure at the periodic health examination: A decision and cost-effectiveness analysis. *Journal of the American Medical Association, 276*, 285–292.

Dannenberg, A.L., Gielen, A.C., Beilenson, P.L., Wilson, M.H., and Joffe, A. (1993). Bicycle helmet laws and educational campaigns: An evaluation of strategies to increase children's helmet use. *American Journal of Public Health, 83*, 667–674.

Deber, R.B. (1994). Physicians in health care management. 7. The patient–physician partnership: Changing roles and the desire for information. *Canadian Medical Association Journal, 151*, 171–176.

Deber, R.B., Kraetschmer, N., and Irvine, J. (1996). What role do patients wish to play in treatment decision making? *Archives of Internal Medicine, 156*, 1414–1420.

DeJong, W. and Hingson, R. (1998). Strategies to reduce driving under the influence of alcohol. *Annual Review of Public Health, 19*, 359–378.

deKoning, K. and Martin, M. (1996). Participatory research in health: Setting the context. In K. deKoning and M. Martin (Eds.) *Participatory Research in Health: Issues and Experiences* (pp. 1–18). London: Zed Books.

Denzin, N.K. (1970). The research act. In N.K. Denzin (Ed.) *The Research Act in Sociology: A Theoretical Introduction to Sociological Methods* (pp. 345–360). Chicago, IL: Aldine.

Denzin, N.K. (1994). The suicide machine. In R.E. Long (Ed.) *Suicide. (Vol. 67, No. 2).* New York: H.W. Wilson.

Dignan, M.B. (Ed.) (1989). *Measurement and evaluation of health education, 2nd edition.* Springfield, IL: C.C. Thomas.

Dockery, G. (1996). Rhetoric or reality? Participatory research in the National Health Service, UK. In K. deKoning and M. Martin (Eds.) *Participatory Research in Health: Issues and Experiences* (pp. 164–176). London: Zed Books.

Donaldson, S.I., Graham, J.W., and Hansen, W.B. (1994). Testing the generalizability of intervening mechanism theories: Understanding the effects of adloescent drug use prevention interventions. *Journal of Behavioral Medicine, 17*, 195–216.

Dressler, W.W. (1993). Commentary on "Community Research: Partnership in Black Communities." *American Journal of Preventive Medicine, 9*, 32–34.

Durie, M.H. (1996). Characteristics of Maori health research. Presented at Hui Whakapiripiri: A Hui to Discuss Strategic Directions for Maori Health Research, Eru Pomare Maori Health Research Centre, Wellington School of Medicine, University of Otago, Wellington, New Zealand.

Eddy, D.M. (1990). Screening for cervical cancer. *Annals of Internal Medicine, 113*, 214–226. Reprinted in Eddy, D.M. (1991). *Common Screening Tests.* Philadelphia: American College of Physicians.

Edelson, J.T., Weinstein, M.C., Tosteson, A.N.A., Williams, L., Lee, T.H., and Goldman, L. (1990). Long-term cost-effectiveness of various initial monotherapies for mild to moderate hypertension. *Journal of the American Medical Association*, 263, 407–413.

Edworthy, J. and Adams, A.S. (1997). *Warning Design*. London: Taylor and Francis.

Elden, M. and Levin, M. (1991). Cogenerative learning. In W.F. Whyte (Ed.) *Participatory Action Research* (pp. 127–142). Newbury Park, CA: Sage.

Emmons, K.M., Thompson, B., Sorensen, G., Linnan, L., Basen-Engquist, K., Biener, L., and Watson, M. (2000). The relationship between organizational characteristics and the adoption of workplace smoking policies. *Health Education and Behavior*, 27, 483–501.

Ende, J., Kazis, L., Ash, A., and Moskowitz, M.A. (1989). Measuring patients' desire for autonomy: Decision making and information-seeking preferences among medical patients. *Journal of General Internal Medicine*, 4, 23–30.

Eng, E. and Blanchard, L. (1990-1). Action-oriented community diagnosis: A health education tool. *International Quarterly of Community Health Education*, 11, 93–110.

Eng, E. and Parker, E.A. (1994). Measuring community competence in the Mississippi Delta: the interface between program evaluation and empowerment. *Health Education Quarterly*, 21, 199–220.

Erdmann, T.C., Feldman, K.W., Rivara, F.P., Heimbach, D.M., and Wall, H.A. (1991). Tap water burn prevention: The effect of legislation. *Pediatrics*, 88, 572–577.

Ericsson, A. and Simon, H.A. (1994). *Verbal Protocol As Data*. Cambridge, MA: MIT Press.

Fawcett, S.B, Lewis, R.K, Paine-Andrews, A., Francisco, V.T, Richter, K.P., Williams, E.L., and Copple, B. (1997). Evaluating community coalitions for prevention of substance abuse: The case of Project Freedom. *Health Education and Behavior*, 24, 812–828.

Fawcett, S.B. (1991). Some values guiding community research and action. *Journal of Applied Behavior Analysis*, 24, 621–636.

Fawcett, S.B., Paine-Andrews, A., Francisco, V.T., Schultz, J.A., Richter, K.P., Lewis, R.K., Harris, K.J., Williams, E.L., Berkley, J.Y., Lopez, C.M., and Fisher, J.L. (1996). Empowering community health initiatives through evaluation. In D. Fetterman, S. Kaftarian, and A. Wandersman (Eds.) *Empowerment Evaluation: Knowledge And Tools Of Self-Assessment And Accountability* (pp. 161–187). Thousand Oaks, CA: Sage.

Feinstein, A.R. and Horwitz, R.I. (1997). Problems in the "evidence" of "evidence-based medicine." *American Journal of Medicine*, 103, 529–535.

Fischhoff, B. (1999a). *Risk Perception And Risk Communication*. Presented at the Workshop on Health, Communications and Behavior of the IOM Committee on Health and Behavior: Research, Practice and Policy, Irvine, CA.

Fischhoff, B. (1999b). Why (cancer) risk communication can be hard. *Journal of the National Cancer Institute Monographs*, 25, 7–13.

Fischhoff, B. and Bruine de Bruin, W. (1999). Fifty/fifty = 50? *Journal of Behavioral Decision Making*, 12, 149–163.

Fischhoff, B. and Downs, J. (1997). Accentuate the relevant. *Psychological Science*, 18, 154–158.

Fisher, E.B., Jr. (1995). The results of the COMMIT trial. *American Journal of Public Health*, 85, 159–160.

Flay, B. (1986). Efficacy and effectiveness trials (and other phases of research) in the development of health promotion programs. *Preventive Medicine*, 15, 451–474.

Flood, A.B., Wennberg, J.E., Nease, R.F.J., Fowler, F.J.J., Ding, J., and Hynes, L.M. (1996). The importance of patient preference in the decision to screen for prostate cancer. Prostate Patient Outcomes Research Team [see comments]. *Journal of General Internal Medicine*, *11*, 342–349.

Florin, P. and Wandersman, A. (1990). An introduction to citizen participation, voluntary organizations, and community development: Insights for empowerment through research. *American Journal of Community Psychology*, *18*, 41–53.

Francisco, V.T., Paine, A.L., and Fawcett, S.B. (1993). A methodology for monitoring and evaluating community health coalitions. *Health Education Research*, *8*, 403–416.

Freire, P. (1987). *Education for Critical Consciousness*. New York: Continuum.

Frick, M.H., Elo, O. Haapa, K., Heinonen, O.P., Heinsalmi, P., Helo, P., Huttunen, J.K., Kaitaniemi, P., Koskinen, P., Manninen, V., Maenpaa, H., Malkonen, M., Manttari, M., Norola, S., Pasternack, A., Pikkarainen, J., Romo, M., Sjoblom, T., and Nikkila, E.A. (1987). Helsinki Heart Study: Primary-prevention trial with gemfibrozil in middle-aged men with dyslipidemia. Safety of treatment, changes in risk factors, and incidence of coronary heart disease. *New England Journal of Medicine*, *317*, 1237–1245.

Friedman, L.M., Furberg, C.M., and De Mets, D.L. (1985). *Fundamentals of Clinical Trials*, *2nd edition*. St. Louis: Mosby-Year Book.

Frosch, M. and Kaplan, R.M. (1999). Shared decision-making in clinical practice: Past research and future directions. *American Journal of Preventive Medicine*, *17*, 285–294.

Gaventa, J. (1993). The powerful, the powerless, and the experts: Knowledge struggles in an information age. In P. Park, M. Brydon-Miller, B. Hall, and T. Jackson (Eds.) *Voices of Change: Participatory Research In The United States and Canada* (pp. 21–40). Westport, CT: Bergin and Garvey.

Gentner, D. and Stevens, A. (1983). *Mental Models (Cognitive Science)*. Hillsdale, NJ: Erlbaum.

Gold, M.R., Siegel, J.E., Russell, L.B., and Weinstein, M.C. (Eds.) (1996). *Cost-Effectiveness in Health And Medicine*. New York: Oxford University Press.

Goldman, L., Weinstein, M.C., Goldman, P.A., and Williams, L.W. (1991). Cost-effectiveness of HMG-CoA reductase inhibition. *Journal of the American Medical Association*, *6*, 1145–1151.

Golomb, B.A. (1998). Cholesterol and violence: is there a connection? *Annals of Internal Medicine*, *128*, 478–487.

Goodman, R.M. (1999). Principles and tools for evaluating community-based prevention and health promotion programs. In R.C. Brownson, E.A. Baker, and L.F. Novick (Eds.) *Community-Based Prevention Programs That Work* (pp. 211–227). Gaithersburg, MD: Aspen.

Goodman, R.M. and Wandersman, A. (1994). FORECAST: A formative approach to evaluating community coalitions and community-based initiatives. *Journal of Community Psychology*, *Supplement*, 6–25.

Goodman, R.M., Steckler, A., and Kegler, M.C. (1997). Mobilizing organizations for health enhancement: Theories of organizational change. K. Glanz, F.M. Lewis, and B.K. Rimer (Eds.) *Health Behavior and Health Education*, *2nd edition* (pp. 287–312). San Francisco: Jossey-Bass.

Gordon, R.L, Baker, E.L, Roper, W.L, and Omenn, G.S. (1996). Prevention and the reforming U.S. health care system: Changing roles and responsibilities for public health. *Annual Review of Public Health, 17*, 489–509.

Gottlieb, N.H. and McLeroy, K.R. (1994). Social health. In M.P. O'Donnell, and J.S. Harris (Eds.) *Health promotion in the workplace, 2nd edition* (pp. 459–493). Albany, NY: Delmar.

Green, L.W. (1977). Evaluation and measurement: Some dilemmas for health education. *American Journal of Public Health, 67*, 155–166.

Green, L.W. and Gordon, N.P. (1982). Productive research designs for health education investigations. *Health-Education, 13*, 4–10.

Green, L.W. and Lewis, F.M. (1986). *Measurement and Evaluation in Health Education and Health Promotion*. Palo Alto, CA: Mayfield.

Green, L.W., George, M.A., Daniel, M., Frankish, C.J., Herbert, C.J., Bowie, W.R., and O'Neil, M. (1995). *Study of Participatory Research in Health Promotion*. University of British Columbia, Vancouver: The Royal Society of Canada.

Green, L.W., Richard, L., and Potvin, L. (1996). Ecological foundations of health promotion. *American Journal of Health Promotion, 10*, 270–281.

Greenfield, S., Kaplan, S., and Ware, J.E. (1985). Expanding patient involvement in care. *Annals of Internal Medicine, 102*, 520–528.

Greenfield, S., Kaplan, S.H., Ware, J.E., Yano, E.M., and Frank, H.J.L. (1988). Patients participation in medical care: Effects on blood sugar control and quality of life in diabetes. *Journal of General Internal Medicine, 3*, 448–457.

Greenwald, P. (1984). Epidemiology: A step forward in the scientific approach to preventing cancer through chemoprevention. *Public Health Reports, 99*, 259–264.

Greenwald, P. and Cullen, J.W. (1984). A scientific approach to cancer control. *CA: A Cancer Journal for Clinicians, 34*, 328–332.

Griffith H.M., Dickey, L., and Kamerow, D.B. (1995) Put prevention into practice: a systematic approach. *Journal of Public Health Management and Practice, 1*, 9–15

Guba, E.G. and Lincoln, Y.S. (1989). *Fourth Generation Evaluation*. Newbury Park, CA: Sage.

Hadden, S.G. (1986). *Read The Label: Reducing Risk By Providing Information*. Boulder, CO: Westview.

Hall, B.L. (1992). From margins to center? The development and purpose of participatory research. *American Sociologist, 23*, 15–28.

Hancock, L., Sanson-Fisher, R.W., Redman, S., Burton, R., Burton, L, Butler, J., Girgis, A., Gibberd, R., Hensley, M., McClintock, A., Reid, A., Schofield, M., Tripodi, T., and Walsh, R. (1997). Community action for health promotion: A review of methods and outcomes 1990–1995. *American Journal of Preventive Medicine, 13*, 229–239.

Hancock, T. (1993). The healthy city from concept to application: Implications for research. In J.K. Davies and M.P. Kelly (Eds.) *Healthy Cities: Research and Practice* (pp. 14–24). New York: Routledge.

Hatch, J., Moss, N., Saran, A., Presley-Cantrell, L., and Mallory, C. (1993). Community research: partnership in Black communities. *American Journal of Preventive Medicine, 9*, 27–31.

He, J., Ogden, L.G., Vupputuri, S., Bazzano, L.A., Loria, C., and Whelton, P.K. (1999) Dietary sodium intake and subsequent risk of cardiovascular disease in overweight adults. *Journal of the American Medical Association, 282*, 2027-2034.

Health Care Financing Administration, Department of Health and Human Services. (1998). *Highlights: National Health Expenditures, 1997* [On-line]. Available: <http://www.hcfa.gov/stats/nhe-oact/hilites.htm>. Accessed October 31, 1998.

Heaney, C.A. and Goetzel, R.Z. (1997). A review of health-related outcomes of multi-component worksite health promotion programs. *American Journal of Health Promotion, 11*, 290–307.

Hingson, R. (1996). Prevention of drinking and driving. *Alcohol Health and Research World, 20*, 219–226.

Himmelman, A.T. (1992). *Communities Working Collaboratively for a Change.* University of Minnesota, MN: Humphrey Institute of Public Affairs.

Hollister, R.G. and Hill, J. (1995). Problems in the evaluation of community-wide initiatives. In J.P. Connell, A.C. Kubisch, L.B. Schorr, and C.H. Weiss (Eds.) *New Approaches to Evaluating Community Initiatives* (pp. 127–172). Washington, DC: Aspen.

Horwitz, R.I. and Daniels S.R. (1996). Bias or biology: Evaluating the epidemiologic studies of L-tryptophan and the eosinophilia-myalgia syndrome. *Journal of Rheumatology Supplement, 46*, 60–72.

Horwitz, R.I. (1987a). Complexity and contradiction in clinical trial research. *American Journal of Medicine, 82*, 498–510.

Horwitz, R.I. (1987b). The experimental paradigm and observational studies of cause-effect relationships in clinical medicine. *Journal of Chronic Disease, 40*, 91–99.

Horwitz, R.I., Singer, B.H., Makuch, R.W., and Viscoli, C.M. (1996). Can treatment that is helpful on average be harmful to some patients? A study of the conflicting information needs of clinical inquiry and drug regulation. *Journal of Clinical Epidemiology, 49*, 395–400.

Horwitz, R.I., Viscoli, C.M., Clemens, J.D., and Sadock, R.T. (1990). Developing improved observational methods for evaluating therapeutic effectiveness. *American Journal of Medicine, 89*, 630–638.

House, E.R. (1980). Evaluating with validity. Beverly Hills, CA: Sage.

Hugentobler, M.K, Israel, B.A., and Schurman, S.J. (1992). An action research approach to workplace health: Integrating methods. *Health Education Quarterly, 19*, 55–76.

Impicciatore, P., Pandolfini, C., Casella, N., and Bonati, M. (1997). Reliability of health information for the public on the world wide web: Systematic survey of advice on managing fever in children at home. *British Medical Journal, 314*, 1875–1881.

IOM (Institute of Medicine) (1999). *Reducing the Burden of Injury: Advancing Prevention and Treatment.* Washington, DC: National Academy

IOM (Institute of Medicine) (2001). *Speaking of Health: Assessing Health Communication. Strategies for Diverse Populations.* C. Chrvala and S. Scrimshaw (Eds.). Washington, DC: National Academy Press.

Israel, B.A. (1994). *Practitioner-oriented Approaches to Evaluating Health Education Interventions: Multiple Purposes—Multiple Methods.* Paper presented at the National Conference on Health Education and Health Promotion, Tampa, FL.

Israel, B.A., and Schurman, S.J. (1990). Social support, control and the stress process. In K. Glanz, F.M. Lewis, and B.K. Rimer (Eds.) *Health Behavior and Health Education: Theory, Research and Practice* (pp. 179–205). San Francisco: Jossey-Bass.

Israel, B.A., Baker, E.A., Goldenhar, L.M., Heaney, C.A., and Schurman, S.J. (1996). Occupational stress, safety, and health: Conceptual framework and principles for effective prevention interventions. *Journal of Occupational Health Psychology, 1*, 261–286.

Israel, B.A., Checkoway, B., Schulz, A.J., and Zimmerman, M.A. (1994). Health education and community empowerment: conceptualizing and measuring perceptions of individual, organizational, and community control. *Health Education Quarterly, 21*, 149–170.

Israel, B.A., Cummings, K.M., Dignan, M.B., Heaney, C.A., Perales, D.P., Simons-Morton, B.G., and Zimmerman, M.A. (1995). Evaluation of health education programs: Current assessment and future directions. *Health Education Quarterly, 22*, 364–389.

Israel, B.A., Schulz, A.J., Parker, E.A., and Becker, A.B. (1998). Review of community-based research: Assessing partnership approaches to improve public health. *Annual Review of Public Health, 19*, 173–202.

Israel, B.A., Schurman, S.J., and House, J.S. (1989). Action research on occupational stress: Involving workers as researchers. *International Journal of Health Services, 19*, 135–155.

Israel, B.A., Schurman, S.J., and Hugentobler, M.K. (1992a). Conducting action research: Relationships between organization members and researchers. *Journal of Applied Behavioral Science, 28*, 74–101.

Israel, B.A., Schurman, S.J., Hugentobler, M.K., and House, J.S. (1992b). A participatory action research approach to reducing occupational stress in the United States. In V. DiMartino (Ed.) *Preventing Stress at Work: Conditions of Work Digest, Vol. II* (pp. 152–163). Geneva, Switzerland: International Labor Office.

James, S.A. (1993). Racial and ethnic differences in infant mortality and low birth weight: A psychosocial critique. *Annals of Epidemiology, 3*, 130–136.

Johnson-Laird, P.N. (1980). Mental models: Towards a cognitive science of language, inference and consciousness *Cognitive Science, No. 6*. New York: Cambridge University Press.

Kahneman D. and Tversky, A. (1983). Choices, values, and frames. *American Psychologist, 39*, 341–350.

Kahneman, D. and Tversky, A. (1996). On the reality of cognitive illusions. *Psychological Review, 103*, 582-591.

Kalet, A., Roberts, J.C., and Fletcher, R. (1994). How do physicians talk with their patients about risks? *Journal of General Internal Medicine, 9*, 402–404.

Kaplan, R.M. (1994). Value judgment in the Oregon Medicaid experiment. *Medical Care, 32*, 975–988.

Kaplan, R.M. (1998). Profile versus utility based measures of outcome for clinical trials. In M.J. Staquet, R.D. Hays, and P.M. Fayers (Eds.) *Quality of Life Assessment in Clinical Trials* (pp. 69–90). London: Oxford University Press.

Kaplan, R.M. and Anderson, J.P. (1996). The general health policy model: An integrated approach. In B. Spilker (Ed.) *Quality of Life and Pharmacoeconomics in Clinical Trials* (pp. 309–322). Philadephia: Lippencott-Raven.

Kasper, J.F., Mulley, A.G., and Wennberg, J.E. (1992). Developing shared decision-making programs to improve the quality of health care. *Quality Review Bulletin, 18*, 183–190.

Kass, D. and Freudenberg, N. (1997). Coalition building to prevent childhood lead poisoning: A case study from New York City. In M. Minkler (Ed.), *Community Organizing and Community Building for Health* (pp. 278–288). New Brunswick, NJ: Rutgers University Press.

Kegler, M.C., Steckler, A., Malek, S.H., and McLeroy, K. (1998a). A multiple case study of implementation in 10 local Project ASSIST coalitions in North Carolina. *Health Education Research, 13,* 225–238.

Kegler, M.C., Steckler, A., McLeroy, K., and Malek, S.H. (1998b). Factors that contribute to effective community health promotion coalitions: A study of 10 Project ASSIST coalitions in North Carolina. American Stop Smoking Intervention Study for Cancer Prevention. *Health Education and Behavior, 25,* 338–353.

Klein, D.C. (1968). *Community Dynamics and Mental Health.* New York: Wiley.

Klitzner, M. (1993). A public health/dynamic systems approach to community-wide alcohol and other drug initiatives. In R.C. Davis, A.J. Lurigo, and D.P. Rosenbaum (Eds.) *Drugs and the Community* (pp. 201–224). Springfield, IL: Charles C. Thomas.

Koepsell, T.D. (1998). Epidemiologic issues in the design of community intervention trials. In R. Brownson, and D. Petitti (Eds.) *Applied Epidemiology: Theory To Practice* (pp. 177–212). New York: Oxford University Press.

Koepsell, T.D., Diehr, P.H., Cheadle, A., and Kristal, A. (1995). Invited commentary: Symposium on community intervention trials. *American Journal of Epidemiology, 142,* 594–599.

Koepsell, T.D., Wagner, E.H., Cheadle, A.C., Patrick, D.L., Martin, D.C., Diehr, P.H., Perrin, E.B., Kristal, A.R., Allan-Andrilla, C.H., and Dey, L.J. (1992). Selected methodological issues in evaluating community-based health promotion and disease prevention programs. *Annual Review of Public Health, 13,* 31–57.

Kong, A., Barnett, G.O., Mosteller, F., and Youtz, C. (1986). How medical professionals evaluate expressions of probability. *New England Journal of Medicine, 315,* 740–744.

Kraus, J.F. (1985). Effectiveness of measures to prevent unintentional deaths of infants and children from suffocation and strangulation. *Public Health Report, 100,* 231–240.

Kraus, J.F., Peek, C., McArthur, D.L., and Williams, A. (1994). The effect of the 1992 California motorcycle helmet use law on motorcycle crash fatalities and injuries. *Journal of the American Medical Association, 272,* 1506–1511.

Krieger, N. (1994). Epidemiology and the web of causation: Has anyone seen the spider? *Social Science and Medicine, 39,* 887–903.

Krieger, N., Rowley, D.L, Herman, A.A., Avery, B., and Phillips, M.T. (1993). Racism, sexism and social class: Implications for studies of health, disease and well-being. *American Journal of Preventive Medicine, 9,* 82–122.

La Puma, J. and Lawlor, E.F. (1990). Quality-adjusted life-years. Ethical implications for physicians and policymakers. *Journal of the American Medical Association 263,* 2917–2921.

Labonte, R. (1994). Health promotion and empowerment: reflections on professional practice. *Health Education Quarterly, 21,* 253–268.

Lalonde, M. (1974). *A new perspective on the health of Canadians.* Ottawa, ON: Ministry of Supply and Services.

Lando, H.A., Pechacek, T.F., Pirie, P.L., Murray, D.M., Mittelmark, M.B., Lichtenstein, E., Nothwehyr, F., and Gray, C. (1995). Changes in adult cigarette smoking in the Minnesota Heart Health Program. *American Journal of Public Health, 85,* 201–208.

Lantz, P.M., House, J.S., Lepkowski, J.M., Williams, D.R., Mero, R.P., and Chen, J. (1998). Socioeconomic factors, health behaviors, and mortality. *Journal of the American Medical Association, 279,* 1703–1708.

Last, J. (1995). Redefining the unacceptable. *Lancet, 346,* 1642–1643.

Lather, P. (1986). Research as praxis. *Harvard Educational Review, 56,* 259–277.

Lenert, L., and Kaplan, R.M. (2000). Validity and interpretation of preference-based measures of health-related quality of life. *Medical Care, 38,*138-150.

Leventhal, H. and Cameron, L. (1987). Behavioral theories and the problem of compliance. *Patient Education and Counseling, 10,* 117–138.

Levine, D.M, Becker, D.M, Bone, L.R, Stillman, F.A, Tuggle II, M.B., Prentice, M., Carter, J., and Filippeli, J. (1992). A partnership with minority populations: A community model of effectiveness research. *Ethnicity and Disease, 2,* 296–305.

Lewin, K. (1951) *Field Theory in Social Science.* New York: Harper.

Lewis, C.E. (1988). Disease prevention and health promotion practices of primary care physicians in the United States. *American Journal of Preventive Medicine, 4,* 9–16.

Liao, L., Jollis, J.G., DeLong, E.R., Peterson, E.D., Morris, K.G., and Mark, D.B. (1996). Impact of an interactive video on decision making of patients with ischemic heart disease. *Journal of General Internal Medicine, 11,* 373–376.

Lichter, A.S., Lippman, M.E., Danforth, D.N., Jr., d'Angelo, T., Steinberg, S.M., deMoss, E., MacDonald, H.D., Reichert, C.M., Merino, M., Swain, S.M., et al. (1992). Mastectomy versus breast-conserving therapy in the treatment of stage I and II carcinoma of the breast: A randomized trial at the National Cancer Institute. *Journal of Clinical Oncology, 10,* 976–983.

Lillie-Blanton, M. and Hoffman, S.C. (1995). Conducting an assessment of health needs and resources in a racial/ethnic minority community. *Health Services Research, 30,* 225–236.

Lincoln, Y.S. and Reason, P. (1996). Editor's introduction. *Qualitative Inquiry, 2,* 5–11.

Linville, P.W., Fischer, G.W., and Fischhoff, B. (1993). AIDS risk perceptions and decision biases. In J.B. Pryor and G.D. Reeder (Eds.) *The Social Psychology of HIV Infection* (pp. 5–38). Hillsdale, NJ: Lawrence Erlbaum.

Lipid Research Clinics Program. (1984). The Lipid Research Clinics Coronary Primary Prevention Trial results. I. Reduction in incidence of coronary heart disease. *Journal of the American Medical Association, 251,* 351–364.

Lipkus, I.M. and Hollands, J.G. (1999). The visual communication of risk. *Journal of National Cancer Institute Monographs, 25,* 149–162.

Lipsey, M.W. (1993). Theory as method: Small theories of treatments. *New Direction in Program Evaluation, 57,* 5–38.

Lipsey, M.W. and Polard, J.A. (1989). Driving toward theory in program evaluation: More models to choose from. *Evaluation and Program Planning, 12,* 317–328.

Lund, A.K., Williams, A.F., and Womack, K.N. (1991). Motorcycle helmet use in Texas. *Public Health Reports, 106,* 576–578.

Maguire, P. (1987). *Doing Participatory Research: A Feminist Approach.* School of Education, Amherst, MA: The University of Massachusetts.

Maguire, P. (1996). Considering more feminist participatory research: What's congruency got to do with it? *Qualitative Inquiry, 2,* 106–118.

Marin, G. and Marin, B.V. (1991). *Research with Hispanic Populations.* Newbury Park, CA: Sage.

Matt, G.E. and Navarro, A.M. (1997). What meta-analyses have and have not taught us about psychotherapy effects: A review and future directions. *Clinical Psychology Review*, 17, 1–32.

Mazur, D.J. and Hickam, D.H. (1997). Patients' preferences for risk disclosure and role in decision making for invasive medical procedures. *Journal of General Internal Medicine*, 12, 114–117.

McGraw, S.A., Stone, E.J., Osganian, S.K., Elder, J.P., Perry, C.L., Johnson, C.C., Parcel, G.S., Webber, L.S., and Luepker, R.V. (1994). Design of process evaluation within the child and adolescent trial for cardiovascular health (CATCH). *Health Education Quarterly*, S5–S26.

McIntyre, S. and West, P. (1992). What does the phrase "safer sex" mean to you? *AIDS, 7*, 121–126.

McKay, H.G., Feil, E.G., Glasgow, R.E., and Brown, J.E. (1998). Feasibility and use of an internet support service for diabetes self-management. *The Diabetes Educator, 24*, 174–179.

McKinlay, J.B. (1993). The promotion of health through planned sociopolitical change: challenges for research and policy. *Social Science and Medicine, 36*, 109–117.

McKnight, J.L. (1987). Regenerating community. *Social Policy, 17*, 54–58.

McKnight, J.L. (1994). Politicizing health care. In P. Conrad, and R. Kern (Eds.) *The Sociology Of Health And Illness: Critical Perspectives, 4th Edition* (pp. 437–441). New York: St. Martin's.

McVea, K., Crabtree, B.F., Medder, J.D., Susman, J.L., Lukas, L., McIlvain, H.E., Davis, C.M., Gilbert, C.S., and Hawver, M. (1996). An ounce of prevention? Evaluation of the 'Put Prevention into Practice' program. *Journal of Family Practice, 43*, 361–369.

Merz, J., Fischhoff, B., Mazur, D.J., and Fischbeck, P.S. (1993). Decision-analytic approach to developing standards of disclosure for medical informed consent. *Journal of Toxics and Liability, 15*, 191–215.

Minkler, M. (1989). Health education, health promotion and the open society: An historical perspective. *Health Education Quarterly, 16*, 17–30.

Mittelmark, M.B., Hunt, M.K., Heath, G.W., and Schmid, T.L. (1993). Realistic outcomes: Lessons from community-based research and demonstration programs for the prevention of cardiovascular diseases. *Journal of Public Health Policy, 14*, 437–462.

Monahan, J.L. and Scheirer, M.A. (1988). The role of linking agents in the diffusion of health promotion programs. *Health Education Quarterly, 15*, 417–434.

Morgan, M.G. (1995). *Fields from Electric Power* [brochure]. Pittsburgh, PA: Department of Engineering and Public Policy, Carnegie Mellon University.

Morgan, M.G., Fischhoff, B., Bostrom, A., and Atman, C. (2001). *Risk Communication: The Mental Models Approach*. New York: Cambridge University Press.

Mosteller, F. and Colditz, G.A. (1996). Understanding research synthesis (meta-analysis). *Annual Review of Public Health, 17*, 1–23.

Muldoon, M.F., Manuck, S.B., and Matthews, K.A. (1990). Lowering cholesterol concentrations and mortality: A quantitative review of primary prevention trials. *British Medical Journal, 301*, 309–314.

Murray, D. (1995). Design and analysis of community trials: Lessons from the Minnesota Heart Health Program. *American Journal of Epidemilogy, 142*, 569–575.

Murray, D.M. (1986). Dissemination of community health promotion programs: The Fargo-Moorhead Heart Health Program. *Journal of School Health, 56*, 375–381.

Myers, A.M, Pfeiffle, P, and Hinsdale, K. (1994). Building a community-based consortium for AIDS patient services. *Public Health Reports, 109,* 555–562.

National Research Council, Committee on Risk Perception and Communication. (1989). *Improving Risk Communication.* Washington, DC: National Academy Press.

NHLBI (National Heart, Lung, and Blood Institute). (1983). *Guidelines for Demonstration And Education Research Grants.* Washington, DC: National Institutes of Health.

NHLBI (National Heart, Lung, and Blood Institute). (1998). *Report of the Task Force on Behavioral Research in Cardiovascular, Lung, and Blood Health and Disease.* Bethesda, MD: National Institutes of Health.

Ni, H., Sacks, J.J., Curtis, L., Cieslak, P.R., and Hedberg, K. 1997. Evaluation of a statewide bicycle helmet law via multiple measures of helmet use. *Archives of Pediatric and Adolescent Medicine, 151,* 59–65.

Nyden, P.W. and Wiewel, W. (1992). Collaborative research: harnessing the tensions between researcher and practitioner. *American Sociologist, 24,* 43–55.

O'Connor, P.J., Solberg, L.I., and Baird, M. (1998). The future of primary care. The enhanced primary care model. *Journal of Family Practice, 47,* 62–67.

Office of Technology Assessment, U.S. Congress. (1981). *Cost-Effectiveness of Influenza Vaccination.* Washington, DC: Office of Technology Assessment.

Oldenburg, B., French, M., and Sallis, J.F. (1999). Health behavior research: The quality of the evidence base. Paper presented at the Society of Behavioral Medicine Twentieth Annual Meeting, San Diego, CA.

Orlandi, M.A (1996a). Health Promotion Technology Transfer: Organizational Perspectives. *Canadian Journal of Public Health, 87,* Supplement 2, 528–533.

Orlandi, M.A. (1996b). Prevention Technologies for Drug-Involved Youth. In J. Inciardi, L. Metsch, and C. McCoy (Eds.) *Intervening with Drug-Involved Youth: Prevention, Treatment, and Research* (pp. 81–100). Newbury Park, CA: Sage Publications.

Orlandi, M.A. (1986). The diffusion and adoption of worksite health promotion innovations: An analysis of barriers. *Preventive Medicine, 15,* 522–536.

Parcel, G.S, Eriksen, M.P, Lovato, C.Y., Gottlieb, N.H., Brink, S.G., and Green, L.W. (1989). The diffusion of school-based tobacco-use prevention programs: Program description and baseline data. *Health Education Research, 4,* 111–124.

Parcel, G.S, O'Hara-Tompkins, N.M, Harris, R.B., Basen-Engquist, K.M., McCormick, L.K., Gottlieb, N.H., and Eriksen, M.P. (1995). Diffusion of an Effective Tobacco Prevention Program. II. Evaluation of the Adoption Phase. *Health Education Research, 10,* 297–307.

Parcel, G.S, Perry, C.L, and Taylor W.C. (1990). Beyond Demonstration: Diffusion of Health Promotion Innovations. In N. Bracht (Ed.), *Health Promotion at the Community Level* (pp. 229–251). Thousand Oaks, CA: Sage Publications.

Parcel, G.S., Simons-Morton, B.G., O'Hara, N.M,. Baranowski, T., and Wilson, B. (1989). School promotion of healthful diet and physical activity: Impact on learning outcomes and self-reported behavior. *Health Education Quarterly, 16,* 181–199.

Park, P., Brydon-Miller, M., Hall, B., and Jackson, T. (Eds.) (1993). *Voices of Change: Participatory Research in the United States and Canada.* Westport, CT: Bergin and Garvey.

Parker, E.A., Schulz, A.J., Israel, B.A., and Hollis, R. (1998). East Side Village Health Worker Partnership: Community-based health advisor intervention in an urban area. *Health Education and Behavior, 25,* 24–45.

Parsons, T. (1951). *The Social System*. Glencoe, IL: Free Press.

Patton, M.Q. (1987). *How to Use Qualitative Methods In Evaluation*. Newbury Park, CA: Sage Publications.

Patton, M.Q. (1990). *Qualitative Evaluation And Research Methods, 2nd Edition*. Newbury Park, CA: Sage Publications.

Pearce, N. (1996). Traditional epidemiology, modern epidemiology and public health. *American Journal of Public Health, 86*, 678–683.

Pendleton, L. and House, W.C. (1984). Preferences for treatment approaches in medical care. *Medical Care, 22*, 644–646.

Pentz, M.A. (1998). Research to practice in community-based prevention trials. Preventive intervention research at the crossroads: contributions and opportunities from the behavioral and social sciences. *Programs and Abstracts* (pp. 82–83). Bethesda, MD.

Pentz, M.A., and Trebow, E. (1997). Implementation issues in drug abuse prevention research. *Substance Use and Misuse, 32*, 1655–1660.

Pentz, M.A., Trebow, E., Hansen, W.B., MacKinnon, D.P., Dwyer, J.H., Flay, B.R., Daniels, S., Cormack, C., and Johnson, C.A. (1990). Effects of program implementation on adolescent drug use behavior: The Midwestern Prevention Project (MPP). *Evaluation Review, 14*, 264–289.

Perry, C.L. (1999). Cardiovascular disease prevention among youth: Visioning the future. *Preventive Medicine, 29*, S79–S83.

Perry, C.L., Murray, D.M, and Griffin, G. (1990). Evaluating the statewide dissemination of smoking prevention curricula: Factors in teacher compliance. *Journal of School Health, 60*, 501–504.

Plough, A. and Olafson, F. (1994). Implementing the Boston Healthy Start Initiative: A case study of community empowerment and public health. *Health Education Quarterly, 21*, 221–234.

Price, R.H. (1989). Prevention programming as organizational reinvention: From research to implementation. In M.M. Silverman and V. Anthony (Eds.) *Prevention of Mental Disorders, Alcohol and Drug Use in Children and Adolescents* (pp. 97–123). Rockville, MD: Department of Health and Human Services.

Price, R.H. (1998). Theory guided reinvention as the key high fidelity prevention practice. Paper presented at the National Institute of Health meeting, "Preventive Intervention Research at the Crossroads: Contributions and Opportunities from the Behavioral and Social Sciences," Bethesda, MD.

Pronk, N.P. and O'Connor, P.J. (1997). Systems approach to population health improvement. *Journal of Ambulatory Care Management, 20*, 24–31.

Putnam, R.D. (1993). *Making Democracy Work: Civic Traditions in Modern Italy*. Princeton: Princeton University.

Rabeneck, L., Viscoli, C.M., and Horwitz, R.I. (1992). Problems in the conduct and analysis of randomized clinical trials. Are we getting the right answers to the wrong questions? *Archives of Internal Medicine, 152*, 507–512.

Raiffa, H. (1968). *Decision Analysis*. Reading, MA: Addison-Wesley.

Reason, P. (1994). Three approaches to participative inquiry. In N.K. Denzin and Y.S. Lincoln (Eds.) *Handbook of Qualitative Research* (pp. 324–339). Thousand Oaks, CA: Sage.

Reason, P. (Ed.). (1988). *Human Inquiry in Action: Developments in New Paradigm Research.* London: Sage.

Reichardt, C.S. and Cook, T.D. (1980). "Paradigms Lost": Some thoughts on choosing methods in evaluation research. *Evaluation and Program Planning: An International Journal 3*, 229–236.

Rivara, F.P., Grossman, D.C., and Cummings, P. (1997a). Injury prevention. First of two parts. *New England Journal of Medicine, 337*, 543–548.

Rivara, F.P., Grossman, D.C., Cummings P. (1997b). Injury prevention. Second of two parts. *New England Journal of Medicine, 337*, 613-618.

Roberts-Gray, C., Solomon, T., Gottlieb, N., and Kelsey, E. (1998). Heart partners: A strategy for promoting effective diffusion of school health promotion programs. *Journal of School Health, 68*, 106–116.

Robertson, A. and Minkler, M. (1994). New health promotion movement: A critical examination. *Health Education Quarterly, 21*, 295–312.

Rogers, E.M. (1983). *Diffusion of Innovations*, 3rd ed. New York: The Free Press.

Rogers, E.M. (1995). *Communication of Innovations.* New York: The Free Press.

Rogers, G.B. (1996). The safety effects of child-resistant packaging for oral prescription drugs. Two decades of experience. *Journal of the American Medical Association, 275*, 1661–1665.

Rohrbach, L.A, D'Onofrio, C., Backer, T., and Montgomery, S. (1996). Diffusion of school-based substance abuse prevention programs. *American Behavioral Scientist, 39*, 919–934.

Rossi, P.H. and Freeman, H.E. (1989). *Evaluation: A Systematic Approach, 4th Edition.* Newbury Park, CA: Sage Publications.

Rutherford, G.W. (1998). Public health, communicable diseases, and managed care: Will managed care improve or weaken communicable disease control? *American Journal of Preventive Medicine, 14*, 53–59.

Sackett, D.L., Richardson, W.S., Rosenberg, W., and Haynes, R.B. (1997) *Evidence-Based Medicine: How to Practice and Teach EBM.* New York: Churchill Livingstone.

Sarason, S.B. (1984). *The Psychological Sense of Community: Prospects for a Community Psychology.* San Francisco: Jossey-Bass.

Schein, E.H. (1987). *Process Consulting.* Reading, MA: Addition Wesley.

Schensul, J.J., Denelli-Hess, D., Borreo, M.G., and Bhavati, M.P. (1987). Urban comadronas: Maternal and child health research and policy formulation in a Puerto Rican community. In D.D. Stull and J.J. Schensul (Eds.) *Collaborative Research and Social Change: Applied Anthropology in Action* (pp. 9–32). Boulder, CO: Westview.

Schensul, S.L. (1985). Science, theory and application in anthropology. *American Behavioral Scientist, 29*, 164–185.

Schneiderman, L.J., Kronick, R., Kaplan, R.M., Anderson, J.P., and Langer, R.D. (1992). Effects of offering advance directives on medical treatments and costs. *Annals of Internal Medicine 117*, 599–606.

Schriver, K.A. (1989). Evaluating text quality: The continuum from text-focused to reader-focused methods. *IEEE Transactions on Professional Communication, 32*, 238–255.

Schulz, A.J, Israel, B.A, Selig, S.M., and Bayer, I.S. (1998a). Development and implementation of principles for community-based research in public health. In R.H. Macnair (Ed.) *Research Strategies For Community Practice* (pp. 83–110). New York: Haworth Press.

Schulz, A.J., Parker, E.A., Israel, B.A, Becker, A.B., Maciak, B., and Hollis, R. (1998b). Conducting a participatory community-based survey: Collecting and interpreting data for a community health intervention on Detroit's East Side. *Journal of Public Health Management Practice, 4*, 10–24.

Schwartz, L.M., Woloshin, S., Black, W.C., and Welch, H.G. (1997). The role of numeracy in understanding the benefit of screening mammography. *Annals of Internal Medicine, 127*, 966–972.

Schwartz, N. (1999). Self-reports: How the questions shape the answer. *American Psychologist, 54*, 93–105.

Seligman M.E. (1996). Science as an ally of practice. *American Psychologist, 51*, 1072–1079.

Shadish, W.R., Cook, T.D., and Leviton, L.C. (1991). *Foundations of Program Evaluation.* Newbury Park, CA: Sage Publications.

Shadish, W.R., Matt, G.E., Navarro, A.M., Siegle, G., Crits-Christoph, P., Hazelrigg, M.D., Jorm, A.F., Lyons, L.C., Nietzel, M.T., Prout, H.T., Robinson, L., Smith, M.L., Svartberg, M., and Weiss, B. (1997). Evidence that therapy works in clinically representative conditions. *Journal of Consulting and Clinical Psychology, 65*, 355–365.

Sharf, B.F. (1997). Communicating breast cancer on-line: Support and empowerment on the internet. *Women and Health, 26*, 65–83.

Simons-Morton, B.G., Green, W.A., and Gottlieb, N. (1995). *Health Education and Health Promotion, 2nd Edition.* Prospect Heights, IL: Waveland.

Simons-Morton, B.G., Parcel, G.P., Baranowski, T., O'Hara, N., and Forthofer, R. (1991). Promoting a healthful diet and physical activity among children: Results of a school-based intervention study. *American Journal of Public Health, 81*, 986–991.

Singer, M. (1993). Knowledge for use: Anthropology and community-centered substance abuse research. *Social Science and Medicine, 37*, 15–25.

Singer, M. (1994). Community-centered praxis: Toward an alternative non-dominative applied anthropology. *Human Organization, 53*, 336–344.

Smith, D.W., Steckler, A., McCormick, L.K., and McLeroy, K.R. (1995). Lessons learned about disseminating health curricula to schools. *Journal of Health Education, 26*, 37–43.

Smithies, J. and Adams, L. (1993). Walking the tightrope. In J.K. Davies, and M.P. Kelly (Eds.) *Healthy Cities: Research and Practice* (pp. 55–70). New York: Routledge.

Solberg, L.I., Kottke, T.E, and Brekke, M.L. (1998a). Will primary care clinics organize themselves to improve the delivery of preventive services? A randomized controlled trial. *Preventive Medicine, 27*, 623–631.

Solberg, L.I., Kottke, T.E., Brekke, M.L., Conn, S.A., Calomeni, C.A., and Conboy, K.S. (1998b). Delivering clinical preventive services is a systems problem. *Annals of Behavioral Medicine, 19*, 271–278.

Sorensen, G., Emmons, K., Hunt, M.K., and Johnston, D. (1998a). Implications of the results of community intervention trials. *Annual Rreview of Public Health, 19*, 379–416.

Sorensen, G., Thompson, B., Basen-Engquist, K., Abrams, D., Kuniyuki, A., DiClemente, C., and Biener, L. (1998b). Durability, dissemination and institutionalization of worksite tobacco control programs: Results from the Working Well Trial. *International Journal of Behavioral Medicine, 5*, 335–351.

Spilker, B. (1996). Quality of Life and Pharmacoeconomics. In B. Spilker (Ed) *Clinical Trials 2nd Edition*. Philadelphia: Lippincott-Raven.

Steckler, A., Goodman, R.M., McLeroy, K.R., Davis, S., and Koch, G. (1992). Measuring the diffusion of innovative health promotion programs. *American Journal of Health Promotion*, 6, 214–224.

Steckler, A.B., Dawson, L., Israel, B.A., and Eng, E. (1993). Community health development: An overview of the works of Guy W. Steuart. *Health Education Quarterly, Suppl. 1*, S3–S20.

Steckler, A.B., McLeroy, K.R., Goodman, R.M., Bird, S.T., and McCormick, L. (1992). Toward integrating qualitative and quantitative methods: an introduction. *Health Education Quarterly, 19*, 1–8.

Steuart, G.W. (1993). Social and cultural perspectives: Community intervention and mental health. *Health Education Quarterly*, S99.

Stokols, D. (1992). Establishing and maintaining healthy environments: Toward a social ecology of health promotion. *American Psychologist, 47*, 6–22.

Stokols, D. (1996). Translating social ecological theory into guidelines for community health promotion. *American Journal of Health Promotion, 10*, 282–298.

Stone, E.J., McGraw, S.A., Osganian, S.K., and Elder, J.P. (Eds.) (1994). Process evaluation in the multicenter Child and Adolescent Trial for Cardiovascular Health (CATCH). *Health Education Quarterly, Suppl. 2*, 1–143.

Stringer, E.T. (1996). *Action Research: A Handbook For Practitioners*. Thousand Oaks, CA: Sage.

Strull, W.M., Lo, B., and Charles, G. (1984). Do patients want to participate in medical decision making? *Journal of the American Medical Association, 252*, 2990–2994.

Strum, S. (1997). Consultation and patient information on the Internet: The patients' forum. *British Journal of Urology, 80*, 22–26.

Susser, M. (1995). The tribulations of trials-intervention in communities. *American Journal of Public Health, 85*, 156–158.

Susser, M. and Susser, E. (1996a). Choosing a future for epidemiology. I. Eras and paradigms. *American Journal of Public Health, 86*, 668–673.

Susser, M. and Susser, E. (1996b). From black box to Chinese boxes and eco-epidemiology. *American Journal of Public Health, 86*, 674–677.

Tandon, R. (1981). Participatory evaluation and research: Main concepts and issues. In W. Fernandes, and R. Tandon (Eds.) *Participatory Research and Evaluation* (pp. 15–34). New Delhi: Indian Social Institute.

Thomas, S.B. and Morgan, C.H. (1991). Evaluation of community-based AIDS education and risk reduction projects in ethnic and racial minority communities. *Evaluation and Program Planning, 14*, 247–255.

Thompson, D.C., Nunn, M.E., Thompson, R.S., and Rivara, F.P. (1996a). Effectiveness of bicycle safety helmets in preventing serious facial injury. *Journal of the American Medical Association, 276*, 1974–1975.

Thompson, D.C., Rivara, F.P., and Thompson, R.S. (1996b). Effectiveness of bicycle safety helmets in preventing head injuries: A case-control study. *Journal of the American Medical Association, 276*, 1968–1973.

Thompson, R.S., Taplin, S.H., McAfee, T.A., Mandelson, M.T., and Smith, A.E. (1995). Primary and secondary prevention services in clinical practice. Twenty years' experience in development, implementation, and evaluation. *Journal of the American Medical Association 273*, 1130–1135.

Torrance, G.W. (1976). Toward a utility theory foundation for health status index models. *Health Services Research, 11*, 349–369.

Tversky, A. and Fox, C.R. (1995). Weighing risk and uncertainty. *Psychological Review, 102*, 269–283.

Tversky, A. and Kahneman, D. (1988). Rational choice and the framing of decisions. In D.E. Bell, H. Raiffa, and A. Tversky (Eds.) *Decision Making: Descriptive, Normative, And Prescriptive Interactions* (pp. 167–192). Cambridge: Cambridge University Press.

Tversky, A. and Shafir, E. (1992). The disjunction effect in choice under uncertainty. *Psychological Science, 3*, 305–309.

U.S. Department of Health and Human Services. (1990). *Smoking, Tobacco, and Cancer Program: 1985–1989 Status Report*. Washington, DC: NIH Publication #90-3107.

Vega, W.A. (1992). Theoretical and pragmatic implications of cultural diversity for community research. *American Journal of Community Psychology, 20*, 375–391.

VonWinterfeldt, D. and Edwards, W. (1986). *Decision Analysis and Behavioral Research.* New York: Cambridge University Press.

Wagner, E., Austin, B., and Von Korff, M. (1996). Organizing care for patients with chronic illness. *Millbank Quarterly, 76*, 511–544.

Wallerstein, N. (1992). Powerlessness, empowerment, and health: implications for health promotion programs. *American Journal of Health Promotion, 6*, 197–205.

Walsh, J.M.E. and McPhee, S.J. (1992). A systems model of clinical preventive care: An analysis of factors influencing patient and physician. *Health Education Quarterly, 19*, 157–175.

Walter, H.J. (1989). Primary prevention of chronic disease among children: The school-based "Know Your Body Intervention Trials." *Health Education Quarterly, 16*, 201–214.

Waterworth, S. and Luker, K.A. (1990). Reluctant collaborators: Do patients want to be involved in decisions concerning care? *Journal of Advanced Nursing, 15*, 971–976.

Weisz, J.R., Weiss, B., and Donenberg, G.R. (1992). The lab versus the clinic. Effects of child and adolescent psychotherapy. *American Psychologist, 47*, 1578–1585.

Wennberg, J.E. (1995). Shared decision making and multimedia. In L.M. Harris (Ed.) *Health and the New Media: Technologist Transforming Personal And Public Health* (pp. 109–126). Mahwah, NJ: Erlbaum.

Wennberg, J.E. (1998). *The Dartmouth Atlas Of Health Care In the United States.* Hanover, NH: Trustees of Dartmouth College.

Whitehead, M. (1993). The ownership of research. In J.K. Davies and M.P. Kelly (Eds.) *Healthy Cities: Research and practice* (pp. 83–89). New York: Routledge.

Williams, D.R. and Collins, C. (1995). U.S. socioeconomic and racial differences in health: patterns and explanations. *Annual Review of Sociology, 21*, 349–386.

Windsor, R., Baranowski, T., Clark, N., and Cutter, G. (1994). *Evaluation Of Health Promotion, Health Education And Disease Prevention Programs.* Mountain View, CA: Mayfield.

Winkleby, M.A. (1994). The future of community-based cardiovascular disease intervention studies. *American Journal of Public Health, 84*, 1369–1372.

Woloshin, S., Schwartz, L.M., Byram, S.J., Sox, H.C., Fischhoff, B., and Welch, H.G. (2000). Women's understanding of the mammography screening debate. *Archives of Internal Medicine,160*, 1434–1440.

World Health Organization (WHO). (1986). *Ottawa Charter for Health Promotion.* Copenhagen: WHO.

Yates, J.F. (1990). *Judgment and Decision Making.* Englewood Cliffs, NJ: Prentice-Hall.

Yeich, S. and Levine, R. (1992). Participatory research's contribution to a conceptualization of empowerment. *Journal of Applied Social Psychology, 22*, 1894–1908.

Yin, R.K. (1993). Applications of case study research. *Applied Social Research Methods Series, Vol. 34*, Newbury Park, CA: Sage Publications.

Zhu, S.H. and Anderson, N.H. (1991). Self-estimation of weight parameter in multi-attribute analysis. *Organizational Behavior and Human Decision Processes, 48*, 36–54.

Zich, J. and Temoshok, C. (1986). Applied methodology: A primer of pitfalls and opportunities in AIDS research. In D. Feldman, and T. Johnson (Eds.) *The Social Dimensions of AIDS* (pp. 41–60). New York: Praeger.

PART THREE

Findings and Recommendations

8

Findings and Recommendations

This report reflects the increasing attention being paid to the behavioral and psychosocial factors that enhance or compromise health. Many behaviors—tobacco use, excessive alcohol consumption and abuse of other substances, unhealthy diet, sedentary lifestyle, and nonadherence to medication regimens—are recognized as health-compromising. Evidence for the effects of social stressors, socioeconomic status, social support, and social capital on health outcomes is growing. First, this chapter explores the interactions of risk factors. Next, it presents the example of tobacco interventions to illustrate an effective multi-level approach and the difficulties in evaluating the interventions. Finally, it presents recommendations for research and practice regarding health and behavior.

INTERACTIONS AMONG RISK FACTORS

Recent decades have seen increasing attention given to the contribution of psychosocial factors, particularly behavior, to promoting or compromising health. The relationship between some behaviors and health status has been recognized since the 1974 Lalonde report. *Healthy People* (U.S. Department of Health, Education, and Welfare, 1979) and *Health and Behavior: Frontiers of Research in the Biobehavioral Sciences* (IOM, 1982) documented the importance of behavior to the burden of illness and disabilities in the United States.

The association of tobacco use with heart disease, a variety of cancers, and poor pregnancy outcomes is perhaps the best known and most dramatic example of the interactions addressed in this report. However, the association of physical activity with fitness and health, dietary nutrients with health or illness, and excessive alcohol consumption with driving fatalities and poor pregnancy outcomes also are recognized widely.

Recently, basic and applied research from a range of disciplines has demonstrated the importance of reciprocal interactions over time among health and biological, psychological, and social factors. Biological factors include genes, neurochemical and hormonal processes, and the functioning of physiological systems. Psychological factors include behavioral, personality, temperamental, cognitive, and emotional variables. Social factors include socioeconomic status, social inequalities, social networks and support, and work conditions. It is now evident that the relationships between health and many behaviors are much more complex than previously thought. Evidence attests that psychosocial factors influence health directly through biological mechanisms and indirectly through an array of behaviors.

Example: Social Status and Health

The role of social status in health and behavior is an example of interactions among biological, psychological, and social factors and health. Lower mortality, morbidity, and disability rates among socioeconomically advantaged people have been observed for hundreds of years, and studies have documented these effects using various indicators of socioeconomic status (SES) and multiple disease outcomes (Kaplan and Keil, 1993). Perhaps the most striking finding is the graded and continuous nature of the association between income and mortality, with differences persisting well into the middle-class range of incomes (Chapter 4). The fact that socioeconomic differences in health are not confined to segments of the population that are materially deprived in the conventional sense argues against an interpretation of socioeconomic differences as simply a function of absolute poverty. Moreover, because causes of death that seem not amenable to medical care show socioeconomic gradients similar to those of potentially treatable causes (Davey Smith et al., 1996; Mackenbach et al., 1989), differential access to health-care programs and services cannot entirely explain socioeconomic differences in health (Wilkinson, 1996).

People who are poor, have low levels of education, or are socially isolated are more likely to engage in risk-related behaviors and less likely to engage in health-promoting behaviors (Adler et al., 1994; Matthews et al., 1989). Behaviors (Chapter 3) occur in specific social contexts. Social environments influence behavior by shaping norms (e.g., the extent to which tobacco use is discouraged or encouraged); enforcing patterns of social control; providing or not providing opportunities to engage in particular behaviors (e.g., safe places to exercise, availability of nutritious foods); and reducing or producing stress, for which engaging in specific behaviors might be an effective coping strategy, at least in the short term (Berkman and Kawachi, 2000).

The stresses associated with environmental and behavioral factors contribute to illness (Cohen and Herbert, 1996; Cohen et al., 1991; Hermann et al., 1995; Kiecolt-Glaser et al., 1996; McEwen, 1998). "Allostatic load" refers to the wear and tear that the body experiences as a result of the repeated activation of the stress response; it also includes contributions of food, alcohol, tobacco, exercise, and sleep through their ability to influence the production of stress hormones (McEwen, 1998; McEwen and Stellar, 1993). The "stress response" triggers and modulates physiological effects that can promote disease including modulation of the immune system (Chapter 2).

BEHAVIOR CHANGE

Producing Behavior Change

Behavior can be changed and those changes can influence health. Interventions can successfully teach health-promoting behaviors or attenuate risky behaviors. Interventions aimed at management of chronic pain, smoking cessation, coping with cancer, and amelioration of eating disorders have been demonstrated empirically to be effective (Compas et al., 1998). Studies show that family or structured-group support, patient education, and behavior-based interventions can increase adherence to prescribed medication regimens (Anderson, 1996). Education aimed at increasing knowledge, control, and confidence (self-efficacy) among diabetics has produced benefits in both attitude and blood glucose management (Anderson et al., 1995). Many studies show that psychological interventions, especially those involving cognitive behavioral methods to enhance coping, are effective in facilitating adaptation to and coping with rheumatoid arthritis (Keefe and Caldwell, 1997; Lorig and Holman, 1993; NIH Technology Assessment Panel, 1996; Parker, 1995).

Studies of support groups, provision of education and information, expression of emotions, and hypnosis suggest the utility of these approaches in the treatment of a range of conditions, including irritable bowel syndrome (Whorwell et al., 1984, 1987), peptic ulcer disease (Klein and Spiegel, 1989), coronary heart disease (Linden et al., 1996), and cancer (improving quality of life and psychological adjustment of cancer patients, possibly affecting health status and survival; see reviews by Andersen, 1992; Compas et al., 1998; Fawzy et al., 1995; Helegeson and Cohen, 1996; Meyer and Mark, 1995). Interventions for insulin-dependent diabetes patients that involved family members meeting together with patients showed an effect on metabolic control (Delamater et al., 1990; Ryden et al., 1994; Satin et al., 1989), but interventions with patients and family members separately did not (McNabb et al., 1994; Thomas-Dobersen et al., 1993). Further research is needed to replicate the results of those studies, determine their efficacy, and identify the conditions under which specific types of psychosocial interventions are most effective.

Maintaining Behavior Change

Maintaining induced behavior change over time and across a variety of settings remains a problem, however, for behaviors as diverse as smoking (Ockene et al., 2000), physical activity (Marcus et al., 2000), diet and weight loss (Jeffery et al., 2000), and adherence to medication regimens. Although interventions can effectively lead to weight loss or smoking cessation, for example, substantial proportions of those who are successful will regain the lost weight or resume smoking. Most studies, though demonstrating the ability to alter behavior, either do not test, or when tested do not demonstrate, sustained behavior change. These factors present major challenges for the research and application of behavioral interventions and point to the need for long-term studies.

Individual behavior has biological underpinnings and consequences and is influenced by the social and psychological contexts in which it occurs. Therefore, changing behavior is generally not simply a matter of personal choice. Instead, interventions are likely to be most effective when they address the individual and the psychological and social contexts in which the behavior occurs. This suggests the utility of intervening at the multiple levels that influence behavior individual (physiological, psychological), family, social networks, organizations, community, and society (state or national population). For example, a person might lose weight as the result of an intervention, but in the months and years after that intervention, the effects of family and friends, eating and offering favorite fatty foods, advertisements for high-calorie treats, exposure to situations in which more nutritious food is not readily available, stress at work combined with little time to seek out nutritious foods, and confusing labeling or messages emphasizing low-fat but not sugar and caloric content are likely to result in weight gain. Interventions that involve family and community members and others with whom an individual has social relationships; community, organizational, and workplace changes; and public policy interventions have all been demonstrated to affect behavior. However, additional research is needed on the functioning and effectiveness of interventions at the levels of family, community, organizations, and public policy, as well as on combinations of them to determine which might be most effective and under what circumstances. Interventions that focus solely on individual attributes, such as self-control or willpower, to change behavior leave many relevant factors to chance and thus are unlikely to be successful over the long term unless other factors (e.g., family and social relationships, work policies, social norms, and individual stress reactivity) happen to be aligned in a way that is conducive to the desired change.

AN INTERVENTION CASE STUDY: TOBACCO

Tobacco use is the leading cause of preventable death in the United States (McGinnis and Foege, 1993), and tobacco control provides a good illustration of the translation of research to application. This example was selected because there is substantial evidence that tobacco use causes ill health (Chapter 3), public health interventions and clinical effectiveness have been evaluated, and cost-effectiveness studies are available.

Clinical Interventions

In 1994, the Agency for Health Care Policy and Research (AHCPR) launched a comprehensive effort to translate research findings on the most effective smoking-cessation strategies into clinical guidelines for health care providers, administrators, and smoking-cessation specialists. AHCPR convened a panel of researchers to summarize the findings of 300 studies into a series of guidelines for clinical practice (USDHHS, 1996; AHCPR, 1996). Primary, secondary, and tertiary prevention strategies were proposed on the basis of meta-analyses of relevant studies:

- A combination of psychosocial counseling and nicotine replacement therapy appeared to be the most effective strategy.
- A dose/response relationship demonstrated that longer counseling sessions (more than 10 minutes) were more effective than were shorter ones (less than 3 minutes) and that more sessions (more than 8) produced better results than did fewer (under 4), but that even fewer or shorter sessions still had a more substantial influence on smoking behavior than did no sessions at all.
- All health-care providers could provide effective counseling that resulted in measurable smoking cessation, but cessation specialists were more effective than were generalists, and multiple providers were more effective than were single providers.

Since that review, new treatments have become available, including nicotine inhalers and nasal spray and bupropion hydrochloride (Hughes et al., 1999). Moreover, the nicotine patch and gum have been made available over the counter. A review of studies of these treatments led to the recommendation that physicians intervene by discussing smoking and potential treatment with every patient who smokes (Hughes et al., 1999). Assessing patients for a combination of behavioral and pharmacotherapeutic approaches also was advised.

The trend in smoking-cessation research has been away from brief interventions studied sequentially to multicomponent interventions that integrate several approaches (Schwartz, 1992). Those programs target smoking at the social, physiological, and psychological levels. They have been found to be more effective in promoting sustained smoking cessation than are single-component approaches (Shiffman, 1993). Recent evidence also suggests that smoking-cessation efforts are more successful when they are tailored to the target population. Specifically, an intervention tailored to specific needs, barriers, and smoking patterns of African Americans resulted in a higher cessation rate at 1 year than did a standard intervention (Orleans et al., 1998).

Opportunities to increase the influence of smoking-cessation strategies are becoming available through managed-care programs in which more aggressive efforts can be undertaken to reach target populations. For example, interactive telephone contact combined with tailored self-help materials (computer-generated recommendations based on questionnaire response patterns; Velicer et al., 1999) and smoking-cessation programs tailored to be responsive to the weight control concerns of women (Suchanek et al., 1999) were provided to substantial portions of the eligible populations and yielded impressive results. Although long-term abstinence rates were low (for instance, around 5–10%), participation of 50–85% produced success rates well beyond what would be expected from a typical reactive program. It should be noted that when success rates were matched to readiness stage (Prochaska, 1997), abstinence significantly improved for those in the preparation stage (to 20–30%) (Velicer et al., 1999), although this stage accounted for only 20% of the sample.

Cost-Effectiveness

A study by Cromwell et al. (1997) evaluated the cost-effectiveness of 15 smoking-cessation interventions endorsed by AHCPR (1996). The entry in Table 7-4 for smoking cessation comes from that study and shows the result for the guidelines as a whole and for each intervention. The authors presented results in terms of cost per quitter, per life-year saved, and per QALY. They also presented sensitivity analyses that included the time that smokers spent in the programs as a cost. (The committee endorses the inclusion of time, a scarce resource, in costs. Recognizing that analysts do not have much experience with this variable, sensitivity analyses might be the way to start.)

The results of the study by Cromwell et al. (1997) show that smoking-cessation programs are a cost-effective way to improve health. More intensive interventions, which involve more counseling or use of nicotine replacement, are more cost-effective (their higher costs are more than offset by greater effectiveness). The total first-year cost of implementing the guidelines was estimated at $6.7 billion (1997 dollars). The return for that investment would be smoking cessation by 1.7 million people at a cost (in 1997 dollars) of about $4,000 per person. In terms of health outcome, the cost would be $2,800 per life-year, or just over $2,000 per QALY.

Evaluating Clinical Interventions

Chambless and Hollon (1998) have proposed a four-component model for the evaluation of health behavior change strategies: efficacy, effectiveness, generalizability, and cost-effectiveness. In a recent review of smoking-cessation interventions using the Chambless and Hollon model, Compas et al. (1998) identified the most efficacious and effective smoking-cessation programs as multicomponent (typically, cognitive/behavioral therapy combined with nicotine patch or gum or such other pharmacologic agents as buproprion [Hurt et al., 1997], nicotine inhalers, social support, and environmental restructuring) and group-based, consisting of 8–12 sessions (Hall et al., 1994; Hill et al., 1993; Stevens and Hollis, 1989), achieving 1-year abstinence rates of 32–34%. Maintenance sessions that included relapse prevention skill training were particularly effective, raising 1-year abstinence rates to 41%. Other studies (e.g., Cinciripini et al., 1995, 1994) have achieved similar 1-year abstinence rates (44%) with the addition of scheduled smoking-reduction strategies. These rates compare favorably with those of earlier studies (e.g., Hunt et al., 1971) in which 20–25% abstinence after 1 year was the norm.

Community-Based Interventions

Chapters 5 and 6 review a number of community, workplace, and school-based interventions targeting the reduction of tobacco use. In the workplace, several programs were successful in reducing smoking among employees through implementation of restrictive tobacco control policies. School-based programs tried to provide educational messages about the health risks of tobacco use and to develop social skills that would allow youths to resist the pressures to smoke. These programs met with varied success, and changes were difficult to sustain.

The study of Altman et al. (1999) illustrates a broad-based community participation approach to reducing tobacco availability and use among adolescents and youths. In that study, four rural communities in Monterey, California, were randomly assigned to treatment or comparison groups. Middle school and high school students in the communities completed questionnaires that evaluated their knowledge, attitudes, and behaviors concerning tobacco use. In the intervention communities, a series of actions were implemented over a 3-year period: widespread community education, training of merchants who sold tobacco, and voluntary policy change. Within the treatment communities, the proportion of stores that sold tobacco to minors dropped from 75% at the baseline assessment to zero at the final evaluation period. There also were reductions in tobacco sales in the comparison communities, but they were much less dramatic (from 64% down to 39%). Although tobacco availability was reduced in the intervention communities, young people still reported that they were able to obtain tobacco from other sources. The strongest effect of the intervention was for younger students (seventh graders). The intervention had only small effects for ninth and eleventh graders.

A recent school-based smoking prevention program (Peterson et al., 2000) calls into question the effectiveness of the social-influences approach to smoking prevention. The Hutchinson Smoking Prevention Project (HSPP), conducted 1984–1999, randomly assigned 40 school districts to experimental or control groups. Students were followed from grade 3 until 2 years after high school. An enhanced social-influence approach to the intervention was used, containing the 15 "essential elements" for school-based tobacco prevention developed by an NCI Advisory Panel (explained in Flay, 1985; Glynn, 1989). Included in the interventions were the following activities. Every year, from grade 3 to grade 10, the students received multiple lessons from trained teachers regarding the strategies for identifying and resisting the influences to smoke, motivating the students not to smoke, and promoting self-confidence in the ability to refuse to smoke. This was supplemented by a biannual newsletter and the availability of materials to help stop smoking. No significant differences between the control and experimental groups were evident at grade 12 or 2 years after high school, suggesting that the intervention had little, if any, impact. The highly controlled, and well-designed nature of the study, including the high follow-up rates, high compliance with the intervention, the maintenance of the randomization by the school districts, well-matched control and treatment groups, and appropriate statistical analysis, strongly suggest that the failure to achieve change was a result of a failed intervention and not poor methodology. This conclusion implies that future interventions need to take a different approach, critically rethinking the interactions of biological, behavioral, and psychosocial risk factors at social and cultural contexts.

Government Level Anti-Tobacco Interventions

The government has adopted multiple strategies to reduce smoking, particularly among children and adolescents. Those interventions are directed toward individual-level behavioral changes using education (e.g., anti-tobacco campaigns), deterrence (e.g., bans on retail sales to minors), and disincentives (e.g., tobacco taxes). They also are directed toward manufacturers (various litigation strategies), information sources (e.g., advertising restrictions), and physical environments (e.g., bans on smoking in the workplace and other public areas). There has been no systematic evaluation of all of the interventions, but researchers have sought to analyze several of the government's anti-tobacco strategies.

Media Campaigns

It has been half a century since the publication of the first evidence that smoking causes lung cancer (Doll and Hill, 1950). Since 1950, knowledge of the health effects of tobacco use has continued to grow systematically. The increasing number of magazine articles on the risks of cancer parallels the increasing knowledge that tobacco use is harmful (Albright et al., 1988) and suggests a positive association between mass-media coverage and public attitudes concerning smoking (Pierce and Gilpin, 1995; Figure 8.1). Although the increase in public knowledge parallels the incidence of smoking cessation in adults (35–50 years old), even in 1990, the cessation rate in the general population was only around 4%. The data on younger adults (20–34 years old) follow a similar but weaker pattern, with

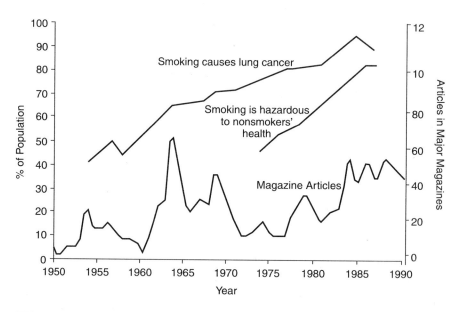

FIGURE 8-1 Dissemination of Health Consequences of Smoking and Population Level of Knowledge, U.S. 1950-1990. SOURCE: Reducing the Health Consequences of Smoking. A Report of the Surgeon General, 1989.

a cessation-rate of about 5% in 1990 (Evans et al., 1995; Gilpin and Pierce, 1997).

The use of the mass-media for anti-smoking campaigns was developed to counter the influence of tobacco industry advertisements promoting smoking. The impact of the media on smoking behavior was most dramatic during the time of the Fairness Doctrine mass-media campaign. In 1967, television networks were required to give equal time to anti-tobacco messages (Pierce and Gilpin, 1995), and per capita cigarette consumption decreased for the first time. In 1972, the tobacco industry voluntarily accepted restrictions on broadcast advertising. Clearly, the use of mass-media can be effective for antitobacco communication.

A major issue of research, policy, and legal debate has been the extent to which tobacco industry communication strategies (cigarette advertising and promotion) encourage teenagers to start smoking (Albright et al., 1988; Gilpin et al., 1997). The tobacco industry's annual budget for advertising and promotional expenditures is upwards of $5 billion. However, a shift is apparent from advertising toward promotional expenditures. In 1995, the tobacco industry reduced its advertising budget and put money into increased incentives to merchants, coupons, and specialty items with visible cigarette brand names or symbols (Emery et al., 1999). Changes in smoking initiation among adolescents can be shown to track with promotional strategies (Pierce et al., 1998a). Joe Camel was introduced in 1985, when smoking initiation by adolescents was at an all-time low (10%), and initiation rates began to rise. With the addition of promotional items like Camel Cash and the Marlboro Miles campaign, and decreases in price, adolescent initiation reached a high of 14% (Evans et al., 1995). Initiation of daily use among minors follows a similar trend. Pierce et al. (1998a) showed that having a favorite brand and being willing to use a promotional item substantially increased the odds that people would move along the smoking-uptake continuum from nonsusceptible never-smoker in 1993 to susceptible or higher in 1996.

Effective antitobacco campaigns have been conducted in Sydney and Melbourne, Australia, and in California (Pierce, 1999). A statewide media-led tobacco control program initiated in Sydney and extended to Melbourne led to a drop in smoking prevalence in both places. The expected delay in effect was observed: Melbourne showed changes after Sydney at the point when the campaign started. The effect was much stronger in males than in females. In California, per capita consumption trends were tracked before, during, and after an antismoking campaign, and smoking behavior was compared with that in the rest of the United States. California showed decreases in per capita consumption and lower consumption overall than the rest of the country. The United States, however, showed a decrease of similar magnitude to that observed in California; no interaction was apparent (Pierce et al., 1998b,c) (Figure 8.2). It is unclear what influence the program had. Similar relationships were observed in measures of smoking prevalence.

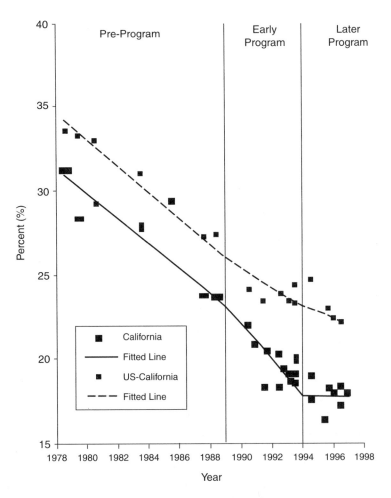

FIGURE 8-2 Smoking Prevalence Among Adults Aged 18 and Older, California vs. U.S. SOURCE: NHIS 1978-80, 1983, 1985, 1987-88, 1990-91, 1993-94; CTS 1990, 1992, 1993, 1996; BRFS.CATS 1991-1995; CPS 1992-93, 1995-96.

Tobacco Taxes

Cigarette excise taxes are an attractive public policy tool for two reasons. First, they generate substantial revenue, whether for a local municipality, a state, or the federal government. Second, there is substantial evidence that, by raising the price of a pack of cigarettes, an excise tax increase will reduce cigarette consumption—some smokers will stop and some will cut down (Chaloupka and Grossman, 1996; Hu et al., 1995; Keeler et al., 1993; Lewit et al., 1981; Manning et al., 1991). These behavioral changes eventually might be reflected in improved population health status (Warner, 1986). But the long-term effectiveness of this intervention has yet to be demonstrated.

Elasticity is the term economists use to measure responsiveness to price changes. It is a unitless measure calculated as the percentage change in overall demand that results from a 1% change in the price of an item. For example, an elasticity estimate of minus 0.40 means that consumption will decrease by 4% in response to a 10% price increase. If fewer people smoke, health benefits are likely. The health benefits, which can be expressed in terms of improved life expectancy and quality of life, are summarized in QALYs. Simulation studies estimate that for a $0.50 tax and an elasticity of minus 0.40, about 25,000 QALYs would result each year. Higher taxes would produce even greater health benefits. The simulations also suggest that the tax has a greater influence each year it is in effect, until a plateau at about 70 years in the future. The reason for the delayed benefit is that youth might be more price sensitive than are older habitual smokers. Thus, the tax could have a greater effect in later years by preventing youths from entering the smoking pool and by inducing current smokers to quit. The analysis suggests that a tobacco excise tax could be among the few policy options that will enhance population health status while raising revenues (Kaplan et al., 2001).

Evaluation Studies

The most encompassing studies have evaluated broad, multidimensional anti-tobacco campaigns initiated in several states. The initiatives differ from one state to another, but they all involve taxation of cigarettes and the use of those revenues for a multipronged approach to reducing smoking. In California, for example, the state mandated funding for health education campaigns, and local health agencies were required to provide technical support and monitor adherence to antismoking laws, community-based interventions, and enhancement of school-based prevention programs (Bal et al., 1990). Evaluation studies in Massachusetts (Abt, 1997), California (Pierce et al., 1998b), and Oregon (Centers for Disease Control and Prevention, 1999) all reported per capita reductions in cigarette consumption.

Despite the promising results shown in the studies, they do have empirical and methodologic limitations. The California study reported a sharp decline in smoking directly after the intervention, but the effect dissipated over time and, ultimately, failed to significantly affect tobacco use (Pierce et al., 1998b). There are several possible explanations. One is that the political and social environment had as much effect as the interventions themselves. Changes in the law, which often are associated with political debate and media coverage, have a "declarative effect" that influences behavior indirectly by changing attitudes. Legal norms reinforce, stimulate, accelerate, or symbolize changes in public attitudes about socially desirable behaviors (Bonnie, 1986). Other possible explanations are temporary reductions in state funding for anti-tobacco programs, political interference with anti-tobacco messages, and industry advertising and pricing policies.

The studies also face challenges in methodology. Most important, public or private funding for evaluation research, including population surveys of smoking behavior, becomes available only after the intervention has occurred. After-the-fact research funding thwarts a comparison of specific behaviors before and after intervention. Even if this important problem could be overcome, however, it would be hard to identify precisely which intervention is having the desired effect. The Massachusetts, California, and Oregon studies, by definition, examined multiple interventions but had no ability to separate the effects of each.

There are, of course, numerous studies of discrete tobacco regulation strategies. Two major interventions that have been studied are programs to prevent youth access to cigarettes and bans on smoking in the workplace and other public places. In the absence of enforcement, banning cigarette sales to minors does not significantly reduce teenage tobacco use. Compliance with the law by retailers is low; youth access studies have demonstrated that most retailers do sell to children. The Tobacco Institute's own "It's the Law" campaign, perhaps predictably, has not been effective (DiFranza and Brown, 1992). Education efforts aimed at retailers have shown an effect, but a small one (Wildey et al., 1995). The most successful legal strategy to reduce youth access imposes civil penalties against store owners (not just clerks), incorporates progressively higher fines culminating in suspension or revocation of the tobacco retailer's license, and forces regular enforcement by using minors in unannounced purchase attempts to monitor compliance. This strategy, implemented by legislation in Woodbridge, Illinois, is successful over time (Jason et al., 1999). Locking devices on cigarette vending machines do not appear to be as effective as outright bans on these machines (Forster et al., 1992).

Legal restrictions on smoking in the workplace and in other public places have demonstrated high conformance with the rule and some reduction in cigarette use. A study of compliance with an indoor clean air act in Brookline, Massachusetts, showed that the law was popular and the incidence of restricted smoking was high (Rigotti et al., 1992). A summary of 19 studies that evaluated the effects of smoke-free workplaces on smoking habits showed that both smoking rates (cigarettes smoked during a 24 hour period) and smoking prevalence (proportion of workers who smoke) decreased as a result of the indoor smoking bans. The authors estimate an annual reduction of 9.7 billion cigarettes (2%) in the United States as a result of smoke-free workplaces (Chapman et al., 1999).

What is notably absent from the evaluative research are rigorous studies of the effects of tobacco litigation and other forms of litigation. Although tort strategies are much used and publicized—by private parties, classes, and state and federal government—there is considerable debate about the effects. Public health advocates strongly favor the approach, whereas some law and economic scholars are skeptical about the tort system as a useful and cost-effective means of intervention (Rose-Ackerman, 1991; Vicusi, 1992).

The experience with government strategies to reduce cigarette-smoking shows that both the interventions and the behavior are highly complex. Many interventions have not been carefully evaluated, and methodologic difficulties have thwarted some of the studies that have been undertaken. A comprehensive, multipronged approach to smoking reduction appears to work best, but long-term problems still exist.

What Works?

Many approaches have been used to decrease the prevalence of tobacco use. Despite the multitude of interventions, it is still not possible to conclude what works and what does not. Some general conclusions can be drawn.

At the individual level, findings suggest that counseling and pharmacological therapies are effective (AHCPR, 1996; Tobacco Use and Dependence Clinical Practice Guideline Panel, 2000). The U.S. Public Health Service issued a Clinical Practice Guideline (Tobacco Use and Dependence Clinical Practice Guideline Panel, 2000) based upon the recommendations of an expert panel. They reviewed nearly 6,000 peer-reviewed articles and recommended that all tobacco users should be offered treatment since effective treatments exist: institutionalizing consistent identification, documentation, and treatment of all tobacco users; brief treatment is effective; greater intensity of counseling is more effective; three types of counseling and five pharmacotherapies were found to be effective. This approach was evaluated for tobacco cessation, but in modified form might also be effective for prevention.

Many community-based interventions have shown variable success. Many of them have been directed toward youth in the belief that they would have the greatest impact for the future. One exemplary study of school-based smoking prevention, the Hutchinson Smoking Prevention Project (HSPP) (Peterson et al., 2000) sponsored by the National Cancer Institute, is described above. This 15-year study, in 40 school districts of Washington state that were randomly assigned to intervention or control groups, involved 8,388 third graders who were followed to 2 years after high school with 94% follow-up. The authors concluded "there is no evidence from this trial that a school-based social-influences approach is effective in the long-term deterrence of smoking among youth."

Similarly, an assessment of policy interventions in a school setting was found to have limited impact. Based on the observation that organizational smoking policy may be a potentially effective way to influence smoking behavior in worksites (Borland et al., 1990), Bowen et al. (1995) surveyed 239 schools as to their smoking policies. They identified three types of policies: a ban on smoking on school grounds; smoking allowed on school grounds; and smoking allowed in designated areas in the building. Their conclusion was: "current smoking policies may have limited ability to reduce student smoking."

A scholarly review of government level approaches to tobacco use prevention and cessation by the Advocacy Institute (2000) found that although single approaches via clean air laws, price increases, counter-advertising, enforcement of existing laws restricting youth access and others may be effective with some people. However, a combination of these approaches has the greatest possibility of success.

In summary, there is limited evidence that any single step is effective in reducing tobacco use. Although a number of studies have been published, many if not most suffer from design flaws that fail adequately to consider co-factors existing in the community. The conclusion of the committee is that a multi-pronged approach including (but not limited to) education, physician intervention, price increases, restricted access to tobacco, clean air laws, and counter-advertising must be used. In current tobacco users, counseling and pharmacotherapies have the greatest potential.

APPLICATION OF RESEARCH RESULTS

Much research is needed to complete the picture of how individual genetic endowments and physiological processes interact with individual personalities, development, other psychological characteristics and processes, and social status and relationships to affect health status. Simply put, how does the environment "get under the skin" (Taylor et al., 1997), and what can be done to optimize health (Ryff and Singer, 1998)? Such research will require the collaboration and cooperation of multiple disciplines. New research methods are likely to be required as multiple influences are considered simultaneously and as causes and effects are considered dynamically and systemically, rather than linearly.

To develop programs that are effective in modifying health behaviors, expanded efforts in all five phases (NHLBI, 1983) of intervention research are needed. These five phases include hypothesis generation, development of intervention methods, controlled intervention trials, studies in defined populations, and demonstration research (Chapter 7). Systematic clinical trials are needed to evaluate the value of behavioral and psychosocial interventions; in particular, more studies are needed that document the effects of these interventions on health, quality of life, and longevity. Studies suggest that interventions at multiple levels are more effective than interventions at single levels, but well-designed evaluations are necessary. Innovative methods and naturalistic experiments also will be necessary to evaluate community, organizational, and public policy interventions, and particularly multilevel interventions. Those methods will be critically important if knowledge from behavioral and psychosocial research is to be translated into applications in more natural settings.

FINDINGS AND RECOMMENDATIONS

Finding 1: Health and disease are determined by dynamic interactions among biological, psychological, behavioral, and social factors. These interactions occur over time and throughout development. Cooperation and interaction of multiple disciplines are necessary for understanding and influencing health and behavior.

Recommendation 1: Funding agencies should direct resources toward interdisciplinary efforts for research and intervention studies that integrate biological, psychological, behavioral, and social variables. The investigations that will be most productive will reflect an understanding of the complexity and interconnections of disciplines. Collaborations across disciplines need to be encouraged and expanded.

Finding 2: A fundamental finding of the report is the importance of the interaction of psychosocial and biological processes in health and disease. Psychosocial factors influence health directly through biological mechanisms and indirectly through an array of behaviors. Social and psychological factors include socioeconomic status, social inequalities, social networks and support, work conditions, depression, anger, and hostility.

Recommendation 2: Research efforts to elucidate the mechanisms by which social and psychological factors influence health should be encouraged. Intervention studies are needed to evaluate the effectiveness of modifying these factors to improve health and prevent disease. Such intervention studies should span the breadth of all phases of clinical trials, from feasibility studies to randomized double-blind studies. Community-based participatory research should also be conducted. Research should include all levels of intervention, from individual to family, community, and society.

Finding 3: Behavior can be changed: behavioral interventions can successfully teach new behaviors and attenuate risky behaviors. Maintaining behavior change over time, however, is a greater challenge. Short-term changes in behavior are encouraging, but improved health outcomes will often require prolonged interventions and lengthy follow-up protocols.

Recommendation 3: Funding for health-related behavioral and psychosocial interventions should support realistically long-duration efforts.

Finding 4: Individual behavior, family interactions, community and workplace relationships and resources, and public policy all contribute to health and influence behavior change. Existing research suggests that interventions at multiple levels (individual, family, community, society) are most likely to sustain behavioral change.

Recommendation 4: Concurrent interventions at multiple levels (individual, family, community, and society) should be encouraged to promote healthy behaviors. Assessments of coordinated efforts across levels are needed. Such efforts should address the psychosocial factors associated with health status (e.g., access to healthy foods or safe places to exercise) as well as individual behavior.

Finding 5: Initiating and maintaining a behavior change is difficult. Evidence indicates that it is easier to generalize a newly learned behavior than to change existing behavior. The old adage "an ounce of prevention is worth a pound of cure" is valid in the context of behavior and health as well.

Recommendation 5: Resources should be allocated to the promotion of health-enhancing behavior and primary prevention of disease. This should be a priority for public health and health care systems.

Finding 6: The goals of public health and health care are to increase life expectancy and improve health-related quality of life. Many behavioral intervention trials document the capacity of interventions to modify risk factors, but relatively few measured mortality and morbidity. However, ramifications of interventions are not always apparent until they are fully evaluated, and unexpected consequences can result.

Recommendation 6: Intervention research must include appropriate measures (including biological measures) to determine whether the strategy has the desired health effects.

Finding 7: Changing unhealthy behavior is not simply a matter of "willpower." Individual behavior has biological underpinnings and consequences and is influenced by the social and psychological contexts in which it occurs. While biological interventions and exhortations to individuals to change their behaviors are easier to administer, changes in social factors, policies, and norms are necessary for improvement and maintenance of population health. Much can be learned as states change cigarette taxes, create controls on public advertising for various products, and increase or decrease opportunities for exercise during the school day or as communities implement or eliminate walking and bicycle paths.

Such social and policy decisions are rich opportunities for learning about behavior change and health.

Recommendation 7: Program planners and policy makers need to consider modifying social and societal conditions to enable healthy behavior and social relationships. Interventions must be evaluated to enable continuous improvement of programs and policies. Research in these domains should be rigorous and scientific, but method should not dominate substance. Longitudinal research designs, natural experiments, quasi-experimental methods, community-based participatory research, and development of new research methods are necessary to advance knowledge in these areas.

REFERENCES

Abt (1997). *Independent Evaluation of the Massachusetts Tobacco Control Program.* Cambridge, MA: Abt Associates.

Adler, N., Boyce, T., Chesney, M., Cohen, S., Folkman, S., Kahn, R., and Syme, L. (1994). Socioeconomic status and health: The challenge of the gradient. *American Psychologist, 49,* 15–24.

Advocacy Institute (2000) *Making The Case: State Tobacco Control Policy Briefing Papers,* 1707 L St., NW, Suite 400, Washington, DC 20036.

AHCPR (Agency for Health Care Policy and Research) (1996). Smoking Cessation Clinical Practice Guideline. *Journal of the American Medical Association, 275 (16),* 1270–1280

Albright, C.L., Altman, D.F., Slater, M.D., and Maccoby, N. (1988). Cigarette advertisements in magazines: Evidence for a differential focus on women's and youth magazines. *Health Education Quarterly, 15,* 225–233.

Altman, D.G., Wheelis, A.Y., McFarlane, M., Lee, H., and Fortmann, S.P. (1999). The relationship between tobacco access and use among adolescents: A four community study. *Social Science and Medicine, 48,* 759–775.

Andersen, B.L. (1992). Psychosocial interventions for cancer patients to enhance quality of life. *Journal of Consulting and Clinical Psychology, 60,* 552–568.

Anderson, B.J. (1996). Involving family members in diabetes treatment. In B.J. Anderson and R.R. Rubin (Eds.) *Practical Psychology for Diabetes Clinicians* (pp. 43–50). Alexandria, VA: American Diabetes Association.

Anderson, R.M., Funnell, M.M., Butler, P.M., Arnold, M.S., Fitzgerald, J.T., and Feste, C.C. (1995). Patient empowerment. Results of a randomized controlled trial. *Diabetes Care, 18,* 943–949.

Bal, D.G., Kizer, K.W., Felten, P.G., Mozar, H.N., and Niemeyer, D. (1990). Reducing tobacco consumption in California. Development of a statewide anti-tobacco use campaign. *Journal of the American Medical Association, 264,* 1570–1574.

Berkman, L. and Kawachi, I. (Eds.) (2000). *Social Epidemiology.* New York: Oxford University Press.

Bonnie, R. (1986). The efficacy of law as a paternalistic instrument. In G. Melton (Ed.) *Nebraska Symposium on Human Motivation, 1985: The Law as a Behavioral Instrument* (pp. 131–211). Lincoln, NE: University of Nebraska Press.

Borland, R., Chapman, S., Owen N., and Hall D. (1990). Effects of worksite smoking bans on cigarette consumption, *American Journal of Public Health*, 80, 178–180.

Bowan, D.J., Kinne, S., and Orlandi, M. (1995). School policy in COMMIT: A promising strategy to reduce smoking by youth. *Journal of School Health*, 65, 140–144.

Centers for Disease Control and Prevention. (1999). Decline in cigarette consumption following implementation of a comprehensive tobacco prevention and education program—Oregon, 1996–1998. *Morbidity and Mortality Weekly Report*, 48, 140–143.

Chaloupka, F.J. and Grossman, M. (1996). Price, tobacco control policies, and youth smoking. *Working Paper No. 5740*. Cambridge, MA: National Bureau of Economic Research.

Chambless, D.L. and Hollon, S.D. (1998). Defining empirically supported therapies. *Journal of Consulting and Clinical Psychology*, 66, 7–18.

Chapman, S., Borland, R., Scollo, M., Brownson, R.C., Dominello, A., and Woodward, S. (1999). The impact of smoke-free workplaces on declining cigarette consumption in Australia and the United States. *American Journal of Public Health*, 89, 1018–1023.

Cinciripini, P.M., Lapitsky, L., Seay, S., Wallfisch, A., Kitchens, K., and Van Vunakis, H. (1995). The effects of smoking schedules on cessation outcome: Can we improve on common methods of gradual and abrupt nicotine withdrawal? *Journal of Consulting and Clinical Psychology*, 63, 388–399.

Cinciripini, P.M., Lapitsky, L.G., Wallfisch, A., Mace, R., Nezami, E., and Van Vunakis, H. (1994). An evaluation of a multicomponent treatment program involving scheduled smoking and relapse prevention procedures: Initial findings. *Addictive Behaviors*, 19, 13–22.

Cohen, S. and Herbert, T.B. (1996). Health psychology: Psychological factors and physical disease from the perspective of human psychoneuroimmunology. *Annual Review of Psychology*, 47, 113–142.

Cohen, S., Tyrrell, D.A., and Smith, A.P. (1991). Psychological stress and susceptibility to the common cold. *New England Journal of Medicine*, 325, 606–612.

Compas, B.E., Haaga, D.F., Keefe, F.J., Leitenberg, H., and Williams, D.A. (1998). Sampling of empirically supported psychological treatments from health psychology: Smoking, chronic pain, cancer, and bulimia nervosa. *Journal of Consulting and Clinical Psychology*, 66, 89–112.

Cromwell, J., Bartosch, W.J., Fiore, M.C., Hasselblad, V., and Baker, T. (1997). Cost-effectiveness of the clinical practice recommendations in the AHCPR guideline for smoking cessation. *Journal of the American Medical Association*, 278, 1759–1766.

Davey Smith, G., Neaton, J.D., Wentworth, D., Stamler, R., and Stamler, J. (1996). Socioeconomic differentials in mortality risk among men screened for the Multiple Risk Factor Intervention Trial. II. Black men. *American Journal of Public Health*, 86, 497–504.

Delamater, A.M., Bubb, J., Davis, S.G., Smith, J.A., Schmidt, L., White, N.H., and Santiago, J.V. (1990). Randomized prospective study of self-management training with newly diagnosed diabetic children. *Diabetes Care*, 13, 492–498.

DiFranza, J.R. and Brown, L.J. (1992). The Tobacco Institute's "It's the Law" campaign: Has it halted illegal sales of tobacco to children? *American Journal of Public Health, 82*, 1271–1273.

Doll, R. and Hill, A.B. (1950). Smoking and carcinoma of the lung. Preliminary report. *British Medical Journal, 2*, 739–748.

Emery, S., Gilpin, E.A., White, M.M., and Pierce, J.P. (1999). How adolescents get their cigarettes: Implications for policies on access and price. *Journal of the National Cancer Institute, 91*, 184–186.

Evans, N., Farkas, A., Gilpin, E., Berry, C., and Pierce, J.P. (1995). Influence of tobacco marketing and exposure to smokers on adolescent susceptibility to smoking. *Journal of the National Cancer Institute, 87*, 1538–1545.

Fawzy, F.I., Fawzy, N.W., Arndt, L.A., and Pasnau, R.O. (1995). Critical review of psychosocial interventions in cancer care. *Archives of General Psychiatry, 52*, 100–13.

Flay, B.R. (1985). Psychosocial approaches to smoking prevention: A review of findings, *Health Psychology, 4*, 449–488.

Forster, J.L., Hourigan, M.E., and Kelder, S. (1992). Locking devices on cigarette vending machines: Evaluation of a city ordinance. *American Journal of Public Health, 82*, 1217–1219.

Gilpin, E.A. and Pierce, J.P. (1997). Trends in adolescent smoking initiation in the United States: Is tobacco marketing an influence? *Tobacco Control, 6*, 122–127.

Gilpin, E.A., Pierce, J.P., and Rosbrook, B. (1997). Are adolescents receptive to current sales promotion practices of the tobacco industry? *Preventive Medicine, 26*, 14–21.

Glynn, T.J. (1989). essential elements of school-based smoking prevention programs, *Journal of School Health, 59*, 181–188,

Hall, S.M., Munoz, R.F., and Reus, V.I. (1994). Cognitive-behavioral intervention increases abstinence rates for depressive-history smokers. *Journal of Consulting and Clinical Psychology, 62*, 141–146.

Helegeson, V.S. and Cohen, S. (1996). Social support and adjustment to cancer: Reconciling descriptive, correlational, and intervention research. *Health Psychology, 15*, 75–83.

Hermann, G., Beck, F.M., and Sheridan, J.F. (1995). Stress-induced glucocorticoid response modulates mononuclear cell trafficking during an experimental influenza viral infection. *Journal of Neuroimmunology, 56*, 179–186.

Hill, R.D., Rigdon, M., and Johnson, S. (1993). Behavioral smoking cessation treatment for older chronic smokers. *Behavior Therapy, 24*, 321–329.

Hu, T.W., Sung, H.Y., and Keeler, T.E. (1995). Reducing cigarette consumption in California: Tobacco taxes vs. an anti-smoking media campaign. *American Journal of Public Health, 85*, 1218–1222.

Hughes, J.R., Goldstein, M.G., Hurt, R.D., and Shiffman, S. (1999). Recent advances in the pharmacotherapy of smoking. *Journal of the American Medical Association, 281*, 72–76.

Hunt, W.A., Barnett, L.W., and Branch, L.G. (1971). Relapse rates in addiction programs. *Journal of Clinical Psychology, 27*, 455–456.

Hurt, R.D., Sachs, D.P.L., Glover, E.D., Offord, K.P., Johnston, J.A., Dale, L.C., Khayrallah, M.A., Schroeder, D.R., Glover, P.N., Sullivan, C. R., Crogan, I.T., and Sullivan P.M. (1997). A comparison of sustained-released buprorion and placebo for smoking cessation. *New England Journal of Medicine, 337*, 1195–1202.

IOM (Institute of Medicine) (1982) *Health and Behavior: Frontiers of Research in the Biobehavioral Sciences*. D.A. Hamburg, G.R. Elliott, and D.L. Parron (Eds.). Washington: National Academy Press.

Jason, L.A., Berk, M., Schnopp-Wyatt, D.L., and Talbot B. (1999). Effects of enforcement of youth access laws on smoking prevalence. *American Journal of Community Psychology, 21,* 143–160.

Jeffery, R.W., Drewnowski, A., Epstein, L.H., Stunkard, A.J., Wilson, T., and Hill, R. (2000). Long-term maintenance of weight loss: Current status. *Health Psychology, 19,* 5–16.

Kaplan, G.A. and Keil, J.E. (1993). Socioeconomic factors and cardiovascular disease: A review of the literature. *Circulation, 88,* 1973–1998.

Kaplan, R.M., Ake, C.F., Emery, S.L., and Navarro A.M. (2001). Simulated effect of tobacco tax variation on population health in California. *American Journal of Public Health, 91,* 239–244

Keefe, F.J. and Caldwell, D.S. (1997). Cognitive behavioral control of arthritis pain. *Medical Clinics of North America, 81,* 277–290.

Keeler, T.E., Hu, T.W., Barnett, P.G., and Manning, W.G. (1993). Taxation, regulation, and addiction: A demand function for cigarettes based on time-series estimates. *Journal of Health Economics, 12,* 1–18.

Kiecolt-Glaser, J.K., Glaser, R., Gravenstein, S., Malarkey, W.B., and Sheridan, J.F. (1996). Chronic stress alters the immune response to influenza virus vaccine in older adults. *Proceedings of the National Academy of Sciences, 93,* 3043–3047.

Klein, K.B. and Spiegel, D. (1989). Modulation of gastric acid secretion by hypnosis. *Gastroenterology, 96,* 1383–1387.

Lalonde, M.A. (1974). *New Perspectives on the Health of Canadians. A Working Document.* Ottawa: Information Canada.

Lewit, E.M., Coate, D., and Grossman, M. (1981). The Effects of Government Regulations on Teenage Smoking. *Journal of Law and Economics, 24,* 545–569.

Linden, W., Stossel, C., and Maurice, J. (1996). Psychosocial interventions for patients with coronary artery disease: a meta-analysis. *Archives of Internal Medicine, 156,* 745–752.

Lorig, K. and Holman, H. (1993). Arthritis self-management studies; A twelve year review. *Health Education Quarterly, 20,* 17–28.

Mackenbach, J.P., Stronks, K., and Kunst, A.E. (1989). The contribution of medical care to inequalities in health: Differences between socio-economic groups in decline of mortality from conditions amenable to medical intervention. *Social Science and Medicine, 29,* 369–376.

Manning, W.G., Keeler, E.B., Newhouse, J.P., Sloss, E.M., and Wasserman, J. (1991). *The Costs of Poor Health Habits.* Cambridge, MA: Harvard University Press.

Marcus, B.H., Blair, S.N., Dubbert, P.M., Dunn, A.L., Forsyth, L.H., McKenzie, T.L., and Stone, E.J. (2000). Physical activity behavior change: Issues in adoption and maintenance. *Health Psychology, 19,* 32–41.

Matthews, K., Kelsey, S., Meilahn, E., Kuller, L.H., and Wing, R.R. (1989). Educational attainment and behavioral and biologic risk factors for coronary heart disease in middle-aged women. *American Journal of Epidemiology, 129,* 1132–1144.

McEwen, B. (1998). Protective and damaging effects of stress mediators. *New England Journal of Medicine, 338,* 171–179.

McEwen, B.S. and Stellar, E. (1993), Stress and the individual: Mechanisms leading to disease. *Archives of Internal Medicine, 153,* 2093–2101.

McGinnis, J.M. and Foege, W.H. (1993). Actual causes of death in the United States. *Journal of the American Medical Association, 270,* 2207–2212.

McNabb, W.L., Quinn, M.T., Murphy, D.M., Thorp, F.K., and Cook, S. (1994). Increasing children's responsibility for diabetes self-care: The In Control study. *Diabetes Educator, 20,* 121–124.

Meyer, T.J. and Mark, M. (1995). Effects of psychosocial interventions with adult cancer patients: A meta-analysis of randomized experiments. *Health Psychology, 14,* 101–108.

NHLBI (National Heart, Lung, and Blood Institute). (1983). *Guidelines for Demonstration And Education Research Grants.* Washington, DC: National Institutes of Health.

NIH Technology Assessment Panel. (1996). Integration of behavioral and relaxation approaches into the treatment of chronic pain in insomnia. *Journal of the American Medical Association, 276,* 313–318.

Ockene, J.K., Emmons, K., Mermelstein, R., Perkins, K.A., Bonollo, D., Hollis, J.F., and Vorhees, C. (2000). Relapse and maintenance issues for smoking cessation. *Health Psychology, 19,* 17–31.

Orleans, C.T., Boyd, N.R., Bingler, R., Sutton, C., Fairclough, D., Heller, D., McClatchey, M., Ward, J.A., Graves, C., Fleisher, L., and Baum, S. (1998). A self-help intervention for African American smokers: Tailoring cancer information service counseling for a special population. *Preventive Medicine, 27 (5 Pt 2),* S61–S70.

Parker, J.C. (1995). Effects of stress management on clinical outcomes in rheumatoid arthritis. *Arthritis and Rheumatism, 38,* 1807–1818.

Peterson, A.V. Jr., Kealey, K.A., Mann, S.L., Marek, P.M., and Sarason, I.G. (2000). Hutchinson smoking prevention project: long-term randomized tiral in school-based tobacco use prevention—results on smoking. *Journal of the National Cancer Institute, 92,* 1979–1991.

Pierce, J.P. (1999). *The Effectiveness of Various Communication Strategies in Promoting Behavior Change.* Presented at the Workshop on Health, Communications and Behavior of the IOM Committee on Health and Behavior: Research, Practice and Policy, Irvine, CA.

Pierce, J.P. and Gilpin, E.A. (1995). A historical analysis of tobacco marketing and the uptake of smoking by youth in the United States: 1890–1977. *Health Psychology, 14,* 500–508.

Pierce, J.P., Choi, W.S., Gilpin, E.A., Farkas, A.J., and Berry, C.C. (1998a). Tobacco industry promotion of cigarettes and adolescent smoking. *Journal of the American Medical Association, 279,* 511–515.

Pierce, J.P., Gilpin, E.A., and Farkas, A.J. (1998c). Can strategies used by statewide tobacco control programs help smokers make progress in quitting? *Cancer Epidemiology, Biomarkers and Prevention, 7,* 459–464.

Pierce, J.P., Gilpin, E.A., Emery, S.L., White, M.M., Rosbrook, B., and Berry, C.C. (1998b). Has the California tobacco control program reduced smoking? *Journal of the American Medical Association, 280,* 893–899.

Prochaska, J.O. (1997). Revolution in health promotion: Smoking cessation as a case study. In G.A. Marlatt and G.R. Vandenbos (Eds.) *Addictive Behaviors: Readings on Etiology, Prevention and Treatment* (pp. 361–375). Washington, DC: American Psychological Association Press.

Rigotti, N.A., Bourne, D., Rosen, A., Locke, J.A., and Schelling, T.C. (1992). Workplace compliance with a no-smoking law: A randomized community intervention trial. *American Journal of Public Health, 82*, 229–235.

Rose-Ackerman, S. (1991). Tort law in the regulatory state. In P.H. Schuck (Ed.) *Tort Law and the Public Interest* (pp. 105–126). New York: Norton.

Ryden, O., Nevander, L., Johnsson, P., Hansson, K., Kronvall, P., Sjoblad, S., and Westbom, L. (1994). Family therapy in poorly controlled juvenile IDDM: Effects on diabetic control, self-evaluation and behavioral symptoms. *Acta Paediatrica, 83*, 285–291.

Ryff, C.D. and Singer, B. (1998). The contours of positive human health. *Psychological Inquiry 9*, 1–28.

Satin, W., La Greca, A.M., Zigo, M.A., and Skyler, J.S. (1989). Diabetes in adolescence: Effects of multifamily group intervention parent simulation of diabetes. *Journal of Pediatric Psychology, 14*, 259–275.

Schwartz, J.L. (1992). Methods of smoking cessation. *Medical Clinics of North America, 76*, 451–476.

Shiffman, S. (1993). Smoking cessation treatment: Any progress? *Journal of Consulting and Clinical Psychology, 61*, 718–722.

Stevens, V.J., and Hollis, J.F. (1989). Preventing smoking relapse, using individually tailored skills training techniques. *Journal of Consulting and Clinical Psychology, 57*, 420–424.

Suchanek Hudmon, K., Gritz, E.R., Clayton, S., and Nisenbaum, R. (1999). Eating orientation, postcessation weight gain, and continued abstinence among female smokers receiving an unsolicited smoking cessation intervention. *Health Psychology. 18*, 29–36.

Taylor, S.E., Repetti, R.L., Seeman, T. (1997). Health psychology: What is an unhealthy environment and how does it get under the skin? *Annual Review of Psychology, 48*, 411–447.

Thomas-Dobersen, D.A., Butler-Simon, N., and Fleshner, M. (1993). Evaluation of a weight management intervention program in adolescents with insulin-dependent diabetes mellitus. *Journal of the American Dietetic Association, 93*, 535–540.

Tobacco Use and Dependence Clinical Practice Guideline Panel, Staff, and Consortium Representatives. (2000). A Clinical Practice Guideline For Treating Tobacco Use and Dependence: A US Public Health Service report, *Journal of the American Medical Association, 28*, 3244–3254.

United States Department of Health, Education, and Welfare. (1979). *Healthy People.* DHEW Publication Number (PHS) 79-55071. Washington, DC: U.S. Government Printing Office.

USDHHS (U.S. Department of Health and Human Services) (1996). *Clinical Practice Guideline, No 18. Smoking Cessation* . Rockville, MD: Agency for Health Care Policy and Research. Centers for Disease Control and Prevention. AHCPR Publication No. 96-0692.

Velicer, W.F., Prochaska, J.O., Fava, J.L., Laforge, R.G., and Rossi, J.S. (1999). Interactive versus noninteractive interventions and dose–response relationships for stage-matched smoking cessation programs in a managed care setting. *Health Psychology, 18*, 21–28.

Vicusi, W.K. (1992). *Fatal Tradeoffs*. New York: Oxford University Press.

Warner, K.E. (1986). Smoking and health implications of a change in the federal cigarette excise tax. *Journal of the American Medical Association, 255*, 1028–1032.

Whorwell, P.J., Prior, A., and Colgan, S.M. (1987). Hypnotherapy in severe irritable bowel syndrome: Further experience. *Gut, 28*, 423–425.

Whorwell, P.J., Prior, A., and Farragher, E.B. (1984). Controlled trial of hypnotherapy in the treatment of severe refractory irritable bowel syndrome. *Lancet, 2 (8414)*, 1232–1234.

Wildey, M.B., Woodruff, S.I., Agro, A., Keay, KD, Kenney, E.M., and Conway, T.L. (1995). Sustained effects of educating retailers to reduce cigarette sales to minors. *Public Health Rep., 110*, 625–629.

Wilkinson, R.G. (1996). Unhealthy Societies: The Afflictions of Inequality. London: Routledge.

APPENDIX A

Workshop on Health, Communications, and Behavior

IOM Committee on Health and Behavior:
Research, Practice and Policy
January 6, 1999
8:30 a.m. - 1:15 p.m.
Arnold and Mabel Beckman Center, Room 1C
100 Academy Drive, Irvine, CA

AGENDA

8:30 a.m. - 8:40 a.m.   Welcome and Opening Remarks
Edward N. Brandt, Jr., MD, PhD (Committee
Chair)
Member, Committee on Health and Behavior:
Research, Practice and Policy

8:40 a.m. - 8:50 a.m.   Introduction to Workshop
Robert Kaplan, PhD (Workshop Chair)
Member, Committee on Health and Behavior:
Research, Practice and Policy

8:50 a.m. - 9:40 a.m.	"Communication of Health Information to the Public: How and When NIH Communicates to the Public" Anne Thomas, MS, National Institutes of Health
9:40 a.m.- 9:50 a.m.	Discussion
9:50 a.m. - 10:40 a.m.	"Risk Perception and Risk Communication" Baruch Fischhoff, PhD, Carnegie Mellon University
10:40 a.m - 11:20 a.m.	Discussion Lawrence Green, DrPH, (Discussant) University of British Columbia, Canada
11:20 a.m.-11:35 a.m.	Break
11:35 a.m -12:15 p.m.	"The Effectiveness of Various Communication Strategies in Promoting Behavior Change" John Pierce, PhD, University of California, San Diego
12:15 p.m.-12:55 p.m.	"Commercial versus Political Speech: Constitutional Implications for Advertising and Public Health Communication" Lawrence Gostin, JD, LLD Member, Committee on Health and Behavior: Research, Practice and Policy
12:55 p.m -1:15 p.m.	Discussion Lawrence Green, DrPH, (Discussant)

APPENDIX B

Consultants

Richard Bonnie
University of Virginia School of
 Law
Charlottesville, VA

Orville Gilbert Brim
MIDMAC
Vero Beach, FL

Paul D. Cleary
Harvard Medical School
Boston, MA

Graham A. Colditz
Channing Laboratory
Boston, MA

Bruce E. Compas
University of Vermont
Burlington, VT

Susan Czajkowski
National Heart Lung Blood
 Institute, NIH
Bethesda, MD

Glen H. Elder, Jr.
The University of North Carolina
Chapel Hill, NC

Baruch Fischhoff
Carnegie Mellon University
Pittsburgh, PA

Paula Louise Friedenberg
George Washington University
Washington, DC

Lawrence W. Green
Institute of Health Promotion
 Research
University of British Columbia
Vancouver, BC

Jessie Gruman
Center for Advancement of
    Health
Washington, DC

David A. Hamburg
Carnegie Corporation of New
    York
New York, NY

Francis Harper
Dana Foundation
New York, NY

Lawrence Fisher
University of California, San
    Francisco

Catherine A. Heaney
Ohio State University
Worthington, OH

Robert A. Jensen
Southern Illinois University
Carbondale, IL

James L. McGaugh
University of California, Irvine
Irvine, CA

Thomas George Pickering
The New York Hospital - Cornell
    Medical Center
New York, NY

John P. Pierce
University of California, San
    Diego
San Diego, CA

Judith Jane Prochaska
San Diego State University
San Diego, CA

Louise B. Russell
Rutgers, the State University of
    New Jersey
New Brunswick, NJ

Jack Shonkoff
Brandeis University
Waltham, MA

Glorian Sorensen
Dana-Farber Cancer Institute
Boston, MA

Michael Stoto
George Washington University
Washington, DC

Richard S. Surwit
Duke University Medical Center
Durham, NC

Anne Thomas
National Institutes of Health
Bethesda, MD

Karen Weihs
Center for Family Research
Washington, DC

Stephen Weiss
University of Miami, School of
    Medicine
Miami, FL

Rena R. Wing
Western Psychiatric Institute &
    Clinic
Pittsburgh, PA

Index

A

Adaptation, 31

Adherence, in clinical interventions, 192-194

Administrative strategies, 246

Adolescents with chronic disease, 212-218
family therapy for, 217-218
interventions affecting family relationship quality and functioning, 215-217
psychoeducational interventions for, 212-215

Adrenal steroids, 44

Adult weight gain, 96-97

Adults with chronic disease, interventions for, 218-219

Advantage, relative, of innovations, 305-306

Adverse social interactions, 150-151

Advocacy Institute, 346

Affliction, disproportionate, of sexually transmitted infections, 110-112

Agency for Health Care Policy and Research (AHCPR), 335-336

Alcohol consumption, 102-107
early data on, 19
maldistribution in, 106
negative health effects, 103-104
positive health effects, 104-105
quantifying net public health benefit, 105-107
socioeconomic factors in, 102-103

Allostasis and allostatic load, 4-5, 41-42
in the autonomic nervous system, 45
patterns of long-term harm associated with, 46

Alzheimer's disease, 211

American Academy of Pediatrics, 115

American Cancer Society, 107, 117, 119, 203

American College of Obstetricians and Gynecologists, 117

American Heart Association, 115
Heart Partners program, 308

American Medical Association, 115, 117

American Psychiatric Association, 22

American Psychological Association, 281

American Stop Smoking Intervention Study (ASSIST), 203, 308

Neuroendocrine responses, 42
Neurotransmitters, experience and
behavior, 48-49
NHLBI. *See* National Heart, Lung, and
Blood Institute
NIDR. *See* National Institute for Dental
Research
NKCC. *See* Natural killer-cell cytotoxicity
NLMS. *See* National Longitudinal
Mortality Study
NNH. *See* Number needed to harm
NNT. *See* Number needed to treat
North Karelia Project, 201
Number needed to harm (NNH),
calculating, 298
Number needed to treat (NNT),
calculating, 297-298
Nurses Cohort Study, 98

O

Obesity, 92-102
adult weight gain, 96-97
defining, 22, 93-94
prevalence and trends, 93-95
socioeconomic factors in, 95-96
weight and disease, 97-102
Objectives for the Nation, 260
Observability, of innovations, 306
Occupational risk factors, 151-157
job strain, 152-153
retirement, 156-157
threatened job loss, 156
unemployment, 153-156
Occupational safety and health (OSH)
programs, 12, 245-246
OD. *See* Organizational development
Operant-conditioning theory, 184-187
Optimism
a component of psychological well-
being, 5
coping facilitated by, 59
Organisation for Economic Co-operation
and Development (OECD), 156
Organizational change interventions,
potential targets for, 247

Organizational development (OD), 242-
243
Organizational dissemination, 301-304
through medical practices, 303-304
through schools, 301-302
Organizational interventions, 12-13, 241-
273
changing employee health behaviors,
244-245
communities and health, 250-254
community-level interventions, 254-258
lessons from, 250
organizations and health, 241-243
reducing environmental risk factors,
245-249
society and health, 258-260
society-level interventions, 260-264
Organizational readiness, in
disseminations to community-based
groups, 305-306
Organizations and health, 241-243
organizational culture, 242-243
planned-change models, 243
Original learning, *versus* extinction, 185-
186
Osteoarthritis, 101
Outcome measurement, 275-278
choice of measures, 275-276
Outcomes assessment, 22
Overweight. *See* Obesity

P

Panel on Cost-Effectiveness in Health and
Medicine, 278
Pap smear, 117
PAR. *See* Participatory action research
PARR. *See* Physical Activity for Risk
Reduction Project
Participatory action research (PAR), 249
Pawtucket Heart Health Program
(PHHP), 201-202
People, social inequalities of, 157-161
Pessimistic thinking, 5
PHHP. *See* Pawtucket Heart Health
Program